MAYO CLINIC

HEALTHY WEIGHT
for EVERYBODY

Donald D. Hensrud, M.D.

Editor in Chief

Mayo Clinic

Rochester, Minnesota

Mayo Clinic Healthy Weight for EveryBody provides reliable, practical, comprehensive, easy-to-understand information on issues relating to obesity, weight loss and achieving a healthy weight. Much of its information comes from physicians, research scientists and other health care professionals at Mayo Clinic. This book is intended to supplement the advice of your personal physician, whom you should consult about weight concerns and any medical condition that you may have. *Mayo Clinic Healthy Weight for EveryBody* does not endorse any company or product. MAYO, MAYO CLINIC, MAYO CLINIC HEALTH INFORMATION and the Mayo triple-shield logo are marks of Mayo Foundation for Medical Education and Research.

Published by Mayo Clinic Health Information, Rochester, Minn. Distributed to the book trade by Kensington Publishing Corporation, New York, N.Y.

For bulk sales to employers, member groups and health-related companies, contact Mayo Clinic Health Management Resources, 200 First St. S.W., Rochester, MN 55905, or send e-mail to SpecialSalesMayoBooks@Mayo.edu.

Photo credits: Stock photography from Corbis Images, Eyewire, Image Club Graphics, ©Isabelle Rozenbaum/PhotoAlto and Photodisc. The individuals pictured in these photos are models, and the photos are for illustrative purposes only. There is no correlation between the individuals portrayed and the condition or subject being discussed.

Library of Congress Control Number: 2004113207

ISBN-13:   978-1-893005-34-1
ISBN-10:   1-893005-34-8

Printed in the United States of America

First Edition

4 5 6 7 8 9 10

Preface

If you're like many people in the United States and around the world, you're looking for answers to help you lose weight. You may know what you're supposed to do in theory, but just can't put it into practice. You've tried many diets before, each time hoping this would be a success. Some were terrible (how much cabbage soup can one person eat?) and others worked for a little while, but the weight came back. Sound familiar?

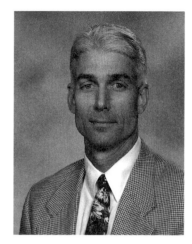

Donald D. Hensrud, M.D.
Editor in Chief

The best approach to long-term weight management is healthy and enjoyable lifestyle changes, and this book can be your guide. Our 12-week Mayo Clinic Healthy Weight Program will teach skills, offer tips and suggest goals to help you establish these permanent lifestyle changes. The Mayo Clinic Healthy Weight Pyramid will guide your decisions, allowing you to eat wonderfully tasty food and manage your weight in the process. And if you experience challenges, like everyone does, our Action Guide to Weight-Loss Barriers will provide strategies to help you stay on track.

Achieving a healthy weight is not impossible. It certainly takes hard work, but the rewards are great. Over time, your efforts will turn into sustainable, healthy lifestyle behaviors that can improve your nutrition and level of physical activity. You'll feel better immediately and reduce your health risks long-term. I truly believe and hope you'll find that a lifestyle that leads to permanent healthy weight should be and can be an enjoyable way for you to live.

Editorial staff

Table of contents

Visual Guide to a Healthy Weight

Section starts following page 128

Action Guide to Weight-Loss Barriers

Mayo Clinic Healthy Weight Program

PART I
What's a healthy weight for you?

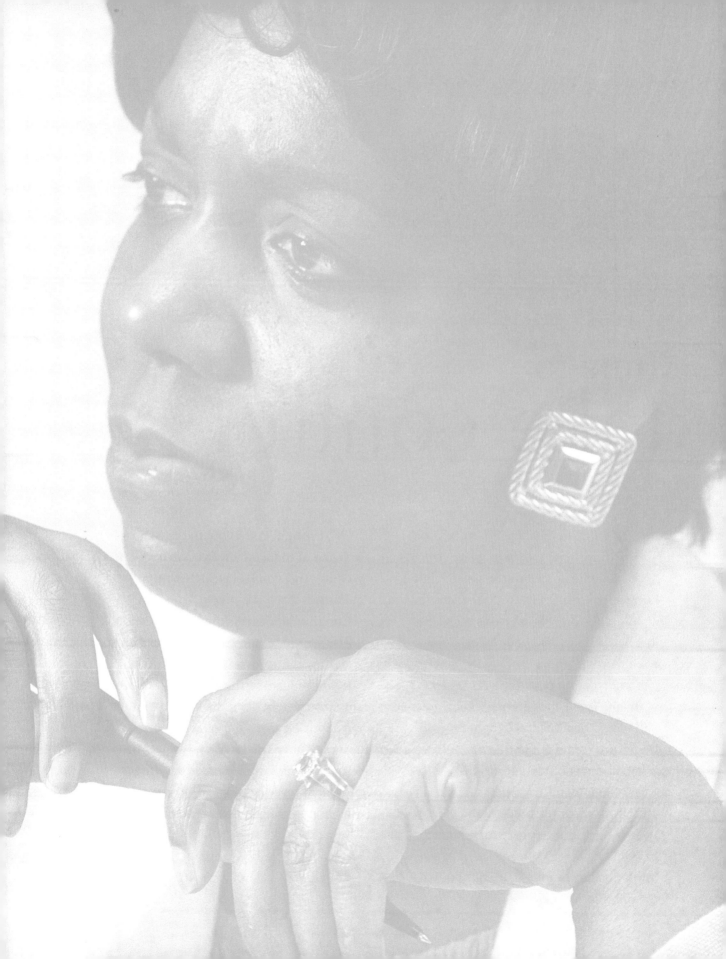

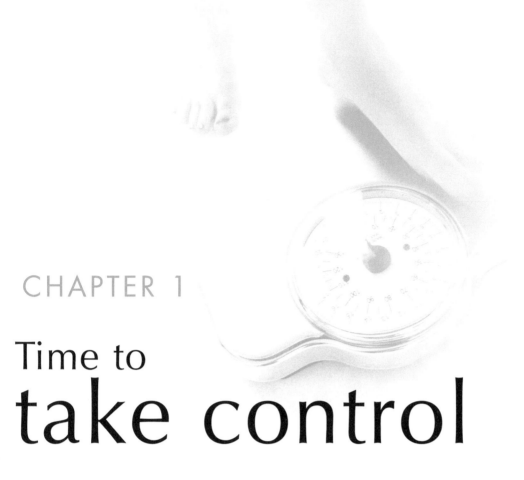

CHAPTER 1

Time to
take control

You go to the refrigerator and stand there with the door open ... *searching* for something to satisfy your hunger. You feel guilty because there shouldn't be any reason to eat more. You just had dinner. And your favorite jeans are already too tight. But you're *hungry*.

Tomorrow's a new day, you say to yourself. You'll start dieting tomorrow — and eating healthier, too. Right now, there's ice cream in the freezer compartment, and it shouldn't go to waste ...

Sound familiar?

Or how about the times right before bed when you raid the pantry for a cookie ... or two ... or three? You're not really even thinking about eating, but your body is on autopilot in search of food.

OK, enough. You know the reasons — or some of them — why you're overweight. And you feel guilty enough already. But what can you *do* about it?

Congratulations! Asking that question is a first step in taking control of your weight and improving your health.

If you're reading this book, you're probably overweight. And most likely you've already tried to do something about it. You may have tried a low-carb approach, or the low-fat, or high-protein, or low-protein approaches. Or the cabbage soup diet. You may have even tried the Mayo Clinic Diet — or what you thought was the Mayo Clinic Diet (more on that later).

But whatever your approach, you're still trying because you haven't had much success. That's not surprising. Most people who diet find it's a never-ending roller coaster ride. That's where this book comes in. It presents a weight-control program that can help you maintain a healthy weight for a lifetime.

NOT JUST ANOTHER DIET

"Weight-control program." Sounds suspiciously like a "diet." You can call it that if you like, but that wouldn't be completely accurate. The word *diet* can refer to what you eat, or it can refer to a special eating plan designed to reduce weight (often, in that usage, it's paired with the word *fad*).

The approach advocated in this book is something more. It's a lifestyle.

Most diets focus only on food — labeling some foods as good and others as bad. The goal is to simply lose pounds. Unfortunately, as you likely know from personal experience, those lost pounds usually come back.

This book, based on Mayo Clinic research and clinical experience, recognizes that successful, long-term weight management needs to focus on more than the food you eat and the pounds you lose. It needs to focus on your health.

Think about that for a moment. Your health is the single most important reason to be concerned about your weight, whether you're obese, overweight or underweight. You may be concerned primarily about your appearance — for many people, appearance plays a major role in self-image and how they feel about themselves. But focusing only on looks can lead to problems. In trying to look like those stick-thin fashion models, you may set yourself up for anxiety and frustration if your goal is unreasonable.

With a focus on improving your health, you'll be motivated to establish clear, reasonable and beneficial goals that will also help you manage your weight. With a healthy weight, you not only can look better but feel better, too.

And the process is far from unpleasant. Achieving a healthy weight doesn't involve special foods, questionable supplements or complicated food combinations. The program presented here simply combines a healthy-eating plan that's easy, filling, tasty — even adventurous — with enjoyable physical activity.

So this "diet," if you want to call it that, is different, and its goal is simple — to help you adopt a long-term lifestyle that allows you to achieve and maintain a weight that's healthy for you.

It's an achievable goal. Mayo Clinic nutritional specialists have seen it in clinical practice — being overweight is something that can be changed. You *can* take control of your weight.

This book is designed to help you do just that. In the following pages, you'll find practical advice on how to reach your healthy weight and, just as importantly, how to maintain it. It's a challenge that takes time and effort, but the results are worth it. Think of this book as your personal coach in a stimulating process.

WHY FOCUS ON HEALTH?

For a moment, put aside thoughts of weight and dieting and looking thin, and think about what it means to simply be healthy. Being healthy allows you to experience an optimum quality of life and to avoid certain health risks. It helps prevent premature aging and enables you to be energetic, strong and active.

Being healthy also gives you a sense of ownership over your body, increasing your confidence and self-respect. It helps you avoid a major source of stress — illness — and it can reduce your risk of incurring large health care costs.

Being overweight can pose a significant threat to your overall health. The more excess fat you carry, the greater your risk of developing certain health conditions. Among these conditions are:

High blood pressure

For men and women alike, high blood pressure is the most common weight-related health condition. Obese individuals are twice as likely to acquire high blood pressure as are individuals who maintain a healthy weight.

Abnormal blood fats

Studies show that being overweight or obese is associated with low levels of high-density lipoprotein (HDL, or "good") cholesterol in your blood. Obesity is also associated with high levels of triglycerides in your blood, which may contribute to cardiovascular disease.

Type 2 diabetes

The most common form of diabetes in the United States is type 2 diabetes. The development of type 2 diabetes is associated with being overweight, specifically weight gain after age 18 in both men and women. In fact, more than 80 percent of adults with type 2 diabetes are overweight or obese.

Cardiovascular disease

The risks of heart-related problems increase with increasing weight. Weight gains of 10 to 20 pounds can increase the risk by 25 percent, and weight gains of 45 pounds or more increase the risk by more than 250 percent.

Research indicates that excess weight also contributes to the risk of ischemic stroke, which occurs when blood supply to part of the brain is cut off and which accounts for 80 percent of all strokes.

Other complications

Your health is at increased risk of other conditions if you're overweight or obese. These conditions include gallstones, osteoarthritis and sleep apnea. Most types of cancer are associated with being overweight. In women, these especially include cancer of the breast, uterus, colon and gallbladder. And overweight men have a higher risk of cancer of the colon and the prostate.

Your health risks from being overweight are even greater if you're physically unfit and inactive. Age is another factor that complicates a weight problem. As you get

A quick start to weight loss

The complete 12-week Mayo Clinic Healthy Weight Program starts on page 180, with supporting material in the accompanying chapters and in the Action Guide to Weight-Loss Barriers. But if you want a quick start on losing weight before reading the entire book, follow these simple guidelines:

- Increase the amount of fruits and vegetables you eat, and make them a larger percentage of the total food you eat.
- Increase your physical activity. Brisk walking is an especially good activity because you can do it virtually anywhere and it's relatively low-stress.

For the full value of the Mayo Clinic Healthy Weight Program, you'll need to advance through the 12 units, learning and adopting the elements presented each week. But moving in the general direction of the program by eating more fruits and vegetables and becoming more physically active will help.

As with any weight-management approach, see your doctor before beginning an eating or exercise program if you have health issues or any questions about your health.

older, your risk of developing weight-related health problems increases.

But even a modest reduction in weight — 5 percent to 10 percent of your total weight — can help prevent or reduce certain health risks. Even if you don't have health problems now, maintaining a healthy weight can boost your energy level, improve your self-esteem and give you a greater sense of independence. These are excellent and often quickly attained payoffs for this challenge.

A PROGRAM THAT WORKS

When it comes to weight loss, there's no shortage of advice. Cruise through any bookstore or peruse any magazine rack and you're bound to come across the lat-est and greatest cure for being overweight. Some even work — for a while.

But what you should be looking for is something that works for a lifetime, and that takes a lifestyle.

The program detailed in this book has that goal — to help you establish a healthy lifestyle to control weight. The tool it uses to get you there is the Mayo Clinic Healthy Weight Pyramid.

Mayo Clinic Healthy Weight Pyramid

The Mayo Clinic Healthy Weight Pyramid is based on the concept of energy density. Simply put, it emphasizes lower-calorie foods that help you feel full.

Research shows that feeling full is determined by the volume and weight of the food you eat. By choosing foods with

Mayo Clinic Diet — myth vs. reality

It seems to be seasonal. Usually in the spring, Mayo Clinic gets deluged with phone calls inquiring about the so-called Mayo Clinic Diet, various versions of which have sprouted up across the country and around the world for decades. The only problem — none of these diets are associated with or have been endorsed by Mayo Clinic.

No one knows the origin of the diet myth, but Mayo dietitians say it's been around since the 1940s. Over the years, the supposed Mayo Clinic Diet has emerged in many forms, but all share a common characteristic: They are "one-size-fits-all" diets. They also limit the variety of foods and promise dramatic weight loss. These are sure signs of a hoax.

If anything comes close to a "real" Mayo Clinic Diet, it would be the healthy-eating principles described in this book.

low energy density (few calories for their bulk), you can consume less calories while still eating the same amount of food you're accustomed to.

The pyramid couples that concept with increased physical activity to help you achieve a healthy weight.

Sounds like a simple plan, and it is. But to take full advantage of this concept, you need the tools to help implement it. Spread throughout the chapters of this book are those tools.

If you want to achieve a healthy weight, it helps to know what that weight might be. Chapter 2 gives you the tools to find your healthy weight.

Knowing your weight goal may tell you where you want to go, but you need to compare it to the weight you're currently at. This allows you to assess your motivation and state of readiness. Chapter 3 will help you measure the challenge that lies ahead and prepare for the changes necessary to achieve your weight goal.

Chapter 4 opens Part 2 of this book, "Building blocks of a weight program," and helps you understand the dynamics of weight control and the basic elements of nutrition. Chapter 5 sets you on the path to healthy eating with a discussion of the Mayo Clinic Healthy Weight Pyramid and how to put it into action.

Action is the focus of Chapter 6, which covers an important element at the core of the Healthy Weight Pyramid — getting and staying physically active.

Chapter 7 coaches you on how to change behavior that affects your weight, while Chapter 8 focuses on your emotional needs, helping you build self-control, self-esteem and a positive outlook.

Part 3 of the book, "Maintaining a weight program," opens with Chapter 9 describing the tools you need for meal planning. Chapter 10 helps you expand your exercise program, while Chapter 11 provides strategies to keep you motivated and sticking with your program.

Part 4 of the book deals with special topics, such as medications and surgery used to achieve a healthy weight.

The Visual Guide to a Healthy Weight provides easy-to-understand visual references to serving sizes and recipes, while the Action Guide to Weight-Loss Barriers, beginning on page 146, tackles common nutritional, behavioral and physical activity-related obstacles to achieving and maintaining a healthy weight.

Capping the book is a 132-page program — the Mayo Clinic Healthy Weight Program — that puts the principles of the Healthy Weight Pyramid into action.

Mayo Clinic Healthy Weight Program

The program section of this book provides you with a 12-week weight-control plan. Along with daily menus, you'll find practical tips from Mayo Clinic dietitians.

Follow the program closely, and you should lose from 12 to 24 pounds over the 12 weeks — a safe, healthy loss of 1 to 2 pounds a week. The more closely you follow the plan, the better your results.

But what then? What do you do after the 12-week program is completed?

By then, you'll be able to answer that question yourself, because embedded in the program are lessons and tips that put into action the principles outlined earlier in the book chapters. These strategies will help you transform key behaviors from unhealthy ones into healthy ones. You won't be "on a program" (or "on a diet"), you'll be living a lifestyle.

IT COMES DOWN TO YOU

If your goal is to lose weight, you can achieve that by eating healthier foods and becoming more physically active. Go for it. You can do it. This book is a good starting point. Your family, your friends and your doctor can help. But in the end, it all comes down to you. Remember to consider your goals from your own perspective, not through the eyes of others. Then make decisions that are best for you.

You've undoubtedly heard statistics about how few people succeed at losing weight and keeping it off. Don't let that discourage you. For one thing, despite the statistics, plenty of people succeed. Sure, you're taking on a tough challenge, possibly one of the hardest you'll ever tackle. But with a little knowledge, a positive attitude and a good plan, you can do it.

The best news is, as you begin to lose weight, feel better and have more energy, as you discover how good it feels to move your body, as you learn the sheer pleasure of eating tasty food that also improves your health, you'll realize how enjoyable a commitment to weight control can be.

Losing weight isn't easy. Quick-fix solutions are rubbish. But if you focus on your health, you'll develop healthy habits. With healthy habits, the pounds will take care of themselves. Even if you don't reach your "ideal" weight, you'll be much healthier than you were before.

Now get ready. This is a lifetime commitment to healthy living. Just wait and see how good you're going to feel.

CHAPTER 2

Finding your healthy weight

The question for many people becomes, "How do I know if I'm at a healthy weight — one that's good for me?" How can you know if your weight reduces your risk of disease and allows you to look and feel good?

Perhaps the best way to assess your weight is to compare it with standards established by doctors, dietitians and other health professionals to help individuals determine whether their weight puts their health at risk. The results indicate where your weight falls within a series of weight categories: underweight, healthy weight, overweight or obese.

This chapter explains what these weight categories mean and will help you identify the category you're in. Whether you

need to lose weight shouldn't be determined only by your desire to fit into a certain swimsuit size. Rather, base your decision on what's healthiest for you.

WHAT MAKES A HEALTHY WEIGHT?

Simply put, a healthy weight means you have the right amount of body fat in relation to your overall body mass. As described in Chapter 1, a healthy weight is one that gives you energy, reduces health risks, helps prevent premature aging and improves your quality of life. Stepping on the scale only tells you your total weight — including bone, muscle and fluid —

not how much of your weight is fat. The scale also doesn't tell you where you're carrying that fat. In determining health risks, both of these factors are more important than weight alone.

The most accurate way to determine how much fat you're carrying is to have a body fat analysis. This requires a professional using a reliable method of estimation, such as weighing a person underwater, or using a X-ray procedure called dual energy X-ray absorptiometry. Either method can be expensive and fairly complicated. A procedure called bioelectric impedance analysis is more widely available, but its accuracy can vary.

Although less certain, the most common method to determine health risk uses estimates of body fat based on your total weight. The National Institutes of Health has adopted a threefold approach to determining a healthy weight. This approach is based on key components:

- Your body mass index
- The circumference of your waist
- Personal medical history

Body mass index

Body mass index (BMI) is a tool for indicating your weight status (see the table on page 18). The mathematical calculation takes into account both your weight and height. BMI equals your weight in pounds divided by your height in inches squared: BMI = (lb / in^2) x 703. Although BMI doesn't distinguish between fat and muscle, it more closely reflects measures of body fat than total body weight does.

Today, most health organizations use BMI values to define healthy weight. BMI is also an international standard recognized by the World Health Organization. This allows for comparison of data from different countries.

Although a BMI number tends to correlate well with an approximate measure of body fat, it's not always a good match. Some people may have a high BMI but relatively little body fat. Many athletes have high BMIs that would seem to classify them as overweight. For example, a professional football player may be 6 feet 3 inches tall and weigh 230 pounds, giving him a BMI of 29 — four points above the classification of healthy weight. But he's not overweight because vigorous athletic training has turned most of his weight into lean muscle mass.

By the same token, there may be some people who have a BMI in the "healthy" range but who carry a high percentage of body fat. For most people, though, the BMI provides a fairly accurate approximation of body fat as it relates to their total weight.

Waist measurement

Many conditions associated with excess weight, such as high blood pressure, abnormal levels of blood fats, coronary artery disease, stroke, diabetes and certain types of cancer, are influenced by the location of fat on your body. Fat distribution can be described in terms of an apple shape or pear shape. If you carry most of your fat around your waist or upper

Body mass index (BMI)

You can determine your body mass index (BMI) by finding your height and weight on this chart. A BMI of 18.5 to 24.9 is considered the healthiest. People with a BMI under 18.5 are considered underweight. People with a BMI between 25 and 29.9 are considered overweight. People with a BMI of 30 or greater are considered obese.

	Healthy		Overweight					Obese				
BMI	19	24	25	26	27	28	29	30	35	40	45	50
Height						Weight in pounds						
4'10"	91	115	119	124	129	134	138	143	167	191	215	239
4'11"	94	119	124	128	133	138	143	148	173	198	222	247
5'0"	97	123	128	133	138	143	148	153	179	204	230	255
5'1"	100	127	132	137	143	148	153	158	185	211	238	264
5'2"	104	131	136	142	147	153	158	164	191	218	246	273
5'3"	107	135	141	146	152	158	163	169	197	225	254	282
5'4"	110	140	145	151	157	163	169	174	204	232	262	291
5'5"	114	144	150	156	162	168	174	180	210	240	270	300
5'6"	118	148	155	161	167	173	179	186	216	247	278	309
5'7"	121	153	159	166	172	178	185	191	223	255	287	319
5'8"	125	158	164	171	177	184	190	197	230	262	295	328
5'9"	128	162	169	176	182	189	196	203	236	270	304	338
5'10"	132	167	174	181	188	195	202	209	243	278	313	348
5'11"	136	172	179	186	193	200	208	215	250	286	322	358
6'0"	140	177	184	191	199	206	213	221	258	294	331	368
6'1"	144	182	189	197	204	212	219	227	265	302	340	378
6'2"	148	186	194	202	210	218	225	233	272	311	350	389
6'3"	152	192	200	208	216	224	232	240	279	319	359	399
6'4"	156	197	205	213	221	230	238	246	287	328	369	410

Modified from National Institutes of Health's *Clinical Guidelines on the Identification, Evaluation, and Treatment of Overweight and Obesity in Adults, 1998*

You can calculate your exact BMI by using this formula:

$$\left(\frac{\text{Weight in pounds}}{(\text{Height in inches}) \times (\text{Height in inches})} \right) \times 703 = \text{BMI}$$

For example, if you weigh 165 pounds and you're 5 feet 10 inches tall, your BMI is 23.9.

$$\left(\frac{165 \text{ pounds}}{(70 \text{ inches}) \times (70 \text{ inches})} \right) \times 703 = 23.9$$

How fat is distributed on your body

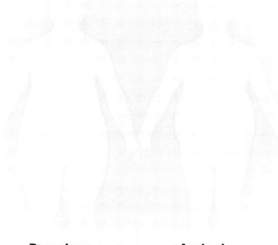

Pear shape   **Apple shape**

body, you're referred to as apple-shaped. If you carry most of your fat around your hips and thighs or lower body, you're referred to as pear-shaped.

In general, when it comes to your health, it's better to have a pear shape than an apple shape. If you have an apple shape, you carry fat in and around your abdominal organs. Fat in your abdomen increases your risk of disease. If you have a pear shape, your risks of these conditions aren't as high.

To determine whether you're carrying too much weight around your middle, you'll need to measure your waist. Find the highest point on each hipbone and measure across your abdomen just above those points. A measurement exceeding 40 inches (102 centimeters) in men or 35 inches (88 centimeters) in women indicates an apple shape and increased health risks. Your risk is even greater if you have a BMI of 25 or higher. The table on page 20 can help you determine whether or not to be concerned about your waistline

Although these cutoffs of 40 and 35 inches are useful guides, there's nothing magical about them. It's enough to know that the bigger the waistline, the greater your health risks.

Medical history

Your BMI and waist measurement numbers don't give you the full picture of your weight status. A complete evaluation of your medical history is also important in determining a healthy weight. Some issues that you and your doctor might consider include:

- Do you have a health condition, such as high blood pressure or diabetes, that would improve if you lost weight?

Is your health at risk?

YOUR BMI	YOUR WAIST MEASUREMENTS			
	Female		Male	
	35 inches or less	Exceeding 35 inches	40 inches or less	Exceeding 40 inches
25 to 29.9	Increased	High	Increased	High
30 to 34.9	High	Very high	High	Very high
35 to 39.9	Very high	Very high	Very high	Very high
40 or higher	Extremely high	Extremely high	Extremely high	Extremely high

If your BMI is between 18.5 and 24.9, your health is likely not at risk from your weight. A BMI of 25 and over may put you at risk of serious health problems.

- Do you have a family history of obesity, cardiovascular disease, diabetes, high blood pressure or sleep apnea? This may mean increased risk for you.
- Have you gained considerable weight since high school? Even people with normal BMIs may be at increased risk of weight-related conditions if they've gained more than 10 pounds since young adulthood.
- Do you smoke cigarettes or engage in little physical activity? These risk factors can compound the risk represented by excess weight.

You can think of the BMI and waist measurement as snapshots of your current health situation. The medical history helps complete the picture by revealing your risk for being overweight or developing weight-related diseases.

What's your healthy weight?

If your BMI shows that you're not overweight (BMI under 25), if you're not carrying too much weight around your abdomen, and if you answered no to all of the medical history questions, there's probably little health advantage to changing your weight. It's probably healthy.

If your BMI is between 25 and 29 or your waist circumference exceeds the healthy guidelines, and you answered yes to one or more of the medical history questions, you'll probably benefit from losing a few pounds. Discuss your weight with your doctor at your next checkup.

If your BMI is 30 or more, you're considered obese. Losing weight will improve your health and reduce your risk of weight-related illnesses.

BEING OVERWEIGHT

Most people, no matter what their BMI, are aware of issues associated with being overweight: Not fitting into clothes you used to wear or having shortness of breath when you exert yourself. What's the line that separates a healthy weight from overweight? Everyone has a different perception. Some people look in the mirror and are convinced they're overweight when they may not be.

Risk factors for being overweight

Being overweight means you're carrying too much body fat in relation to your body mass. Being obese means that your excess body fat is putting you at risk of illness and premature death. A number of factors can increase your risk of becoming overweight or obese.

Lifestyle factors

Many social and economic factors contribute to unhealthy eating habits and lack of activity. These include increased consumption of high-calorie foods, eating larger portions of food, more sedentary jobs, and the increased use of technology and labor-saving devices.

Genetic factors

Evidence suggests that obesity runs in some families, but the role that genes play remains unclear. A few, rare genetic mutations are known to cause obesity. But scientists believe that obesity is more likely the result of a complex interaction between genes and the environment.

It's true that children of obese parents have a higher risk of becoming obese adults than children of lean parents do. But it could be argued that children simply follow the eating and exercise patterns of their parents.

This means that although you may have a genetic predisposition to being overweight, it's not an inescapable fate. Ultimately, your weight is determined by how you interact with many physical and social factors in your environment.

Psychological factors

People overeat to cope with problems in their lives or to deal with emotions such as boredom, sadness and frustration. In some people, a psychiatric illness called binge eating disorder may contribute to obesity. Binge eating is characterized by frequent episodes of compulsive eating, accompanied by feelings of guilt and lack of control.

Other factors

Other factors may contribute to excessive weight gain but generally aren't enough in and of themselves to lead to obesity.

Age. As you get older, the amount of muscle in your body tends to decrease, and fat accounts for a greater percentage of your weight. In addition, people tend to be less active and their metabolism decreases as they get older. These changes reduce the amount of calories that their bodies can use without gaining weight.

Stopping smoking. Some smokers gain weight, usually no more than a few pounds, after they give up cigarettes and their metabolic rate readjusts to presmoking levels. But the benefits of stopping smoking usually outweigh whatever health costs may result from the slight weight gain they experience.

Pregnancy. Some women may gain more weight than recommended during a pregnancy, and they may retain that excess weight after the pregnancy.

Medications and illnesses. Certain drugs, such as corticosteroids, tricyclic antidepressants, anticonvulsants, insulin and hormones, may cause weight gain.

Recognizing an eating disorder

If you suspect that someone you know has an eating disorder, consult a doctor for advice. Eating disorders can be life threatening and require prompt professional help. Warning signs to watch for include:

- Continued weight loss
- Excessive exercise
- Skipping meals or eating alone
- Keeping food hidden
- Being extremely fussy about food or going on strange diets
- Anxious or ritualistic behavior at meals
- Extreme preoccupation with weight, shape and body image
- Frequent trips to the bathroom, especially during or after a meal
- Evidence of laxative use

These medications often can be adjusted to avoid excessive weight gain. In rare cases, obesity can be traced to a medical cause, such as low thyroid function or Cushing's syndrome. A medical problem also can cause you to be less active and therefore more likely to gain weight.

BEING UNDERWEIGHT

A body mass index lower than 18.5 means that you're probably underweight. According to a survey by the Centers for Disease Control and Prevention, only about 2 percent of people in the United States are underweight. Women are four times as likely to be underweight as men, and being underweight is more common among young adults (18 to 24 years) and older adults (65 and over).

Some people are naturally thin and may have trouble putting on weight despite a full diet and healthy lifestyle. In develop-ing countries, being underweight is often caused by malnutrition. In countries such as the United States, eating disorders often are a cause of being underweight. Eating disorders are psychiatric illnesses characterized by severe disturbances in eating behavior and a preoccupation with weight. The two most common eating disorders are anorexia nervosa and bulimia nervosa.

Anorexia nervosa

People with anorexia nervosa generally have an intense, irrational fear of being overweight. They often have a BMI less than 18, although they also may be within the healthy weight range. They refuse to eat and they lose weight by self-starvation, vomiting, abuse of laxatives, use of diuretics or strenuous exercise. Anorexia nervosa may be associated with menstrual irregularities, fatigue, depression, irregular heart rate, lightheadedness, mild anemia, and brittle nails and hair.

Bulimia nervosa

Bulimia nervosa is also known as bingeing and purging. A person with this disorder eats large amounts of food in a short time, then uses vomiting or laxatives to purge the food. Periods of bingeing and purging may alternate with periods of extreme dieting. Weight may stay constant but also can fluctuate. People with bulimia nervosa often feel a lack of control over their eating habits. Other signs and symptoms include dehydration, fatigue, depression, irritability, dry skin, damaged teeth and gums and an irregular heartbeat.

Eating disorders appear to involve many factors, including genetics, family behavior, social pressures and, sometimes, the abnormal function of brain systems that govern mood and appetite. Part of the answer may also be the media messages sent to young adults that equate being attractive with being thin.

Risk factors for eating disorders

Many factors may increase the risk of an eating disorder:

- Teenage girls and young women are more likely than teenage boys and young men to develop eating disorders.
- Eating disorders are much more common during the teens and 20s, although they can occur in midlife.
- Individuals who feel insecure or overly criticized in their family relationships are at higher risk of eating disorders.
- Eating disorders may be more common in people who have close family members with eating disorders.

- People with depression, anxiety disorders and obsessive-compulsive disorder are more likely to have eating disorders.
- Highly competitive athletes are at greater risk of developing an eating disorder.

Treatment of eating disorders

An eating disorder requires prompt medical attention. Someone who is undernourished needs to get back to a healthier weight before other aspects of treatment can begin. Medications may be prescribed to reduce bingeing and preoccupation with food. A person with severe anorexia may need to be hospitalized immediately in order to rehydrate the body.

ACCEPTING YOUR HEALTHY WEIGHT

Be realistic. Don't accept media portrayals about what's a normal weight and what's an ideal body image. Listen to your doctor, who can help you — either directly or through referral to a dietitian or nutrition specialist — to find the weight that best suits your body type and enhances your long-term health.

Keep in mind that the information presented here is designed to help you make educated decisions about your healthy weight. This information applies to most people, but it can't take into consideration all of the factors that may affect your weight and health. See your doctor or dietitian if you feel you would benefit from an individual assessment.

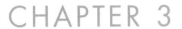

CHAPTER 3

Measuring the challenge

So you've decided that it's time to lose weight. Maybe it's because you're concerned about your health, or your doctor has advised you to lose a few pounds because you're overweight and your family has a history of diabetes. Or maybe you struggle to bend over, and short walks quickly leave you out of breath. Maybe your desire to lose weight has to do with your appearance. You've looked in the mirror and you don't like the size and shape of your waist. Or perhaps you simply want to weigh the same as you did when you finished college.

There are a thousand reasons why people try to lose weight. Take a few minutes to consider your reasons. It's important to start a weight program with an under-standing of what your motivations are. They bolster your commitment to losing weight and sustain your effort to make enduring changes in your life.

It's also critical that you're physically and emotionally prepared to start a weight program: Do you feel that your life is under control, or are you undergoing a lot of stress right now? Are there other health concerns or social problems demanding your attention? Are you committed to losing weight, no matter what it takes, or do you worry, in the back of your mind, that this attempt could end up being just another diet failure?

An honest assessment of your readiness will help guide your plans for weight loss. It provides a context for the personal goals you set for how much weight you'd like to lose, how quickly you'd like to lose it and when you want to get started.

WHAT'S YOUR MOTIVATION?

Motivation is an emotional incentive to take action. It's the likely reason why you're looking at this book right now. Motivation pushes you to do more than read the familiar diet dictums of "eat less" and "exercise more," and actually try to put them into practice.

Before you start a weight program, it's helpful to examine your motivations. Your chance of success is greater if your motivations to lose weight are based on what you want for yourself — for example, to be healthier and feel better about yourself — and not on what others expect of you. Take time to consider your motivations in relation to the weight category indicated for you by the body mass index (BMI) table (see table on page 18).

Then try this: List all the benefits you expect from weight loss, such as having more energy, improving your health, wearing clothes that are a better fit, and feeling more confident. Write down every benefit you can think of.

Now list all of the barriers you can think of that might prevent you from losing weight. These may include having to give up favorite foods, having to watch what you eat and having no time for exercise. Consider the emotional angles, too. For example, does being overweight

make you feel safe in some way? Are you discouraged about weight-loss experiences from the past? Write down everything that comes to mind, no matter how trivial or far-fetched the notion may seem.

Compare your benefits list with your barriers list and note which list is longer. Identify strategies that can help you overcome these barriers. Write down specific solutions and consider whether you can regularly put them into practice.

Here are strategies that can get you started and increase your chances of weight-loss success:

- **Make a commitment.** Focus on the good things about losing weight, such as increased energy and improved health.
- **Prioritize.** Don't set yourself up for failure by trying to lose weight while distracted by other concerns. Resolve those other problems first.
- **Be realistic.** Healthy weight loss is slow and steady over time. Aim to lose no more than 1 to 2 pounds a week. Quick weight loss is usually followed a short time later by quick weight gain.
- **Beware of dietary gimmicks.** Over-the-counter diet pills and special food combinations aren't the answer to long-term weight control. You want to incorporate healthy-eating behaviors permanently into your life.
- **Get active and stay active.** Regular walks four or five days a week can make you more fit and invigorate your weight program. Exercise sensibly by starting out slowly and then gradually increasing the duration and intensity.

ARE YOU READY TO START?

Losing weight requires a full commitment and all of your mental and physical energy. Success depends on your readiness to meet this challenge, and you can't afford to be distracted by other concerns. Before jumping into a weight program, consider whether now is the right time to start. Your timing is crucial. If you're not ready, you may be setting yourself up to fail. Ask yourself the following questions to determine your state of readiness:

How motivated am I to make lifestyle changes right now? Be honest. Knowing you need to make changes in your life and feeling up to the challenge are two different things. Success depends on your willingness to take action.

What's going on in my life over the next several months? The distraction of other problems, whether they involve relationships, jobs or finances, diminishes your chances of success. Allow your life to calm down before you start.

Am I being realistic about my weight-loss goals? Start small. Work on losing 5 pounds at a time. If you reach that goal and still want to lose weight, set another goal for 5 pounds. Try achieving a comfortable weight that you maintained easily as a young adult.

Do I truly believe that slower is better? Weight loss of 1 to 2 pounds a week is the best. That may seem like an agonizingly slow pace, but if improving your health is a long-term goal, the speed of your weight loss won't matter.

Do I have time to keep records of my food intake and my physical activity? Studies show that keeping records increases your chance of success.

Do I have family and friends to support my efforts? You need to have someone in your corner. If you don't, then consider joining a group weight-loss program that's professionally run.

Do I want to improve my health, or am I just interested in looking better? Either choice can be a legitimate reason to lose weight, if your expectations are realistic.

Do I believe I can change my eating behaviors? Sounds easy to do in theory but in practice, it can be difficult. It's hard to cast aside established behaviors.

Am I willing to find ways to be more physically active? Moving more is essential to successful weight control, but the demands of your lifestyle can interfere.

Do I have an eating disorder or other emotional issues that I need to contend with before I start? If you have a tendency to binge and purge, or to starve and overexert when you exercise, or if you're depressed or anxious, then you may want to seek professional help.

Am I willing to look at my past successes and failures with weight loss and with other areas of my life? Be optimistic. Learn from the past about what motivates you. Keep working to resolve barriers that might prevent success.

Do I believe that a healthy weight is a lifelong commitment? There's no going back to your old behaviors. Are you ready to make a permanent change?

Can I view a healthy weight program as a positive experience? If you're losing weight because you want to and not because you think it's expected of you, you'll quickly appreciate the benefits that come from weight loss.

There are a lot of issues to consider in this assessment. And there's often no definitive "yes" or "no" to many of these questions. Nevertheless, if you feel positive about most of your responses, you should consider starting your weight-loss program now. If you're uncertain about many of the questions, you may want to consider waiting for a better time. But don't let other problems hold you back for long. Think of ways to resolve your concerns, then reassess your readiness to lose weight as soon as you can.

Keep these perspectives in mind as you make your decision:

Pick the right time. If you're going through a difficult phase in your life, for example, you just lost your job, are in the midst of a divorce or are caring for a sick parent, this may not be a good time to make the lifestyle changes required for weight loss. Everyone's life includes stress, but stress does ebb and flow. Some times are tougher than others. If you're coping with a life crisis, it might be wise to postpone — but not cancel — weight loss until things ease up a bit. You may not have the energy you need just now.

Persistence pays off. At the same time, don't trick yourself into thinking you can wait until everything's calm, because life is rarely calm. And once you've started a weight program, don't use life's ups and downs as an excuse to quit. If you get hit with the unexpected — you can count on that happening — cut yourself some slack if you need to, but stick with your program. For example, try to maintain your current weight but not work at losing more weight until the crisis passes. Whatever you do, stay motivated and keep sight of your long-term goals.

Discovering your barriers to weight loss

Everyone will encounter barriers in his or her path that can stop a weight program in its tracks. Some of these barriers are external — like holiday parties — and others are internal — like poor body image — but they're always slightly different for each person. It's important to identify what your personal barriers are and to learn to cope with them. You can develop responses that ease problem situations as they develop. For example, you can make your appearance at office holiday parties brief or you can involve yourself in planning and operating the festivities so that you'll be occupied (and not eating) during the party.

Some of the common barriers that people face when they try to lose weight are listed in the Action Guide to Weight-Loss Barriers on pages 146 to 179. If one or more barriers apply to you, review the accompanying Action Guide strategies on how to respond to them.

MEET REALISTIC EXPECTATIONS

No one can make you lose weight. In fact, external pressure — often from people close to you — may only make matters worse. Likewise, losing weight to satisfy someone else rarely works. You must want to change your diet and be more active in order to please yourself.

Of course, this doesn't mean you have to do it alone. Your doctor or another health care professional can help you develop a weight program. And be certain to ask for support from your spouse, partner, family and friends. These people know you best and are likely to provide the sort of encouragement you need.

When you're thinking about what to expect from a weight program, be realistic. Remember that healthy weight loss comes slow and steady. Don't aspire to an impractical ideal. Instead, try to achieve a healthy weight for you, focused on improving your health. If you've always been heavy, then aim for a weight that causes your blood pressure, cholesterol levels, energy and sleep to improve.

Always be willing to examine the underlying assumptions you make about weight loss. For example, maybe you thought losing weight would be easier or faster, or that your life would change in significant ways. Perhaps you thought you'd receive more compliments and more social engagements. These underlying assumptions can negatively affect your attitude and self-esteem, not to mention the success of your program.

GOAL SETTING

Goal setting is a way to meet your expectations. It puts your thoughts into action. But your ability to reach weight goals is closely tied to how realistic your expectations are. You can exercise regularly and avoid dessert for a month of Sundays, but if your expectation is to get back to your high-school weight in time for a big reunion next summer, it's probably not going to happen. If your expectation is to gradually improve healthy behaviors that help you control your weight, your chance of success is greater.

Your weight goals should be challenging but achievable in a reasonably short period of time. Always be mindful of how much weight you'd like to lose and how fast it should come off. Your overall weight goal can be met through a series of smaller goals that build on each other. Goals that are unrealistic or too long-term just make you feel frustrated and disappointed when you don't meet them.

As you start to develop a weight program, consider two types of goals — performance goals and outcome goals. A performance goal measures specific activity that you can do and includes factors over which you have control. Often, people set more than one performance goal. You might decrease the number of servings of high-fat foods in your diet and increase your intake of fresh fruits and vegetables. You might begin walking or jogging a specific number of miles each week. You might start keeping a daily food and activity diary. At the end of the time you've set for yourself, you gauge your success on how well you've stuck to your plan rather than on how many pounds you may have lost.

On the other hand, an outcome goal measures the end result but doesn't assess how you achieve that result. An outcome goal is generally longer term than is a performance goal and involves a measure or level that you want to achieve, for example, a goal to lose 20 pounds.

When an outcome goal is made with little regard to performance goals, it can sometimes lead to failure. For example, you decide that you'll lose 12 pounds in a month. Your focus is on that end-of-the-month goal, not on the individual steps you may take to lose weight. At the end

of the month, you weigh yourself and find that you've lost only 4 pounds. At first, this may prompt you to try harder, but after several more tries, you begin to feel frustrated and give up the program.

Both performance goals and outcome goals should work together in support of your weight program. Performance goals help you focus on specific activities, and success is measured by your mastery of each activity. Outcome goals help you focus on the desired result and keep you moving ahead.

When you struggle with your weight program, always be willing to reassess and adjust goals. Make sure they're your goals and not anyone else's. Keep them realistic. You will lose the weight. Your life will change. But it takes time.

Be SMART about goals

Goal setting isn't as simple as it may sound. You don't identify a couple of goals you want to achieve and then expect them to occur like magic. You'll be setting yourself up for disappointment. The key to successful weight control is to set goals that are SMART — specific, measurable, attainable, realistic and trackable:

Specific. State exactly what you want to achieve, how you're going to do it and when you want to achieve it. It's helpful to plan a series of small goals that build on each other instead of one big, all-encompassing goal.

Measurable. Be sure you can tell whether you've achieved a goal or not. For example, if your goal is to walk for 30 minutes a day, a watch will let you know when you've achieved it.

Attainable. Ask yourself whether a goal is reasonable before you set it. Are you allowing sufficient time and resources? Start slowly and work your way up to larger goals.

Realistic. Set goals that are within your capabilities, and take into account your limitations. Do you really want to be a size 8 when you were never that size before, even in high school?

Trackable. Look for ways to record your progress, such as a food diary or exercise log. Tracking your effort helps keep you motivated.

PART II

Building blocks of a weight program

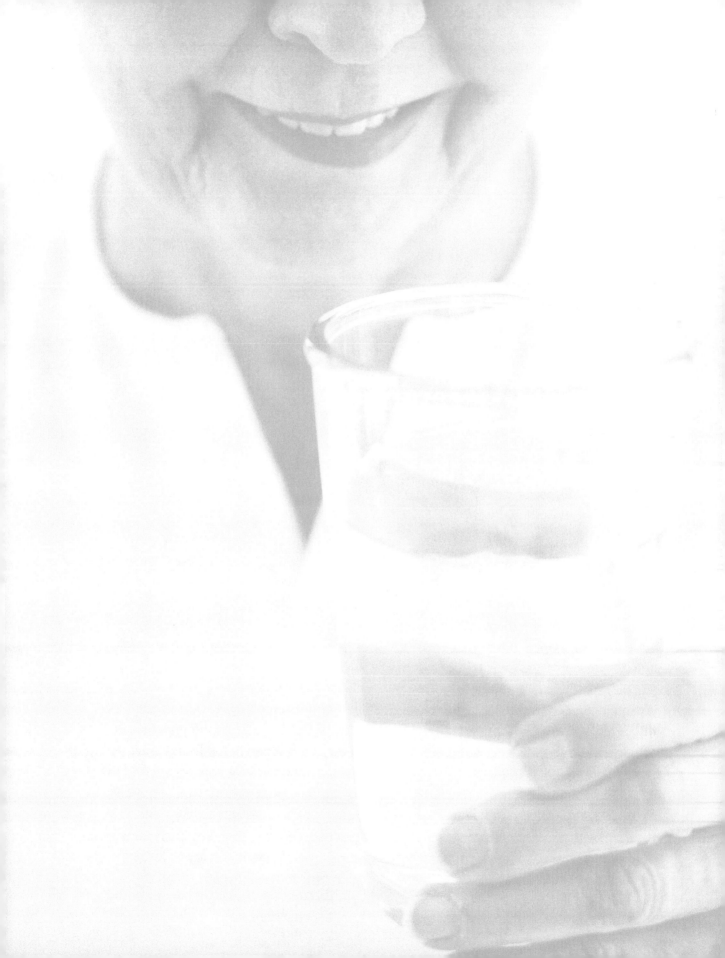

CHAPTER 4

Understanding weight control

H ere's something you may not associate with weight control: energy. All living things need energy to grow and develop, to function properly and, in short, to survive. Your body has a constant demand for energy. You replenish lost energy with the food you eat. Weight is all about the balance you maintain between energy added through diet and energy burned through activity. This energy balance is a basic principle of weight control.

Food energy is measured in units called calories. It's easy to find lists of foods and the calories they contain. Other lists show how many calories you can burn by doing certain activities. This knowledge is helpful in assessing your own energy balance

and maintaining a healthy weight. At first, it may seem overwhelming to keep track of your calorie intake and expenditure. But try to focus on the overall situation, not on exact totals. With practice, you may get to the point where the task becomes second nature.

This chapter provides you with some of the science behind the energy balance. Do you have to know everything there is to know about different foods and exact calorie amounts? Will you be expected to do rigorous exercises that you're not prepared for? No to both questions, but a general understanding will guide your decisions about diet and activity. Your success with weight control is all about making informed choices.

DIETARY SOURCES OF ENERGY

There's truth to the saying, "You are what you eat." Food provides much more than energy for your body to function. Food draws people together — the kitchen is frequently the hub of home life. Food can be adventurous, a means of exploring other customs and cultures. Food preparation can be an exquisite form of art.

Food also elicits many emotions. Some people eat when they're sad, others when they're happy. Most associate food with celebrations and special moments in their lives. Food appeals to our senses of taste, smell, sound, sight and touch.

With so many cultural, social and emotional associations, is it any wonder that controlling what you eat is one of the most difficult aspects of controlling your weight? Food can be healthy and enjoyable for you, but food that's too high in calories or of too large a portion can cause you to be overweight and put you at risk of disease. In this age of abundance, convenience and automated efficiency, the healthy enjoyment of food takes more planning than you may think.

Elements of nutrition

The food you eat supplies many types of nutrients, which provide the energy your body needs in order to grow and function. These nutrients include carbohydrates, fats, proteins, vitamins and minerals. Food is also a source of water and fiber, both of which are essential to your good health.

What's a calorie?

Calories can be used to measure any kind of energy but people most often associate the term with nutrition. One calorie is the amount of energy required to raise the temperature of 1 gram of water by 1 degree Celsius (1.8 F). Because that's such a small unit of measure, food energy is actually measured in terms of kilocalories (1,000 calories). Nevertheless, the numbers you see on nutrition labels are still marked as calories. In nutrition, the terms *calorie* and *kilocalorie* have become synonymous.

Carbohydrates

Carbohydrates can be simple or complex. Simple carbohydrates are the sugars found in fruits, honey and milk. They're absorbed quickly into the body for energy. Complex carbohydrates, also known as starches, are found primarily in whole grains, pasta, potatoes, beans and vegetables. Digestion is required to change complex carbohydrates into simple sugars.

Complex carbohydrates, such as whole-grain products, contain many vitamins and minerals as well as fiber. Through processing, complex carbohydrates are refined, meaning most of these important benefits have been removed.

Fats

Fats are a natural component of various foods, and they come in different forms. The oils used in cooking are a form of fat.

Fats are also found in foods of animal origin, such as meat, dairy, poultry and fish, and in such common foods as avocados, nuts and olives.

Proteins

Proteins build and repair body structures, produce body chemicals, carry nutrients to your cells and regulate body processes. They're composed of basic elements called amino acids. There are two types of amino acids: those that your body can generate (nonessential amino acids) and those that can be obtained only from the food you eat (essential amino acids).

Vitamins

Many foods contain vitamins, such as A, B, C, D, E and K. Vitamins help your body process carbohydrates, fats and proteins. They also help produce blood cells, hormones, genetic material and chemicals for the nervous system. Vitamin deficiencies lead to various diseases. Fresh, natural foods usually contain more vitamins than do processed foods.

Minerals

Minerals such as calcium, magnesium and phosphorus are important to the health of your bones and teeth. Sodium, potassium and chloride, commonly referred to as electrolytes, help regulate the water and chemical balance in your body. Your body needs smaller amounts of minerals such as iron, iodine, zinc, copper, fluoride, selenium and manganese, commonly referred to as trace minerals.

Water

It's easy to take water for granted, but it's a vital nutritional requirement. Many foods, especially fruit, contain a lot of water. Of course, the most direct way to get water into your system is to drink it. Water plays a role in nearly every major body function. It regulates body temperature, carries nutrients and oxygen to cells via the bloodstream and helps carry away waste. Water also helps cushion joints and protects organs and tissues.

Fiber

Fiber is the part of plant foods that your body doesn't absorb. The two main types of fiber are soluble and insoluble, and fiber-rich foods usually contain both. Foods high in soluble fiber include citrus fruits, strawberries, apples, legumes, oatmeal and oat bran. Soluble fiber helps lower blood cholesterol and adds bulk to stools. Insoluble fiber is found in many vegetables, wheat bran, and whole-grain breads, pasta and cereals. Insoluble fiber stimulates the gastrointestinal tract, helping to prevent constipation.

Where the calories come from

Carbohydrates, fats and proteins are the types of nutrients that contain calories and thus are the main energy sources for your body. The amount of energy each nutrient provides varies, as well as the mechanism by which the energy is supplied. *Empty calories* is a term applied to sugar and alcohol. They contribute calories, but no other essential nutrients.

Carbohydrates are the nutrients in the food you eat that get used up first. During digestion, they're released into your bloodstream and converted into glucose, or blood sugar. When there's a demand, the glucose is absorbed immediately into your body's cells to provide energy. If there's no immediate demand, glucose can be stored in your liver and muscles. When these storage sites become full, excess glucose is converted into fatty acids and stored in fat tissue for later use.

Fats are an extremely concentrated form of energy and pack the most calories. When digested, they're broken down into fatty acids, which can be used immediately for energy or for other body processes. If there's an excess of fatty acids, a small quantity can be stored in your muscles, but most of them are stored in fat tissue. There's virtually no limit to how much fat your body can store.

Proteins have many responsibilities in your body but can also supply energy for physical activity if your body runs out of carbohydrate power. This can happen if you consume too few calories or if you're involved in prolonged physical activity. Any excess calories from protein, of course, are also stored in fat tissue.

Vitamins, minerals, water and fiber don't contain calories. Although these nutrients may not provide energy, they're still vital to your health and well-being. When they're lacking from your diet, you increase your risk of serious illness. Other substances in food, such as cholesterol, don't provide calories either.

Food sources of energy

Fats supply more calories per gram than do carbohydrates and proteins combined. Many people are surprised that alcohol can be such a high source of calories.

Nutrient	Calories (per gram)
Fats	9
Alcohol	7
Carbohydrates	4
Proteins	4

YOUR ENERGY ACCOUNT

Imagine that the energy needs of your body are like a bank account. Lots of transactions go on in this account. You have daily deposits, and you have daily withdrawals. Your deposits are food, with three nutrients providing the bulk of your energy: carbohydrates, fats and proteins. When you eat, you're adding to your energy account — in the form of calories.

Withdrawals on this account can be made in three ways, each of which burn calories. The most obvious type of withdrawal is when you exert yourself by doing physical activity. But your body also withdraws energy to meet its basic needs, such as breathing, blood circulation, hormone adjustments, and cellular growth and repair. Even when you're in a state of complete rest, your body is using energy. This energy use at rest is called your basal metabolic rate (BMR). Your body also makes an energy withdrawal when it digests and absorbs food.

Your BMR is responsible for the greatest demand on your energy account — generally, one-half to two-thirds of your total energy expenditure. The energy needs of your BMR and for digestion remain relatively steady and aren't easy to change. The best way to increase your energy withdrawal — in other words, to burn more calories — is to increase the amount of physical activity you do.

Influences on your energy account

If everyone were physically and functionally identical, it would be easy to determine the standard energy needs for all kinds of activity. But other factors affect your energy account. Obviously, people differ in many ways and their energy needs vary accordingly. Some of the factors that influence your BMR and your overall energy needs are age, body size and composition, and sex.

Age

Children and adolescents, who are in the process of developing their bones, muscles and tissues, need more calories per pound than adults do. In fact, infants need the most calories per pound of any age group because of their rapid growth and development. As hormone levels and body composition change with age, so does a person's BMR. By the time you reach adulthood, your BMR and energy needs are declining, generally at a rate of 2 percent a decade.

Daily calorie needs

It takes calories to keep your body functioning throughout the day, even when you're not moving. Keeping your heart, brain and other organs working and staying warm requires a certain amount of energy. This amount of energy is called your basal metabolic rate (BMR), or basal energy expenditure.

Your body also requires energy to digest, absorb, transport and store the food you eat. This is known as the thermic effect of food. It takes about 10 percent of your total energy expenditure — considerably more than you might think.

Daily tasks such as getting dressed, brushing your teeth, and walking to work also require energy. These actions increase your energy expenditure by about 20 percent. When you add in planned physical activities — such as jogging, hiking or playing a round of golf — your body demands even more calories to keep going. That's why your energy requirements, or how many calories you need to consume to maintain a given weight, depend on how sedentary or active you are.

Body size and composition

In order to function properly, a bigger body mass requires more energy, and thus more calories, than does a smaller body mass. In addition, muscle burns more calories than fat does, so the more muscle you have in relation to fat, the higher

Calories and energy

A typical candy bar contains about 270 calories. If you were to set that candy bar on fire and burn it completely, the process would produce exactly 270 calories of energy.

Your body also burns calories to create energy, but the process is a result of chemical reactions rather than of heat.

your BMR. Based on this principle, you can slightly increase your BMR and the amount of energy you burn by building up your muscle mass through regular physical activity.

Sex

Men usually have less body fat and more muscle than do women of the same age and weight. This is why men generally have a higher BMR and higher energy requirements than women do.

Balancing your account

Your body weight is a physical reflection of your energy account. Daily fluctuations of your weight indicate the daily changes in your account. If you withdraw from the account approximately the same amount of energy as you deposit, your weight stays the same. If you expend more from the account than you deposit, you lose weight.

There's a magic number in this energy equation. Because 3,500 calories equals about 1 pound of body fat, you'd need to

consume 3,500 excess calories to gain a pound, and conversely, you'd need to burn 3,500 calories more than you take in to lose a pound. This knowledge may seem impractical on a daily basis but it does generally indicate what it takes to reach your weight goal.

Many people prefer keeping their energy accounts balanced — meaning there's just enough calories in the accounts to meet their energy needs but no more. The tricky part is that energy needs vary from day to day. The amounts of food that people eat also vary. So the balance between calories consumed and calories expended is constantly shifting.

Tracking these shifts would require a bit of old-fashioned accounting — tallying up all the sources of energy income

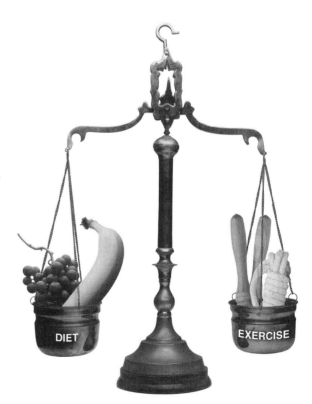

(dietary consumption) and all the forms of energy expenditure — including your BMR and your energy needs for digestion. Who has the time and resources to make this daily effort?

It's easier to think about weight control in terms of general principles. One thing you can be sure of is that losing weight requires an energy deficit. You create this deficit by eating fewer calories, increasing the number of calories burned through physical activity, or doing both. Reducing calories tends to figure more prominently than physical activity does during the initial stages of weight loss. But as you work toward a healthy weight, you'll find that physical activity is more and more essential to reaching your goal.

HEALTHY WEIGHT CONTROL

Do you have to eat carrots and celery sticks and avoid even the sight of chocolate for the rest of your life in order to maintain a healthy weight? Not really. In terms of energy balance, you can see that it's possible to eat any food you like and lose weight as long as the total calories you consume are less than the total calories you burn. It's liberating to know that it's not necessarily the kinds of food you eat that make you gain weight. It's more about the amounts of food and the number of calories they contain.

Suppose you could choose one item to eat from among the following choices: a candy bar, six slices of bacon, 20 cups of salad greens or four apples. Regardless of what you choose, you would be consuming around 270 calories. The fact is, you'd probably be hungrier an hour later if you ate the candy bar than if you ate 20 cups of salad greens. So if you're counting calories, the types of food you eat can affect the volume of food you eat.

Clearly, and you can probably see this one coming, the types of food you eat also affect your overall health. Consider this: If the bulk of your diet consists of foods that are high in saturated fat, such as bacon and candy bars, you run the risk of increasing your low-density lipoprotein (LDL, or "bad") cholesterol levels, narrowing your arteries and restricting blood flow, which could potentially result in a heart attack. Evidence also links diets high in refined carbohydrates and low in fiber, such as in highly processed or prepackaged foods, to conditions such as diabetes and cardiovascular disease.

In addition, if you're lacking vegetables and fruits in your diet, you're missing many health benefits such as:

- Vitamins and minerals needed for vital body processes and for defending against certain bone conditions (vitamin D and calcium deficiencies) and anemia (iron deficiency)
- Phytochemicals, a group of compounds that may help prevent chronic diseases, such as cardiovascular disease and diabetes, and cancer
- Antioxidants, substances that slow down oxidation, a natural process that leads to cell and tissue damage

STICKING TO PRINCIPLES

So, there really is true science behind a part of your life that you may consider routine and ordinary. The everyday decisions you make regarding the food you eat and the activity you do and, ultimately, the weight you carry, relate to what's called the first law of thermodynamics. This law states that energy must remain constant — it can neither be created nor destroyed, merely transferred or converted to different forms.

Thus, the calories you eat can either be converted to physical energy, or they can be stored within your body, but they can't magically disappear. Unfortunately, there is no silver bullet or magic potion for weight loss. All unused calories in your body become fat, regardless of where they come from. Unless you use these stored calories, either by reducing calorie intake so that your body must draw on reserves for energy or by increasing physical activity and the amount of energy you expend, this fat will remain on your body.

In theory, the energy balance equation is simple. In practice, as you may know already, reaching a healthy weight can seem complex. But as you grasp the concept of energy balance, weight control may become easier to understand. A healthy weight can be achieved in a way that allows you to enjoy food as well as long-term health.

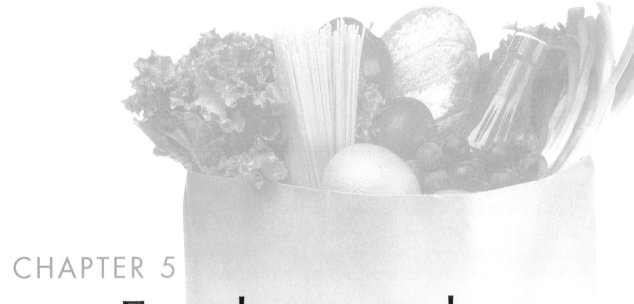

CHAPTER 5

Fundamentals of healthy eating

Achieving a healthy weight may require you to cut back on some favorite foods and change your eating habits. But that doesn't mean you'll be sacrificing delicious meals, dining satisfaction or convenience in the kitchen.

You can make the necessary changes to your diet while eating foods that are good tasting, healthy and practical. Being open to variety in the kinds of foods you eat and the manner in which they're prepared can help you achieve your weight goals and maintain your interest. Healthy eating means enjoying great taste as well as great nutrition.

Healthy eating involves a diet emphasizing vegetables, fruits and whole grains. This approach will reduce your risks of certain diseases. Heart disease, high blood pressure and many cancers are linked most notably to diets high in saturated fat and refined carbohydrates. So even if weight loss isn't your primary goal, adopting a healthier approach to eating can be beneficial.

Maintaining a healthy weight over your lifetime involves an eating plan that you enjoy and never tire of. That means no severe restrictions, no extreme hunger and no unrealistic expectations are placed on you. You don't want to become disillusioned or bored with your dietary routine. A healthy approach that allows you to eat a wide variety of foods and not feel as if you're starving yourself involves the concept of energy density.

WEIGHT LOSS AND ENERGY DENSITY

In Chapter 4 you learned about the energy balance equation. To maintain your body weight, the amount of energy you take in (calories consumed) must equal the amount of energy you expend (calories burned), often through activity.

To lose weight, you need to create an energy deficit, by decreasing your energy intake or increasing your energy expenditure or both. For example, eliminating one 12-ounce soft drink each day from your diet can decrease your energy intake by around 140 calories. To burn the same amount of calories, you'd need to take a brisk 30-minute walk. Doing both — eliminating the soft drink and taking a walk — works best. Both are healthy actions and you eliminate twice the calories.

Regardless, losing weight almost always requires you to cut down on the number of calories you consume. If just thinking about reducing calories brings hunger pains, believe it or not, it's possible to lose weight and still be satisfied with the amount of food you eat. The key is to replace foods that are high in calories with ones that are low in calories.

Think volume

All foods contain a certain number of calories in a given amount (volume). For example, 1 cup of raw vegetables contains about 25 calories. Of course, the number of calories per unit of volume varies from one type of food to the next.

Some foods contain many calories in just a small portion. They're described as high in energy density — remember that calories are your body's primary energy source. Foods that are high in energy density include most high-fat foods, simple sugars, alcohol, fast foods, sodas, candies and processed foods. For example, a regular candy bar generally contains 270 calories. Eating one candy bar may provide a lot of the calories you allow for yourself each day but it doesn't fill your stomach. This could spell trouble if you're trying to lose weight because your calorie intake could quickly exceed calorie expenditure.

Foods such as vegetables and fruits have fewer calories in a greater volume. These types of foods are considered low in energy density. In contrast to the 270 calories in a regular candy bar, a cup of cubed cantaloupe has about 60 calories. So if you choose to eat a generous portion of cantaloupe instead of a candy bar, you can consume fewer calories and walk away from the table feeling full.

Different foods and energy densities

	Calories
1 cup raw vegetables	25
1 cup fresh melon	60
1 cup fat-free milk	90
1 cup cooked pasta	160
1 cup regular salad dressing	720

Two factors play important roles in what makes food less energy dense and more filling: water and fiber.

- **Water.** Most fruits and vegetables contain a lot of water, which provides volume and weight to what you eat but not calories. Grapefruit, for example, is about 90 percent water and has just 39 calories in a half-fruit portion. Carrots are about 88 percent water and have only 52 calories in 1 cup.
- **Fiber.** Fiber is the part of plant-based foods that your body doesn't absorb. The high fiber content in foods such as vegetables, fruits and whole grains provides bulk to your diet, so it makes you feel full sooner. The fiber also takes longer to digest, making you feel full longer. The recommended daily amount of fiber for adults is 20 to 35 grams but on average, most adults consume between 10 and 15 grams each day.

Feeling full on fewer calories — it sounds like one of those diet gimmicks. But the energy density concept makes sense. Research suggests that feeling full is strongly determined by the volume and weight of food in your stomach, not necessarily by the amount of calories you eat. By choosing foods with a low energy density, you can consume fewer calories while eating similar amounts of food as you did before. See pages A2-A3 of the Visual Guide for a visual example.

Scientists at Pennsylvania State University and the University of Alabama at Birmingham, as well as at Mayo Clinic, have tested the concept of energy density.

Participants in several studies who switched to a diet of low energy density foods were able to lose significant amounts of weight. More importantly, they were able to keep a good deal of the weight off over time, decreasing their risk of weight-related diseases, by sticking with a low energy density diet.

NEW APPROACH TO HEALTHY WEIGHT

An effective diet to control weight may require you to reduce calories, but it should not be at the cost of good health, taste and practicality. Shopping, cooking and eating practices should be simple and inexpensive. Otherwise, you won't stay with the plan. A diet that's enjoyable and satisfying is vital to the long-term success of your healthy weight program.

Welcome to the Mayo Clinic Healthy Weight Pyramid. The pyramid is based on the concept of energy density and it promotes a plant-based diet, represented by the organization of the pyramid — the vegetables and fruits groups share the base of the pyramid, and the carbohydrates group is located just above them.

The Mayo Clinic Healthy Weight Pyramid can help you improve your health and achieve your weight goals. It's an easy-to-use guide to what you need to eat daily from each of six food groups.

You may be wondering, Why another food pyramid? The U.S. Department of Agriculture (USDA) has already developed the USDA Food Guide Pyramid to help implement its dietary guidelines. Although the Mayo Clinic Healthy Weight Pyramid is similar to the USDA pyramid, a closer look will reveal that it differs in several ways:

- The Mayo Clinic Healthy Weight Pyramid is geared toward losing weight as well as maintaining weight. The USDA pyramid does not emphasize weight loss.

- The Mayo Clinic Healthy Weight Pyramid emphasizes health-promoting choices within each food group.

- The foundation of the Mayo Clinic Healthy Weight Pyramid are the vegetables and fruits groups. Mayo's approach incorporates an unlimited allowance of fresh vegetables and fruits into your diet — this allowance does not apply to dried fruits and fruit juices, which are healthy but have many more calories.

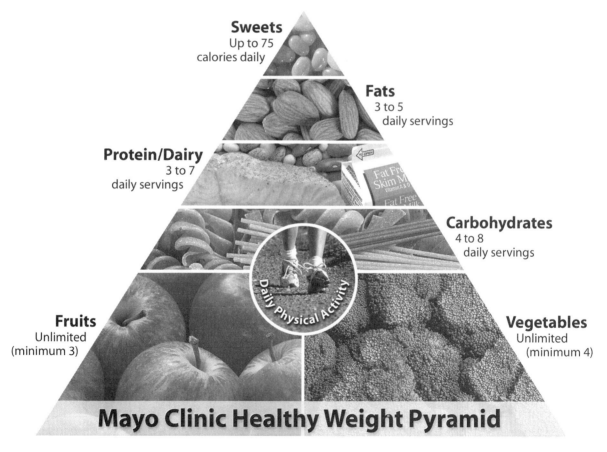

Sweets
Up to 75
calories daily

Fats
3 to 5
daily servings

Protein/Dairy
3 to 7
daily servings

Carbohydrates
4 to 8
daily servings

Daily Physical Activity

Fruits
Unlimited
(minimum 3)

Vegetables
Unlimited
(minimum 4)

Mayo Clinic Healthy Weight Pyramid

© Mayo Foundation for Medical Education and Research.
See your doctor before you begin any healthy weight plan.

A LOOK AT THE FOOD GROUPS

The six food groups of the Mayo Clinic Healthy Weight Pyramid are vegetables, fruits, carbohydrates, protein and dairy, fats, and sweets. Most of the foods we eat fall into one of these groups.

Does the organization seem confusing at first? After all, vegetables and fruits are types of food while, as you learned in Chapter 4, carbohydrates, protein and fats are nutrients found in many different types of food. For example, vegetables and fruits contain carbohydrates and some contain proteins and fats. Sweets are sources of carbohydrates and fats.

Well, it's a fact that foods, no matter how you organize them, don't fall neatly into categories. The food groups of the Mayo Clinic Healthy Weight Pyramid are based on several factors. For one thing, the food groups differ in their levels of energy density — and foods with the lowest energy density are at the base of the pyramid. Foods within each group also share common health benefits to your overall diet. The group breakdown is also practical in terms of your ability to select and prepare the different foods.

Vegetables and fruits

Vegetables and fruits share many attributes. In fact, some foods that we term *vegetable* are technically fruits. Both offer a wide array of flavors, textures and colors. They not only provide sensory pleasure but also many disease-fighting nutrients. Most vegetables and fruits are low in energy density because they have a high content of water and fiber, which provide no calories. You can improve your diet without reducing the amount of food you eat by eating more vegetables and fruits in place of foods that have more calories.

Vegetables

Vegetables include roots such as carrots and beets, tubers such as potatoes, members of the cabbage family, and salad greens such as lettuce and spinach. Other plant foods, such as tomatoes, peppers and cucumbers, are included in this group, although technically they're fruits.

One serving of vegetables contains about 25 calories. In general, vegetables have less sugar (and therefore have fewer calories) and are less sweet tasting than fruits are. Vegetables contain no cholesterol, are low in fat and sodium, are high in dietary fiber and in essential minerals, such as potassium and magnesium, and contain beneficial plant chemicals known as phytochemicals.

Fresh vegetables are best, but frozen vegetables are good, too. Most canned vegetables are high in sodium because sodium is used as a preservative in the canning process. If you use canned vegetables, look for labels that indicate that no salt is added, or be sure to rinse them.

Fruits

Any food that contains seeds surrounded by an edible layer is generally considered a fruit. In North America, fruits such as apples, oranges, peaches and plums, and

Setting the record straight

Carbohydrates don't make you fat; excess calories do. Recently, many diets have promoted low-carbohydrate foods for weight loss. These diets claim that carbohydrates stimulate insulin secretion, which promotes body fat. So, the logic goes, reducing carbohydrates will reduce body fat. As a matter of fact, carbohydrates do stimulate insulin secretion immediately after they're consumed, but this is a normal process that allows carbohydrates to be absorbed into cells. People who gain weight on high-carbohydrate diets do so because they're eating excess calories. Excess calories from any source, whether it contains a lot of carbohydrates or only a few, will cause weight gain.

Furthermore, some low-carbohydrate diets restrict grains, fruits and vegetables and emphasize the consumption of protein and dairy products, which can be high calorie and loaded with saturated fat and cholesterol. Plant-based foods not only are low in saturated fat and cholesterol-free but also are loaded with vitamins, minerals and other nutrients. These nutrients play a protective role in fighting serious diseases such as cancer, osteoporosis, high blood pressure and heart disease.

So be skeptical of the low-carbohydrate claims. Many carbohydrate-containing foods are healthy and can be an important part of a weight-loss plan. For more on low-carbohydrate diets, see Chapter 12.

slightly more exotic fruits such as mangos and papayas, are commonly available. These foods taste sweet or sweet-tart and are often eaten for snacks or desserts.

Like vegetables, fruits are great sources of fiber, vitamins, minerals and other phytochemicals. One serving equals about 60 calories and is virtually fat-free, so fruits can help you control your weight and reduce your risk of weight-related diseases. Fresh fruit is best, but frozen fruits with no added sugar and fruits canned in their own juice or water are also excellent. Use fruit juice and dried fruits, such as raisins and prunes, sparingly because they're a concentrated source of calories. That is, they have a higher energy density.

Carbohydrates

Carbohydrates include a wide range of foods that are a major source of energy for your body. Most carbohydrates are plant-based. These include grain products such as cereal, bread, rice and pasta. Carbohydrates may also come from other food groups, including starchy vegetables such as potatoes, corn, sweet potatoes and winter squash. Dairy products are the only animal-based foods that supply substantial carbohydrates.

Carbohydrates provide a variety of nutrients and are generally low in fat and calories. One serving equals approximately 70 calories. Carbohydrates vary in energy density, depending on whether they're simple or complex. The more complex carbohydrates — for example, grains and grain products — have a moderately low energy density. They're often high in fiber. Be aware that grain products such as croissants and dessert breads include ingredients that are high in fat and calories, making them high in energy density.

When choosing grain products, look for the word *whole*, as in whole wheat, on the packaging and in the ingredients list. Whole grains contain the bran and germ, which are sources of fiber, vitamins and minerals. When grains are refined, some of the nutrients and the fiber are eliminated. As a rule, the less refined a carbohydrate, the better it is for you.

Protein and dairy

Proteins are essential to human life — every cell in your body contains them. Your skin, bone, muscle and organ tissues are made up of proteins, and they're found in blood, hormones and enzymes. Proteins are also vital nutrients in many foods. One serving of protein equals approximately 110 calories.

Foods rich in proteins and relatively low in fat and saturated fat include legumes, fish and lean meat. Whole-milk dairy products are good sources of proteins and calcium but are high in fat, especially saturated fat. Low-fat or skim milk, yogurt and cheese have the same nutritional values as the whole-milk varieties but without the fat and calories. They're relatively low in energy density, too, because they contain a lot of water.

Fats

Many people are surprised to hear that certain fats are essential to the life and function of the body's cells. Along with providing reserves of stored energy, these fats play a role in the immune system, help maintain cell structure, and play a role in the regulation of many body processes. Deposits of fat tissue protect and insulate vital body organs. In short, you need some fat in your diet.

Fats (lipids) are substances that don't dissolve in water. The fats group includes oils, margarine, butter, salad dressings and mayonnaise, but almost every food has some fat, at least in very small amounts. Avocados, olives, seeds and nuts are placed in this food group because of their high fat content. Animal products — meats, dairy products and eggs — are the main sources of fat in the American diet. Fruits, vegetables and grains are relatively low in fat.

There are several different kinds of fat in the food you eat, including saturated, polyunsaturated, monounsaturated and trans fats. In terms of healthfulness, not all fats are equal. The healthier fats are the monounsaturated varieties, including olive oil and canola oil. But all fats contain approximately 45 calories a serving, and are a high-energy-density food. For that reason, all fats, including the healthier ones, should be consumed sparingly.

Saturated fat

Saturated fat is the main dietary culprit in raising blood cholesterol and increasing the risk of disease in your body's coronary arteries. Foods high in saturated fat include red meats and most dairy products, as well as butter, lard, and coconut, palm and other tropical oils. Limit these fats and choose low-fat dairy products.

Polyunsaturated fat

This type of fat helps lower your blood cholesterol but is susceptible to a harmful process called oxidation. Safflower, corn, sunflower and soy oils are high in polyunsaturated fat. Cold-water fish such as salmon provide a heart-healthy form of this fat — omega-3 fatty acids.

Monounsaturated fat

Monounsaturated fat helps reduce low-density lipoprotein (LDL) cholesterol and is more resistant to oxidation than the polyunsaturated fats. It also helps clear arteries by maintaining high-density lipoprotein (HDL) cholesterol. Nuts, avocados, canola oil, olive oil and peanut oil are sources of monounsaturated fat. These are the healthier fats to consume in your diet.

Trans fat

Also referred to as partially hydrogenated vegetable oil, this type of fat may be even more harmful to your health than saturated fat. Trans fat raises "bad" LDL cholesterol levels and lowers "good" HDL cholesterol, along with other effects. The most common sources of trans fat include margarine or shortening, and any products made from them, such as cookies, crackers and deep-fried foods.

Sweets

Foods in the sweets group include candies, cakes, cookies, pies, doughnuts and other desserts. And don't forget the table sugar you add to cereal, fruit, and beverages. Sweets are a high source of calories, mostly from sugar and fat, and are high in energy density, yet they offer little in terms of nutrition. You don't have to give up these foods entirely. But be smart about your selections and portion sizes. The pyramid recommends limiting sweets to 75 calories a day. Where possible, select better dessert choices, such as fig bar cookies and low-fat frozen yogurt.

DAILY CALORIE GOALS

The best way to regulate calorie consumption is to know how many calories you should eat each day. If you meet this daily calorie goal on a regular basis, you should be able to reach your overall weight goal.

Let's return to the discussion of your body's calorie needs from Chapter 4. The total amount of calories you burn in a day is typically the sum of three different processes: calories burned at rest (basal metabolic rate, or BMR), calories burned during the digestive process, and calories burned during physical activity. Physical activity is the best way for you to increase or decrease your calorie expenditure.

Theoretically, if what you eat contains the same number of calories as what you burn each day, you'll maintain your weight because you're eating exactly as many calories as your body requires. For most people, this ranges from 1,600 to 2,400 daily calories. Daily calorie goal levels are calculated in general increments of 200 calories, for example, 1,600, 1,800 and 2,000 calories a day. The table on this page indicates, on average, the daily calorie goals for individuals seeking to maintain their weight. Although these recommendations should work, in practice they often don't. Usually, people eat more calories than they realize.

Figuring out the exact number of calories you need in a day can be complex and highly individualized. If your goal is weight loss, subtracting 500 calories a day from your daily calorie goal should promote losing about a pound a week, because 3,500 calories (500 calories x 7 days) equals one pound of body fat. But this approach will require exacting records and calculations.

Here's a simpler approach: It's recommended that an average woman who wants to lose weight should set her daily calorie goal at 1,200 calories. The average man should set his daily calorie goal at 1,400 calories. These calorie goals are good starting points for most people who begin their weight-control programs at or below 250 pounds. These goals will put less stress on the body than does a drastic cut in calorie intake.

If you weigh more than 250 pounds, refer to the chart on page 184 to learn your calorie level. Daily calorie goals under 1,200 for women and 1,400 for men generally aren't recommended. If your calorie goals are too low, you may not be getting enough of the nutrients you need for good health. Although it's tempting to starve yourself to lose weight quickly, this is not a healthy long-term strategy.

The recommendations of the Healthy Weight Pyramid serve as a general guide for everybody's situation and need to be adapted to many different needs. Over time, people's calorie goals will change based on their age, sex, health risks and activity level. Their daily calorie goals can be adjusted to higher levels if they become too hungry during the day or if they've reached their target weight and want to stop losing pounds.

Daily calorie goals for maintaining weight

On average, daily calorie goals for people seeking to maintain their weight are as follows:

Calories	
1,600	Children ages 2 to 6, most women and some older adults
2,000	Average adult
2,200	Older children, teenage girls, active women and most men
2,400	Teenage boys and active men

ALL ABOUT SERVINGS

In learning about diet and nutrition, you're sure to come across the term *servings*. Here, an important clarification needs to be made. A serving isn't the amount of food you choose to eat or the amount that's put on your plate. This is called a portion. A serving is a specific amount of food, defined by standard measurements such as cups, ounces or pieces — for example, medium or small pieces of fruit.

The U.S. Department of Agriculture Food Guide Pyramid is based on the number of servings from each food group, as is the Mayo Clinic Healthy Weight Pyramid. Your ability to monitor the number of servings you eat at meals is key to meeting your daily calorie goal.

Due to the variation in calorie content, serving sizes vary from one food group to the next. The average serving sizes for the different food groups are shown on page A6 of the Visual Guide.

You need to be aware that there's also some variation in serving sizes within a single food group. For example, due to the different calorie content, a small apple, medium orange and large peach are all equivalent to one fruit serving. One-half cup of carrot, one cup of broccoli, and two cups of shredded lettuce are all a single vegetable serving. An extended list of the serving sizes for different food groups can be found on pages A7 to A11 of the Visual Guide.

All of the different measurements may seem overwhelming but don't panic and throw your hands up in frustration just yet! Serving sizes aren't as complex as they seem at first. Remember that you don't have to have the entire serving-size list memorized in your head. You'll be surprised at how quickly you'll retain knowledge of the foods you use frequently and how adept you'll become at gauging the total number of servings you eat in a day. But it takes practice.

Average serving sizes

Below are the average serving sizes for food groups in the Mayo Clinic Healthy Weight Pyramid.

Food group	Average serving size	Calories per serving
Vegetables	2 cups leafy or 1 cup solid	25
Fruits	1/2 cup sliced or one medium piece	60
Carbohydrates	1/2 cup grain or 1 slice of bread	70
Protein and dairy	1/2 cup beans, 3 oz. fish, 1 cup skim milk or 1 1/2 to 2 oz. meat or hard cheese	110
Fats	1 tsp. oil or 2 tbsp. nuts	45

Daily serving recommendations for calorie levels

Food group	Starting calorie goals				
	1,200	1,400	1,600	1,800	2,000
Vegetables	4 or more	4 or more	5 or more	5 or more	5 or more
Fruits	3 or more	4 or more	5 or more	5 or more	5 or more
Carbohydrates	4	5	6	7	8
Protein/Dairy	3	4	5	6	7
Fats	3	3	3	4	5

Very often, a portion of food you eat will contain several servings of different food groups. For example, a portion of chicken casserole may contain various servings of vegetables, protein and dairy, and carbohydrates. Your best estimate of the different serving sizes is usually sufficient. You may be able to refer to a recipe or ingredients list on the package. Be on the lookout for what are known as hidden calories — the extra calories from ingredients you may not be aware of in sauces, spreads, gravies and condiments.

Recommended servings

Once you've established a calorie goal — for example, 1,200 calories a day — you can monitor your food intake by sticking to the number of servings recommended for that level. Recommended servings for common daily caloric goals are listed in the table on this page. These servings are spread out over several meals and snacks during the course of your day. If you eat the recommended number of servings daily, you should be getting about the right number of calories to meet your weight goal. You don't have to count the calories, except for when you eat sweets.

The recommended numbers of servings from the carbohydrates, protein and dairy, and fats groups are limits — you shouldn't exceed them. Servings from the vegetables and fruits groups, on the other hand, are minimums. You should eat *at least* the recommended number of fresh vegetables and fruits listed for your calorie level, and there's no worry if you exceed them.

THE BIG PICTURE

The idea behind the Mayo Clinic Healthy Weight Pyramid is to focus your diet on vegetables, fruits and whole grains. If you're hungry — eat! Starving yourself is not part of this program. Choose from the base of the pyramid and reach for more fruits or vegetables.

It's possible that the amount of calories you eat each day will be higher than the level you're aiming for, especially because

What if you have special health concerns?

You feel like a snack and there's an orange handy. But you've avoided fruit because you've got diabetes, and you're concerned about what that orange will do to your blood sugar. What should you do?

That depends on you. If you're overweight, closely following the calorie and activity guidelines of this book will have you losing excess pounds. And if you're losing weight, eating fruit won't necessarily affect your blood sugar in a negative way. Likely, you'll be just fine following the eating principles of the Mayo Clinic Healthy Weight Pyramid, which allows unlimited fruits and vegetables. But, you need to monitor your blood sugar to see how eating by the principles of the pyramid affects you.

The Mayo Clinic Healthy Weight Pyramid fits well for the vast majority of people, including most people with health concerns such as diabetes, high triglycerides or irritable bowel syndrome. But, as with any valid eating program, it's not a one-size-fits-all approach. You need to adapt it to your specific health situation or needs — you need to individualize it.

The Mayo Clinic Healthy Weight Pyramid has enough flexibility to allow that, so work with your doctor or a registered dietitian to find out how to apply the principles of the pyramid in a way that works best for you.

you're allowed unlimited vegetables and fruits and up to 75 calories a day from the sweets group. But that's OK. That's been taken into consideration. The Mayo Clinic Healthy Weight Pyramid still will enable you to manage your weight while improving your health.

If you're extremely hungry during the day, despite eating lots of vegetables and fruits and drinking enough water, consider advancing to the next higher calorie level. For example, if you're a woman and your weight is 175 pounds and you're following the 1,200-calorie plan, you might switch to the 1,400-calorie plan. A 260-pound man following the 1,600-calorie plan might switch to 1,800 daily calories.

You should also advance to the next higher calorie level if you're losing weight too quickly — more than three pounds a week after the first couple of weeks. Once you've reached a healthy weight and you want to maintain it, advancing one calorie level higher should be sufficient.

The recommendations of the Mayo Clinic Healthy Weight Pyramid can provide you with the nutrients you need for a healthy weight. The emphasis on vegetables and fruits makes your program high in fiber, vitamins and minerals. It's also low in fat, saturated fat, cholesterol and sodium. The program provides enough protein for proper tissue growth, repair and maintenance, and enough fat to meet your body's essential requirements. The selection of low-fat dairy foods helps ensure adequate calcium intake.

CHAPTER 6

Staying physically active

When you're physically active, your body uses energy to work, helping to balance the calories you take in with food. To keep the pounds off, you have to do more than transform your eating habits. You have to make physical activity an integral part of your day. If you don't move much, the energy balance usually tips toward an excess of calories and extra pounds.

Simply put, to lose weight you can eat less, get more active or both. The evidence suggests that doing both is best.

It's human nature to be efficient and seek step-saving measures. But to improve health and manage weight, you'll need to do just the opposite — look for excuses to get more active. Think of physical activity as a positive approach to weight control. You're acting — adding to your life — rather than avoiding or taking something away. The walk you take after dinner will not only burn calories but also improve your digestion, boost your energy level and help you relax.

Of course, while being more active sounds simple enough, in practice it isn't so easy. Most Americans just aren't moving enough. A majority of adults in the United States aren't physically active on a regular basis, and many aren't active at all. Part of the problem is more efficient technology and the shift to more sedentary jobs. Another part is personal: lack of time or motivation, boredom with exercise and concerns about being hurt.

START WHERE YOU ARE

Anyone can become more physically active. It's never too late to start, regardless of age, weight, fitness level and health condition. But adding more activity to your life, if you haven't been active in the recent past, can be a big change. Many people start an exercise program but don't stick with it, often because they try to do too much too soon. An all-or-nothing mentality is a recipe for discouragement, not to mention possible injury.

As you think about getting more active, take into account your personal fitness level, health concerns, available time and motivation. Tailoring your expectations to your personal situation can help you set achievable goals and stay active.

How fit are you?

Being physically fit allows your heart, lungs and muscles to perform optimally. Fitness is an individual quality that's influenced by your age, sex, genetic makeup, eating habits and level of physical activity. Although you can't change the first three factors, the last two are certainly within your control.

You know you're fit if you can:

- Carry out daily tasks without getting overly tired and still have energy to enjoy leisure pursuits
- Walk a mile or climb a few flights of stairs without becoming winded or feeling heaviness or fatigue in your legs
- Carry on a conversation during moderate exercise such as brisk walking

When you're not physically active, you become unfit (deconditioned.) Signs of deconditioning include feeling tired much of the time and fatiguing quickly. You're unable to keep up with others your age and you avoid certain activities because you know you'll soon tire.

If you find that you're unfit, don't fret. Studies show that even the most inactive people can gain considerable health benefits just by adding a few minutes more of physical activity each day.

Better together

All physical activity burns calories — and the longer and more intense your activity, the more calories you'll burn. Exercise also raises your metabolism, not just during the activity but following it as well. The longer and harder the activity, the longer your metabolism remains elevated.

When you lose weight by eating fewer calories, without raising your activity level, you lose lean tissue (muscle) as well as body fat. Loss of lean tissue makes it harder to keep weight off because your body responds to this change by burning fewer calories. This sets the stage for regaining weight. But when you combine reduced calorie consumption with exercise, you still lose body fat but less lean tissue than if you weren't active. Physical activity keeps you burning calories nearer to the same level as you did before reducing your calorie intake.

If you've been leading a sedentary life, start by just trying to move around more. Set a goal of increasing the time you spend gardening or housecleaning, or use the stairs instead of the elevator. Remember to start out slowly. Choose less strenuous activities, such as walking at a comfortable pace. As you become fit, you can start doing more strenuous activities.

Health concerns

If you have a chronic medical condition or a physical disability, you'll want to stay physically active in ways that give you the most benefits with the least chance of discomfort or injury. Research has shown that physical activity improves the health of people with conditions such as diabetes, osteoporosis and cardiovascular disease. Your doctor can help you design an activity program that's right for you.

Obese people face certain challenges in trying to be active. It can be difficult to move or bend, and they often feel self-conscious exercising in front of others. Exertion can leave them out of breath, and aggravate joint problems.

If you're obese and wish to start moving more, start slowly and add repeated small amounts of gentle activity. If you're uncomfortable being active around other people, keep in mind that you have just as much right to be healthy and active as anyone else. If your feet or joints hurt when you stand for periods of time, choose nonweight-bearing activities, such as swimming or water aerobics.

Finding the time

Physical activity is a lifelong pursuit. It needs to be as natural and routine a part of your life as bathing or brushing your

Do you need to see a doctor?

If you're middle-age or older, are significantly overweight, or have been inactive for several years, talk to your doctor before increasing your activity level. You and your doctor can choose activities that are safe and beneficial for you.

If any of the following statements apply to you, consider consulting your doctor:

- You have a heart condition and your activity should be medically supervised.
- You have a family history of heart-related problems before age 55.
- You have a medical condition requiring a doctor's care.
- You smoke.
- You get breathless or experience chest pain after mild exertion.
- You have frequent dizzy spells.
- You have severe muscle, ligament or tendon problems.
- You've been told to reduce your physical activity for any reason.
- You're taking medications, such as insulin, that may require adjustment if you exercise.

teeth. The important thing is to do what you can to get up and move.

Of course you're busy. And the time you might consider for physical activity is time you're probably spending on other demands right now. Chances are, though, if you monitor your daily activities throughout the week, you'll find several 15- or 30-minute blocks of time for activity. Can you give up an hour of television or get out of bed half an hour earlier?

Try to plan activity for times when you'll have little chance to cancel or interrupt the session. If you save it for your spare time, you'll probably never get around to exercising.

It's helpful to schedule physical activity just as you would a doctor's appointment or business meeting. Exercising regularly in the hour before the evening meal provides a change of pace and helps you let go of the day's tensions. Early morning also works well for many people. You may feel more alert and energetic during the day if you work out in the morning.

You can also squeeze extra movement into activities that you already do in the day. Instead of seeking shortcuts and step savers, look for ways to use your body more. Walk an extra block when you're out exercising your dog, or get off at an earlier stop when riding the bus or subway and walk the rest of the way to your destination. Next time you're on an escalator, continue walking instead of standing still. A few minutes here and there adds up. Get the whole family involved

Get fit, get healthy

The sooner you start being more physically active, the healthier you'll feel. You can achieve most of these benefits with 30 to 60 minutes of physical activity — either continuous or in small chunks of time throughout the day — on most days of the week.

Weight control is just one of many health benefits associated with regular physical activity. Others include:

- Lower risks of heart disease, diabetes, osteoporosis and some types of cancer
- Lower cholesterol, blood pressure and blood sugar levels
- Reduced risk of premature death
- More energy, vitality and stamina
- Stronger bones, muscles and joints
- Better balance and coordination
- An improved immune system
- Better sleep
- Less stress, anxiety and depression
- An improved quality of life and sense of well-being

in more active pursuits. Hold a business meeting during a walk or round of golf.

If you're finding it tough to eke out any time at all for physical activity, take a close look at your priorities. Is everything you're doing necessary or worthy of your time? Ask yourself what's most important. Remember that physical activity provides high priority benefits on just about everyone's list, such as improved health, more energy and a longer life.

Getting motivated

For many people, the mere thought of getting more active brings bad memories of high school gym class or of aching, sore muscles. You may find yourself besieged with negative thoughts: "It's too hard," "I'm not athletic," "I'll get hurt," "I'm too old … fat … uncoordinated … tired." Such thoughts are normal, but they don't have to be the last word. Anyone can get motivated to be more active. Motivation is a process, not a thing.

Motivation to change a behavior — like getting more active — is influenced by many factors, including your values, beliefs, emotions and past experiences, as well as other people's opinions and behaviors. A key to successfully adopting a new behavior is believing that the benefits you'll get from the change will outweigh the disadvantages.

If your motivation comes from within, you're doing the activity for yourself — because you enjoy it, because you want to look better, because you want to get healthier or feel better about yourself. Even if it's your doctor telling you that you need to lose weight, you'll be more motivated if you can find a way to embrace physical activity as something you want to do for yourself.

That's not to say that external motivators have no place in changing your behavior. An occasional reward, such as a new pair of shoes, for meeting an exercise goal may be just the boost you need. Encouragement from family, friends and co-workers can also keep you going.

Here are other motivational tips:

Set goals. Setting a goal gives you something to work toward. It's best to start simple. Set goals that are specific, realistic and measurable. For example, instead of just saying you'll walk more, set a goal of walking 30 minutes at least four days a week.

A realistic goal is something you can achieve within a fairly short time. If you've been inactive in the past, running five miles on your first day probably isn't a very realistic goal.

Build flexibility into your goal. For example, if your goal is to walk mornings but you oversleep on one day, plan to walk in the evening instead. Change your goals as your fitness improves and to keep things interesting.

Choose activities you enjoy. People stick with exercise when they enjoy it. Choose activities that you look forward to, not dread. Maybe you can become reacquainted with a sport you enjoyed when you were younger. Perhaps you can enroll in a class to learn a new activity that you've always wanted to try.

Discover your barriers to exercise. Common barriers that keep people from exercising include boredom, fear of injury, lack of skill or coordination, guilt over being away from the family, lack of time, lack of energy, self-consciousness, cost, and feeling too old or unathletic. It's important to try and identify your personal barriers. This allows you to start working toward solutions. See pages 159-168 for strategies to common barriers.

LIVING THE ACTIVE LIFE

Physical activity occurs from the moment you slip out of bed in the morning until you crawl back into bed at night. At the most basic level, physical activity simply means moving — every motion of your body burns calories.

Exercise is a more structured approach to physical activity that's focused on increased fitness. Fitness includes several components, including aerobic conditioning and strength training. Exercise in longer sessions is more efficient at burning calories and brings even greater health benefits than the physical activities of daily living.

But any activity that gets you moving, even for a few minutes at a time, is a healthy start to becoming more fit. Studies indicate that informal physical activity — also referred to as lifestyle activity — can provide similar health benefits to structured exercise. Walking to the store, weeding the garden, washing the car and cleaning the house all count. All movement is good, whether or not it falls in the category of exercise.

Activity doesn't have to be condensed into one chunk of time in your busy schedule. The cumulative effect of physical activity throughout the day is what matters. To achieve health benefits, aim to accumulate at least 30 to 60 minutes of moderately intense physical activity each day. As a general rule, for walking to be moderately intense, a person should be able to speak in short sentences but not be able to sing a song. You can add time and intensity to your workouts as your body becomes more fit.

How active is your lifestyle?

Your body constantly uses energy for tasks such as digesting food, keeping your heart and lungs working, and staying warm. The energy demands of your internal body systems rarely change.

Day-to-day actions such as getting dressed, straightening up the house and running errands also require energy. You can control this energy demand. Depending on how much you move, deliberate physical activity may account for anywhere between 15 percent and 50 percent of the total calories you burn.

To add more activity to your life, start by assessing your daily routine. Write down what you do each day for several days and analyze the results. Do you find that you often drive to work, park a few feet from the office door, take the elevator, sit at a desk for hours, drive home and then watch television in the evening? That adds up to a pretty sedentary life. This type of assessment often provides a direction on how to change your routine.

Another way to measure your activity is to buy a pedometer, which counts the number of steps you take. Establish a baseline number of daily steps and try to increase that total — for example, your goal might be to regularly add 1,000 steps to your baseline. Once you've become accustomed to that level, increase the new baseline by another 1,000 steps.

Adding activities to your day

Take advantage of every chance you have to get up and move around. The following offers simple ways to get more activity in your day, no matter where you are (see also pages 200 and 238):

At home

- Stretch, walk on a treadmill or use an exercise bike while watching television.
- Manually wash your car.
- Use hand tools instead of power tools.
- Rake leaves.
- Vacuum your carpets and furniture.
- Go for a short walk before breakfast. Or schedule dinner 30 minutes earlier and walk afterward.

At work

- Take the stairs, not the elevator, at least for a few floors.
- Walk during your lunch hour.
- Get up and visit your co-workers instead of e-mailing them.

- Do stretching exercises at your desk.
- Take an activity break. Get up to stretch and walk around.

Out and about

- Park a little farther from your destination and walk.
- Bike or walk to the store.
- Join a local recreation center.

While traveling

- Take a walk around the terminal while you're waiting for your flight.
- Do abdominal crunches, push-ups and stretching exercises in your hotel room.
- Stay at hotels with workout facilities.
- Get up early and walk the neighborhood around your hotel.

A family affair

If you're a parent, one of the best ways to incorporate physical activity into your daily routine is to involve your kids. Developing the habit of being active with

Are you a fidgeter?

Some people have a built-in mechanism for keeping weight off through their everyday movements. Studies show that people who fidget burn extra calories. Fidgeting appears to help them control their weight, even when they overeat.

In a Mayo Clinic study on weight management, people who gained the least weight were those with the most calories burned due to normal activities of daily living, such as fidgeting, moving around and changing posture. The researchers labeled this factor nonexercise activity thermogenesis.

The study provides an optimistic message, even if you're not a fidgeter. Every calorie you burn by moving counts. Even browsing in a store takes twice as much energy as sitting in a chair. If you can increase the calories you burn, you'll tend to stay leaner than if you sit still.

your children adds enjoyment to your life and helps them establish a pattern of behavior they will benefit from throughout their lives. Studies show that children whose parents participate in physical activity are more likely to be active than children of sedentary parents. Play with your kids instead of watching them play. Free-play activities such as hide-and-seek, hopscotch and jumping rope are great for burning calories and improving fitness. Also consider these tips:

- Plan a family activity at least three times a week. This could be basketball in the driveway or a bike ride. If you can't block out 20 to 30 minutes at one time, break the time into smaller segments.
- Limit how much time family members can spend in front of a television or computer screen.
- Incorporate more activity into family outings. Take a family walk after dinner.
- Plan vacations that involve physical activities such as hiking, swimming, canoeing and skiing.

AEROBICS FUNDAMENTALS

Regular exercise, combined with lifestyle activities, provides greater fitness and health benefits. One of the simplest and safest forms of exercise — and a great place to start if you're new to exercise — is aerobic activity.

Aerobic means "with oxygen," as opposed to *anaerobic*, "without oxygen." Aerobic workouts, such as low to moder-

ately intense walking and swimming, increase your breathing and heart rates. These activities make you breathe harder as you continuously move your muscles at a regular, even pace. If sustained for a period of time, aerobic exercise burns a lot of calories and is, therefore, an excellent activity for meeting weight goals.

Exercises that are considered anaerobic, such as lifting weights or sprinting, work muscles in a way that builds strength and speed. But the demands on the muscles can fatigue them quickly. That's one reason why anaerobic activity is usually of short duration. These exercises are described in more detail in Chapter 10.

Aerobic benefits

From a health standpoint, regular aerobic exercise is about as close as you can get to a magic potion. For one, it improves your cardiovascular fitness — the health of your heart, lungs and circulatory system. This increases your ability to use oxygen, referred to as aerobic capacity. A higher aerobic capacity gives you more endurance and allows you to work at a more intense level for a longer time. This makes it easier for you to do household chores and climb stairs without shortness of breath. You can spend an afternoon gardening without getting too tired.

Long-term benefits of regular aerobic exercise include a reduced heart rate and lower blood pressure. It can also result in reduced body fat and blood fat levels and a lower risk of diabetes, cardiovascular disease and other conditions.

Types of aerobic activities

Brisk walking is great aerobic exercise. It increases your aerobic capacity, puts little strain on your joints and involves most of the major muscle groups.

If regular, brisk walks don't appeal you, you can choose from other activities that, if done at a moderate intensity, provide excellent aerobic benefits. Consider an activity that interests you because you're more likely to stick with the exercise when it's fun and convenient. Activities you may consider include:

- Jogging
- Bicycling
- Swimming
- Exercising with machines
- Water aerobics
- Racket sports
- Rowing
- In-line skating or ice skating
- Cross-country skiing

How much and how often?

No matter what activity you choose to do, your muscles and joints need time to get accustomed to the different demands. If you've been inactive, start with five- or 10-minute periods of activity at a time. Build up gradually in one-minute increments, with an eventual goal of 30 to 60 minutes. Increasing the time gradually minimizes your risk of injury.

At first, try to exercise three times a week. Add more days slowly, after you've gotten in the habit of exercising. For best weight control, you'll eventually want to be active most days of the week.

Borg exertion scale

6	no exertion at all
7	extremely light
8	
9	very light
10	
11	light
12	
13	somewhat hard
14	
15	hard (heavy)
16	
17	very hard
18	
19	extremely hard
20	maximal exertion

Copyright 1998 Gunnar Borg

How hard you exercise is referred to as intensity. For aerobic exercise, intensity reflects the amount of oxygen your body uses, which translates into how hard the exercise feels to you. While working out, you should be able to speak in brief sentences. If you're out of breath, your body isn't getting the oxygen it needs.

The Borg ratings of perceived exertion scale (see the table above) is one way to estimate activity intensity. The scale ranges from 6 to 20 with 6 representing your body at rest and 20 representing maximal effort. Moderate activity may range from 12 to 14. At a moderate level, you feel the physical effects of the activity but the effort isn't excessive or extreme.

Your rating on the Borg exertion scale is based on the physical sensations you experience while exercising. These include heart rate, breathing rate, perspiration and muscle fatigue. How your body feels allows you to adjust the intensity.

Your perception of intensity is more important than the absolute level of exertion. For example, brisk walking at three to four miles an hour might be perceived as light exercise by a young, physically fit person. But to an older, unfit person, the same level of activity might feel strenuous. Both people can benefit from exercising at what they perceive as moderate intensity, even though they won't be walking at the same pace. For more on exercise intensity, see page 100.

A WALKING PROGRAM

On average, a walk at moderate intensity burns about 250 to 340 calories in one hour. This expenditure will vary, depending on your weight and level of fitness.

Start a walking program with slow, short walks and gradually increase your time. If you haven't been active, begin with a five-minute stroll around the block. As you increase your physical effort, your body will respond by increasing its aerobic capacity. Gradually extend the length of time you walk. Your ultimate goal is to walk a total of about four hours a week.

Walk at an even, comfortable pace that you can maintain. If you're getting short of breath, slow down. Once you've reached a point where you can walk a few miles without much strain, you can vary the intensity by walking hills, lengthening your stride, swinging your arms more or increasing your speed.

Below is an example of a 12-week walking program. Notice how the four-hour goal is reached by gradually adjusting the duration and frequency of the walks.

You may, of course, vary this program to suit your needs and preferences. For example, you can choose to walk three to four days a week instead of five or six, but walk for longer periods of time.

12-week walking program

Weeks	Total time (min.)	Days	Approximate hours per week
1	20	3	1
2	20	3	1
3 – 4	25	3	$1\frac{1}{4}$
5 – 6	30	3 – 4	$1\frac{1}{2}$ – 2
7 – 8	35	3 – 4	2 – 3
9 – 10	40	4 – 5	3 – $3\frac{1}{2}$
11 – 12	40	5 – 6	$3\frac{1}{2}$ – 4

These tips can help make your walking program safe and enjoyable:

Practice good walking posture (see page A4 of the Visual Guide). Walk with your back comfortably straight, head up, eyes forward and shoulders relaxed. Let your arms swing freely and your feet roll from heel to toe.

Choose a pleasant place to walk. Vary your path occasionally. When you're ready, try routes with inclines and hills.

Find a walking partner to go with you. A companion helps keep you motivated.

Music can energize your walk, but if you wear a headset outdoors, keep the volume low and watch for traffic.

Find alternate walking routes when the weather is unpleasant, such as an indoor mall or community center.

Reward yourself for reaching milestones in your program. Treat yourself to an evening with friends, a new pair of walking shoes or a massage.

ACHES AND PAINS

Forget the saying, "No pain, no gain." Exercise shouldn't be painful. But anyone who's physically active is bound to feel soreness, stiffness, or minor aches and pains occasionally. If you've been inactive for a long time, you'll likely feel at least mild discomfort when you start to exercise. Rest assured, you probably haven't injured yourself. It's just your body meeting a new challenge.

Muscle soreness following exercise is common, especially if you've been seden-

Exercise red flags

Moderate activity shouldn't cause discomfort. You'll breathe faster and feel like you're working, but you shouldn't feel pain or be exhausted. If any of the following signs or symptoms occur while exercising, stop and consult your doctor:

- Chest pain or tightness
- Dizziness or faintness
- Pain in an arm or your jaw
- Severe shortness of breath
- Bursts of rapid or slow heart rate
- Irregular heartbeat
- Excessive fatigue
- Severe joint or muscle pain

tary or trying a new activity. This type of soreness usually means that your muscles are growing stronger. The discomfort should disappear in a day or two. Rest combined with continued gentle activity will help. Take a leisurely stroll, for example, or ride an exercise bike with no resistance. Mild aches may also be relieved with ice, massage and over-the-counter pain medications.

Pain during exercise sends a different signal — it can be a warning sign of impending injury. Most injuries that occur during physical activity result from trying to do too much, too hard, too soon or with too little preparation. It's important to start out slowly and progress gradually. Stop exercising and consult a doctor if you experience any of the signs and symptoms from the table above.

Here are other ways to minimize your chance of injury and stay safe:

Warm-up and cool-down

Warming up prepares your body for exercise. A warm-up often involves doing your activity at a slower pace, for example, easy walking. This will gradually increase your heart rate, body temperature and blood flow to your muscles. Cooling down is the process in reverse. Slowing your pace allows your heart rate to gradually return to normal and your body temperature to cool.

Wear proper gear

Wear comfortable clothing suitable for the activity, weather and place where you exercise. In cold weather, dress in layers. In hot weather, wear lightweight, loose-fitting clothes that wick away moisture. Don't skimp on footwear and protective gear such as a bike helmet.

Drink fluids

To replenish lost fluids, drink a glass of water before and after your activity. Carry a bottle of water with you if you'll be exercising for more than 45 minutes.

Be cautious about medications

Follow your doctor's recommendations for the medications you're taking. Pain relief medications, including aspirin and ibuprofen, can mask pain that would normally warn that you're overdoing it. You may overexert and damage your muscles, ligaments or tendons without realizing it.

At the same time, pain relievers can ease mild pain after exercise or allow someone with a condition such as arthritis to stay active without pain. But if the pain increases, check with your doctor about using the medications during exercise.

Be flexible

When you're sick with a cold, the flu or another illness, consider taking a break from exercise, especially if the signs and symptoms are below the neck — which means that your lungs have probably been affected by the illness. Resume when you're feeling better. If the break has been more than a week, make sure to start out slowly again.

ON YOUR WAY

Stick with your goal to be more active, even if you don't perceive immediate benefits from your effort. Within a few weeks, you'll start to feel more energy and vigor. Over eight to 12 weeks, you'll likely notice an improvement in your fitness level. You'll be able to do more and feel better doing it. You may find it easier to lose weight and keep it off.

No need to rush the process. Slow, steady changes make the difference. And remember that the benefits of fitness are the sum of all your daily activity, not just exercise.

CHAPTER 7

Learning healthy behaviors

How often do you find yourself putting food into your mouth when you're not hungry? Do you prefer to relax in the evening by watching television or going for a walk? These questions relate to your behavior. Behavior is the way you react to specific situations or to changes in your environment or within your body.

Many behaviors that you may feel you were born with are actually ones you've learned how to do. For example, newborn babies are remarkably direct about food intake. When they're hungry, they cry for food. When they're full, they refuse to take in a drop more. You probably don't act that way now. Chances are that over time you've learned eating habits in res-

ponse to factors other than hunger, factors often triggered by a preoccupied brain rather than an empty stomach. The same thing goes for activity. How active you are is the result of practices you may have learned from your parents or friends.

The only proven formula for achieving and maintaining a healthy weight — eat less and move more — sounds simple. But anyone who's overweight and who has tried to follow the formula knows it's more challenging than it sounds. What gets in the way? Often, it's learned behaviors. The good news is that these behaviors, if they're contributing to weight gain, can also be unlearned over time.

Many factors, among them physical symptoms, emotions, social pressure, conditioned thinking and lack of awareness, influence behaviors. It's those factors you need to target, not just what you eat or do. Your behavior and your weight aren't isolated from each other. They're integral parts of who you are. You'll need to address all aspects of your lifestyle if you want to make lasting changes.

Changing behavior involves changing your approach to eating and activity, which means changing how you think and feel. Sound tough? It often is. It takes concentration and effort. It requires commitment. That's why weight control is so challenging. But have confidence you'll succeed. This chapter describes strategies that are effective in helping you change.

FIRST THINGS FIRST

One of the most important steps to successful weight control is to have realistic goals and expectations. If you set your expectations too high or hold yourself to impossible goals, you're setting yourself up for failure. If you understand what's possible in the context of your everyday life and work within those parameters, you're more likely to succeed.

It's also important that you enjoy and find satisfaction in the changes you're making to your lifestyle. A study of individuals who successfully managed their weight after completing a medically supervised weight-loss program showed that satisfaction with the amount and quality of daily activities was an impor-

tant factor in success. If you don't like what you're doing to lose weight, it's unlikely you'll stay with the program.

Which brings us back to expectations. Most people are rarely satisfied when it comes to weight loss. If they lose 2 pounds, they wish it were 5. If they lose 5 pounds, they wish it were 20. And if they don't reach their unrealistic goal, they're ready to throw in the towel completely.

It's all about attitude

Here's a typical scenario: You get on the scale and you're dismayed by the number you see. Your immediate reaction is panic. "Oh my gosh," you think, "I've gained more weight." The panic is often accompanied by negative thoughts: "I'm a blimp." "I'll never lose weight."

The panic and negative thoughts are followed by one of two reactions. One is a feeling of hopelessness. You turn to food for comfort. You go to the kitchen and, oversized serving spoon in hand, wrap yourself around a quart of ice cream. "What's the use?" you ask yourself, "I'm destined to be fat."

The other reaction is fierce determination. You tell yourself you've had it. You're going to live on water and carrot sticks and walk 10 miles a day until you weigh what you weighed as a teenager. This intense approach can cause medical problems. It can also result in feelings of deprivation and burnout.

Thus, both of these reactions are self-defeating. Neither will result in any useful changes that lead to long-term weight control. Both will leave you frustrated and even more discouraged about controlling your weight. So what do you do?

When people start a weight-control program, they frequently don't think through the long-term commitment that's involved. This lack of anticipation can lead to dropout. Unfortunately, dropout only reinforces the self-defeating attitude and strengthens the belief that you just can't lose weight successfully. This reaction often sends you to — you guessed it — the refrigerator or pantry for comfort.

If you're serious about achieving a healthy weight, you'll need to approach weight control as you would any major, long-term goal. You'll be facing obstacles and finding ways to overcome them. You'll be to setting goals that are practical and realistic. You'll be determining what help you need and how to get it. In other words, you'll need a plan.

SMALL CHANGES CAN ADD UP

We tend to be comfortable with our behaviors and habits, even if they're not always enjoyable or beneficial. They're familiar. They give order and stability to our lives. Our actions express who we are, and it's not always easy to define ourselves otherwise. That means most of us are reluctant to change the way we're used to doing things. It may feel like we're changing our very essence.

Although change can be difficult, it's not impossible. Most people underes-

timate their ability to change. And changing behaviors in many small ways can add up to a big difference in lifestyle.

Here's a common dietary example: Many people have switched from drinking whole milk to skim milk. Maybe they tapered off gradually, or maybe they switched from one to the other in one bold leap. Either way, they made what they thought was an impossible change. Skim milk probably seemed watered-down at first. Now that these people are used to skim, whole milk probably tastes too thick and rich. It's a small change, but when combined with other small dietary shifts, it all adds up to a healthier diet.

Take a moment to think about big changes you've faced in your life — finishing school, getting married, moving, starting a new job — and how you adjusted, sometimes in many small ways. The fact is, you got through it. The strengths you relied on then may help you now.

YOU NEED CONFIDENCE

Changing old behaviors doesn't mean you just replace them with new ones. You have to change the beliefs that support the old behaviors. Say you're convinced that fat is in your genes. And you also believe that if you could only be thin, you'd be happy. Merge these two beliefs and what do you have? — an assumption that you're destined to be unhappy.

Yet, hope springs eternal, so you go on diet after diet. You lose weight, only to hit a plateau or a challenge that destroys your motivation. You regain the weight, and, of course, you're miserable. Not only have you reinforced the belief that you're destined to be fat and unhappy, you've also made a habit of failing at weight loss.

What would happen if you could change those underlying beliefs? True, that's easier said than done. But what would happen if you tried? Here's what could change:

- "I'm destined to be overweight" instead becomes "I can develop new behaviors for eating and physical activity that will help me control my weight."

- "If I were thin, I'd be happy" becomes "I need to change what's making me unhappy so I can be happy with my life. I can learn to accept myself regardless of my weight and meet my needs other than through food."

To change your outlook, maybe you should seek outside help, such as a professionally led support group. Perhaps you need to keep a journal, which can make you aware of negative beliefs and help you stop them whenever they enter your head. Maybe you need to motivate yourself more with small rewards for accomplishment. Only you can judge.

As for the cycle of going on and off diets, be aware of how easily this can become a habit. No matter how hard you try to succeed with your actions, if you believe in the back of your mind that you'll fail because you always have in the past, your chances of achieving long-term weight control are minimal. Be aware of your negative attitudes and tell yourself they just aren't true anymore. This is a new day and a new you.

PREPARING FOR CHANGE

Because everyone's environment is complex and his or her needs are different, changing a behavior is a highly individualized process. The method, timing and pace of change vary from one person to the next. As you contemplate making a change in your life, here are general principles to guide you:

- **It's not a race.** The first rule of change is to not change too quickly. You're trying to develop a new lifestyle. This doesn't happen overnight. It takes time and dedication to unlearn unhealthy behaviors and develop new, healthy ones.

- **Forget the scale.** Don't use daily numbers on the scale as a measure of your success. You can control what you eat and what you do more than you can control the numbers. So concentrate on those actions as your goal. Keep your motivation sharp and focus on feeling healthier and more energized.

- **Anticipate a lapse.** There will be days when you eat more or move less than you intended. That's what's called a lapse, and it's inevitable that you'll occasionally lapse. But it's important not to use a lapse as an excuse to give up. Have a plan for such occasions. You ate a slice of pizza that you hadn't planned on? You were too busy to exercise this morning? Think about what triggered the lapse and learn from it. Keep in mind that a healthy weight results from long-term commitment, not from a single event.

Studies show that most people stay on a diet for only a week or two before giving up. Often, they've been unable to change unhealthy behaviors that weaken their commitment. They may have been unable to resist favorite high-calorie foods. They may have become quickly bored with their walking program.

To achieve a healthy weight, you'll need to identify your unhealthy behaviors and change them permanently. To beat the odds, you may need to strengthen your commitment to change before you start taking action.

First, consider and write down all the good things that losing weight can do for you, such as improving your health, giving you more energy and making you look and feel better. Then write down the negatives of trying to control your weight, such as having to add exercise to an already busy schedule or getting your family to go along, at least partially, with dietary changes. Focus on the positives of weight loss, and try to come up with solutions for the negatives.

Decide on a positive phrase that reflects you and what you're trying to accomplish. "I'm improving my eating and exercise habits," "I'm creating a new me," or "I'm working toward good health" might better express your effort and the long-term attitude you're choosing.

As you consider taking action toward weight control, realize that willpower alone won't be enough. Discarding a behavior, or adopting a new one, can take anywhere from three to 30 tries. There's no magic formula that everyone can follow. Different techniques work for different people. You'll need to discover what's effective and satisfactory for you.

STRATEGIES FOR CHANGE

A general strategy to change behavior is described on pages 248-249 in the Healthy Weight Program. Here are other strategies that you may consider to help change unhealthy behaviors:

Keep a food diary

It helps to understand what causes a behavior before you try to change it. One of the best ways to do that is to keep a diary that records not just what you eat, but what triggers your eating, even when you're not hungry.

Keeping a diary takes some effort, but it's often one of the success tools used by people who reach and maintain their weight goals. Several studies suggest that keeping a diary causes people to reduce their food intake, probably by increasing their awareness of eating behavior.

You can combine your diary with a food record (described in Week 3 of the Healthy Weight Program). In addition to recording the types of food and amounts of food you eat, your diary may include:

- Feelings (bored, anxious, stressed)
- Social interaction (with friends, alone)
- Environment (potluck at work, passed by a bakery)
- Level of hunger (from extremely hungry to not hungry at all)
- Rate of eating (fast, slow, moderate)

Start your diary without altering your regular routine. After several days, you may be able to discern behaviors that affect your weight. Maybe every time you get upset you find yourself reaching for cookies. Or you're afraid to hurt a friend's feelings, so you take food even if you don't want to eat. Whatever the patterns, you can work on changing them.

Enjoy your food

When you eat, keep your mind focused on the pleasure of what you're doing. Be aware of every bite. To stay focused, you can't be doing anything else — don't read, don't watch television, just savor your food. Remember, eating should give you pleasure, not just fuel your body.

If you've ever consumed a quart of ice cream without realizing you were eating, you know what it's like to eat without awareness. There's little pleasure in it, and you feel guilty afterward. Eating with awareness may take practice, but it's worth the effort. You'll enjoy food more and be satisfied with eating less.

Stick to your schedule

If your diary indicates that you eat many times during the day, having a meal schedule can give you a better sense of control. This doesn't necessarily mean the traditional three meals of breakfast, lunch and dinner. Create a schedule that's convenient and enables you to eat when you're hungry. You can build flexibility into the schedule by defining half-hour or hour time frames for eating rather than sticking to exact times.

You may find that eating three meals and two snacks works best for you. Or perhaps six mini-meals suit your schedule better. The important thing is to stick with a routine. But don't go more than four or five hours without eating because you could become extremely hungry, causing you to overeat. If you find yourself craving a snack 20 minutes before your scheduled meal, see if you can wait it out. If you can't wait, at least appease your hunger with something small and healthy.

Have a plan

Try to plan what you're going to eat for the day at least one day in advance. Your decisions will depend, in part, on your daily calorie goal. Planning ahead means you'll have the ingredients on hand at mealtimes and can start preparing food without delays. This helps keep you from grabbing a slice of leftover pizza when you arrive home hungry.

Planning ahead also means packing your lunch, snacks or even your breakfast to take to work. This saves you from relying on vending machines or fast-food fare and from making impulsive food choices. Once you get in the habit of brown-bagging, you may find it saves time during the workday because you don't have to constantly seek out food.

Of course, the best plans can go astray. A good rule of preparedness is always to have something ready that's healthy to munch on, such as low-calorie popcorn, cut-up vegetables or fruit. That way, you'll always have a backup if an unexpected deadline keeps you working through the lunch hour, or you're running errands at dinnertime.

Find your eating place

Designate an appropriate place in the house for eating, preferably at a dining table. Set the table, even if you're eating alone. Make the environment as pleasant as possible. And remember, don't be distracted at meals. By eating in one place, you begin to associate that place, and that place only, with eating. If you stop eating in the recliner while watching television, you'll be less likely to get a sudden craving for food whenever you sit in a recliner or turn on a television. It's that simple. And it's that difficult. You still may want to get food while watching television but you're slowly changing the habit.

Shop from a list

The practice of making a shopping list goes along with planning meals ahead of time. Following a list will help keep you from impulse buying. Along the same lines, don't shop when you're hungry — you'll be tempted to grab anything that looks vaguely appetizing. While you're at it, read the labels on food packages. Don't

assume something's healthy for you just because it appears to be. If the product has more chemicals than real food in it, do you want it in your body?

Manage food problems

You might trick yourself into believing that bag of chocolate-covered peanuts you tossed into your shopping cart is for a special occasion, but once it's in the house, can you resist sampling them? Do yourself a favor. Don't buy high-calorie foods that tempt you to snack.

That doesn't mean you have to give up sweets and junk food entirely. Just consider not having them in your home. Besides, plenty of foods can satisfy a sweet tooth and provide needed nutrients.

If you have time, look for recipes in cookbooks that emphasize a healthy, low-calorie diet. Or shop in stores that offer nutritious alternatives to high-calorie, low-fiber concoctions that line the typical supermarket shelves. Beware of products, including baked goods, that claim to be low fat. They often have as many or more calories and more sugar than do their high-fat counterparts.

Keep in mind that as you acquire new eating habits, your tastes will change. Foods that once seemed dreamy eventually may taste too sweet or too fatty. Believe it or not, you can unacquire a taste.

Out of sight, out of mind

Keep tempting foods where you can't see them, especially if your diary reveals that your urge to eat is triggered by visual cues. Put the food at the back of the cupboard or refrigerator, where it won't catch your eye when you enter the kitchen or prepare food. Have water, fruits and vegetables at the front of your refrigerator.

Eat from hunger

Food is comforting, so many people reach for food when they may need something else to resolve a problem. Eating can be an irresistible urge when you're tired, lonely or sad, when you're angry or frustrated. Unfortunately, eating can't satisfy any long-term emotional needs. And eating for reasons other than hunger will almost certainly provide you with too many calories.

People do forget what real hunger feels like. Don't eat for a few hours and see how you feel. If what you experience isn't physical hunger, don't try to comfort yourself with food. If you're tired, then rest or meditate. If you're thirsty, drink a glass of water. If you're anxious, take a walk. Stop making eating your all-purpose response to every concern or situation. When you have an urge to eat but you're not sure whether you're hungry, wait 15 to 30 minutes and see how you feel. Here's a clue: If you can't decide what you want to eat, chances are you're not very hungry.

Stop when you're full

Brace yourself for a shock: No matter what you heard from your parents as a child, you don't have to finish all the food on your plate. Even if you served yourself what you considered a reasonable portion, how do you know before you start eating how much food will satisfy your hunger? Eat slowly, savor every bite and stop when you're full.

If you belong to the clean-plate club, try to change this behavior by leaving a dab of food at every meal — just to signal your brain that it's OK. As you become more adept at identifying when you're hungry and when you're satisfied, it will become easier not to overeat. Keep in mind that eating to the point of feeling stuffed is likely to trigger feelings of guilt and negative self-thoughts.

Reduce your stress level

Eating is often associated with stress. If you have a deadline to meet and you're feeling fidgety, eating may seem like the best way to help you focus. Or if your mind is preoccupied with relationship problems, you may eat to soothe your nerves. Eating to ease stress almost always results in overeating. Finding other ways to cope with stress may prevent a relapse and unnecessary weight gain. Instead of automatically heading to the refrigerator, consider these suggestions for lowering your stress level (see also pages 299 and 301):

- Eat a healthy diet with regular meals to help avoid out-of-control snacking.
- Prioritize, plan and pace your activities.
- Spend time with people who have a positive outlook and sense of humor.
- Get enough sleep to help clear your mind and make you ready for the day.

Lifestyle changes

I was a couch potato with an international reputation. Friends from coast to coast — and in Europe and Asia, too — knew that I would go to great lengths to avoid exercise, and that I was even proud of my slothful status.

Shortly after my 40th birthday, however, I realized my clothes seemed to have become tighter. When I caught a glimpse of myself in a full-length mirror shortly after a shower, I knew I had a problem.

My desk job required that I take decisive action. I wasn't going to lose 20 pounds with my daily activities, of which there were pitifully few. So, with my husband's encouragement, we joined a university recreation center less than a mile from our home.

We started getting up at 5:30 a.m. I would immediately dress in my workout togs, even though we would spend the next hour reading the newspaper and drinking coffee. That way, I had no excuses when the appointed time came to head to the gym.

My routine was simple. I walked on an indoor track every day, Monday through Friday, for one hour. At first, my pace was on the slow side, but as I saw other walkers speeding by, I learned to pick up my pace. I read a few books on walking and discovered that I'd do best if I could walk at least a 15-minute mile. It was hard, but I managed it within a month.

By the time I lost the 20 pounds, six months later, I knew I would be walking for the rest of my life. I realized that losing the weight was nice, but the overall health benefits were even better. I had more energy and more stamina than ever before, and my hips had slimmed down enough that I could wear the same size top and bottom — for the first time in my life.

As I've learned more about physical activity, I've added 15 minutes of weightlifting twice a week. When the weather gets nice, from March through October, I walk outside, sightseeing through the neighborhoods in our vicinity.

It's been nearly six years since I launched my fitness program, and it's one of the best decisions I ever made. I believe it has added years of health and enjoyment to my life.

Linda
Kansas City, Mo.

- Organize work spaces so that you know where things are.
- Get plenty of exercise.
- Take stretch breaks throughout the day.
- Do something good just for yourself or for somebody else.
- Don't feel guilty if you're not productive every minute of every day.
- Learn to delegate responsibility.
- Take a day off with no set plans.
- Learn to accept things you can't control.

Get support

Support from others can be very helpful as you attempt to control your weight. Look for a confidant you feel comfortable with but be careful whom you enlist. We all have our own agendas, and they're not always ones we're conscious of. So not everyone in your circle of friends can empathize with you or be happy that you're losing weight. Pick someone who you're certain wants only the best for you and will encourage you.

An ideal support person might be someone who's also trying to lose weight. It could be your spouse, co-worker or friend. Some people fare better with professional support, such as a physician, nurse, dietitian or personal trainer. Others like the group support they get from organizations such as Weight Watchers or Overeaters Anonymous.

There are also many individuals who like to work alone and don't want to ask for others' help. Do whatever works for you, but keep in mind that different approaches fit different needs.

KITCHEN DUTY

Your kitchen is an obvious place to consider when you're thinking about behavior change. That's where the food in your house is stored and prepared, right? It's also the room where you may eat. A little reorganization of your kitchen may affect how you function there, and ease some difficult behavior changes.

Your primary goal in reorganizing your kitchen is to be able to prepare healthy meals in a short amount of time. (This includes reducing the number of times you need to run to a store at the last minute for ingredients.) This will save you hard work, money, stress and waste. It also reduces situations involving poor food choices and hurried meals.

The best way to achieve your goal is to always have a supply of basic foods and kitchen tools on hand, and to know where to find them. A well-stocked kitchen includes what are known as staples, the ingredients that you regularly use when you cook. While some staples are fairly standard — for example, salt or canned tomatoes — the full list of staples will vary, depending on your tastes and talent for cooking. Many of these items have a long shelf life and can be stored until they're needed. The staples necessary for the Mayo Clinic Healthy Weight Program are listed on page 187.

An efficient kitchen also requires tools. This doesn't mean equipping your kitchen with expensive gadgets. Just a few high-quality basics will do: a couple of good knives, frying pan, sauce pan, mixing bowl, measuring cups, mixing spoon, spatula and vegetable peeler are sufficient to prepare many healthy recipes.

Besides being able to work efficiently in your kitchen, you also need to feel at ease there. Here are guidelines that can help put a personal stamp on your kitchen:

- Create work areas for specific tasks, such as food preparation, mixing and baking. Store tools that you use for these tasks at the designated areas. For example, knives and cutting boards in the food preparation area, and bowls and measuring cups in the mixing area.
- Organize storage spaces so you'll know where to find ingredients. Consider grouping items that are commonly used together. For example, certain seasonings such as basil, oregano and thyme, or cans of broth, tomatoes and beans.
- Reduce clutter in your kitchen. Keep your countertop working spaces clear. Put seasonal or infrequently used items in storage when not in use. Clean out your refrigerator weekly.
- Keep a place for reminders, such as a pad of paper or a small whiteboard, where you can note menu plans, ingredients for recipes and grocery lists.

POTENTIAL PROBLEMS

Weight control should bring about positive changes in your life — ones that make you feel better about yourself, both physically and emotionally. But for some

people, the preoccupation with weight becomes so severe that it evolves into a complex mental disorder. Eating disorders involve abnormal eating habits, including not eating enough, extreme dieting and exercising, eating excessive amounts of food, or purging food from the body through deliberate use of laxatives or by vomiting. They often occur along with disorders such as depression, substance abuse and anxiety disorders.

People with eating disorders such as anorexia nervosa and bulimia often are underweight, but those with bulimia can also be overweight. Women and girls experience eating disorders far more often than do men and boys. These conditions are described in Chapter 2. Other common problems that can derail weight programs are binge eating and overexertion.

Binge-eating disorder

Binge-eating disorder is characterized by frequent episodes of unrestrained eating, in which a person eats large amounts of food very quickly and usually alone or in secret. During the binge episode, the person feels out of control of his or her eating. After the binge episode, the person often feels ashamed, depressed or guilty about what has taken place.

Unlike an eating disorder such as bulimia, there is no self-induced purging or vomiting after binge eating. People with binge-eating disorder are more likely to be overweight. Feelings of self-disgust and shame can lead to further overeating episodes, creating a cycle of binge eating.

Many adults experience some episodes of binge eating, but when they occur more than two days a week or are a source of distress, professional help may be needed.

Overexertion

If you include regular exercise as part of your weight-loss program, you're to be commended. However, keep in mind that moderation is important. Pushing too hard with exercise may lead to overexertion, which is counterproductive to reaching your weight goal. Too much exercise can also be an indication of an eating disorder or having a poor body image.

It's normal to feel tired after a workout, but if your fatigue persists beyond your normal recovery time, then you could be overdoing it. Signs and symptoms of overexertion include early fatigue during workouts, decreased performance, loss of coordination, increased heart rate with less effort, headache, gastrointestinal problems and decreased ability to ward off infection.

If you suspect overexertion, take a break. Do light workouts that are less demanding. Or try a new activity that's not too strenuous. If you continue to feel fatigued, have injured yourself from overexertion, or feel compulsive about exercising every day, talk with your doctor about your exercise level.

CHAPTER 8

Addressing your emotional needs

As you begin a weight-control program, your physical needs are undoubtedly on your mind. You're improving your diet, starting to exercise and changing unhealthy behaviors. But how's your confidence?

When it comes to weight control, caring for your emotional needs is as important as meeting your physical needs. You'll be more successful if you feel good about yourself and what you're doing.

Even with the best of intentions, you'll likely run into roadblocks along the way. Frustration and negative feelings may undermine your commitment. The choices you make to lose weight may fail you, and there may be times when your goals seem unattainable.

These obstacles and unexpected developments can test you. But if you face them with openness, honesty and a positive attitude, you can overcome them. Use this chapter as your road map for overcoming emotional challenges.

ASSESSING YOUR BODY IMAGE

You may have picked up this book in search of the perfect body. You imagine having a thin waist, toned legs, washboard abs — a body you'll be proud to take to the beach. Sounds good, doesn't it? A perfect vision. And that's exactly what it is — a vision — because a perfect body is nearly impossible to attain.

Most of us aren't supermodels or professional bodybuilders. We're real people with real bodies — complex in their wonders and flaws. Unfortunately, it's the gulf between the ideal and reality that causes unhappiness and discouragement.

In a recent survey, 56 percent of women and 43 percent of men said they weren't happy with their bodies. When it came to weight, the numbers increased to 66 percent and 52 percent, respectively.

How do you break from a negative mind-set? Start by accepting that every body is different, influenced by genetics and environment that help to determine body size and weight. Even if everyone ate the same food and did the same exercises for a lifetime, people's bodies would still come in all shapes and sizes.

Don't rely completely on charts, graphs, formulas and tables to decide what your ideal body shape or weight should be. Focus on what makes you feel good about your body. If you're eating balanced meals, getting exercise and have the energy to do the things you want to do, you're on the right track. Trust that you'll get to the best weight for you.

Are you being realistic?

How you view your body plays a role in the success of your weight-control program. Some degree of dissatisfaction with your body is normal and may even be beneficial because it motivates you to eat better and exercise more. But having a poor body image can lead to eating disorders, depression and low self-esteem.

When it comes to body image, you may be tougher on yourself than anyone else is. You may overemphasize features that you don't like. You see the imperfections, the wrinkles, the extra weight — and not the positive attributes.

Unrealistic standards can make you feel bad about yourself and keep you from doing things you'd like to do, such as swimming at the beach, going dancing or exercising at the gym. You fear you look too fat in your swimsuit, too jiggly on the dance floor and too ridiculous in your gym clothes to be seen in public. You let your perceptions dictate how you live your life. You may overcome such obstacles with these suggestions:

- Realize it's your own discomfort stopping you, not what others are thinking.
- Replace "I can't" with "I can." Instead of, "I can't go to the beach with this extra weight," think, "I can go to the beach if I use relaxation techniques to help put me at ease."
- Be realistic. If you go to the pool, a dance or the gym, will yours be the only imperfect body there? Of course not. Remember that most people respect others for their efforts to exercise and keep fit, regardless of appearance.
- Think about how empowered and in control you'll feel when you do something you've been afraid to do.

Being happy with who you are

There's a saying that goes, "Happiness comes not from what you have, but from how you regard what you have."

You have the power

Losing weight is no easy task. So when you do well and meet your goals, congratulate yourself on your effort and self-control. Don't give your weight program the credit. You did it. The program just gave you directions for getting it done. So cheer yourself on!

Celebrate reaching short-term as well as long-term goals. Consider what you've already accomplished, whether it's changing your diet, getting more exercise, going down one size in clothing or being able to walk a flight of stairs without getting winded. These are positive changes. Reward yourself with a fun day-trip, a new CD or simply time to relax.

If you get discouraged, make a list of the ways you feel better as a result of your weight loss. Look at the ways you've succeeded in changing your eating and activity habits, and remember that this will likely bring health benefits you may not even realize. Pat yourself on the back for every time you've chosen fruits or vegetables over junk food, and for every hour spent walking instead of sitting in front of the television. Have confidence in yourself to achieve a healthy weight.

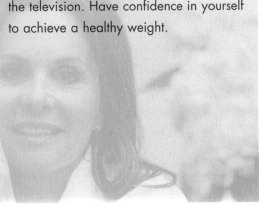

What does this have to do with your weight program? Well, you likely spend a lot of time comparing how you think you look with how you want to look. You may judge your looks based on images you see on television and in magazines, and on people you come in contact with every day — your size 4 neighbor, your co-worker with the broad shoulders and muscular biceps. The resulting envy and barrage of critical thoughts aren't healthy for you. They won't change the way you look and they negatively impact how you view your body. These comparisons will just leave you upset about your appearance and yourself.

You can counteract those feelings and learn to be happy with what you have. Try these suggestions:

- Think of a skill, talent or personality trait that you take special pride in. Then fill in the blank: "I like the fact that I have (or can do) _____."
- Give yourself a break. Hop off the scale and stop bad-mouthing yourself. Avoid negative "double takes" of yourself. Appreciate what you see in the mirror.
- Play up the positives. There's a lot to like about you. Remind yourself that there's more to you than clothing size.
- Accept compliments. Don't push away kind words with a knee-jerk response like, "You need to have your eyes checked." Practice saying thank you.
- Wear what you like. Don't worry about what's appropriate for your age, status or body type. If you like bright colors and eye-catching jewelry, wear them.

- Pick friends wisely. Associate with people who accept you as you are.
- Give yourself time. You didn't develop a negative body image overnight. Don't expect an instant about-face.

SELF-CONTROL VS. WILLPOWER

You may think that you can reach a healthy weight if you just exert enough willpower. You just won't eat those foods that cause you to gain weight. Unfortunately, this well-intentioned plan only sets you up to fail as your willpower inevitably cracks. So what's the fix? Admit that willpower doesn't work, and focus instead on self-control.

Think of it this way. Say that before you start your weight program, you know that you have a terrible sweet tooth. You can approach the problem in two ways. One is to figure out how to fit occasional sweets into your diet without destroying your overall plan. Two is to tell yourself you'll avoid sweets entirely — although you'll continue to buy sweets so others can enjoy them. If you choose the second approach, you'll have to exert tremendous willpower. You'll likely feel deprived when you can't have sweets, and deprivation can lead to binge eating.

So tell yourself that you can eat small amounts of certain sweets. But what if, even then, you know that you can never eat just one small piece of cheesecake. Here's a trick. Instead of using willpower to avoid the cheesecake, use self-control.

What's the difference? Self-control is, "It's hard for me to control my eating of cheesecake, so I'm not going to keep it in the house, but I may have an occasional piece when I dine out." Willpower is, "I'm going to buy my favorite cheesecake, but I'm not going to eat it. I'll prove to myself how strong my willpower is." The first approach is sensible planning. The second may be torture. And because the lifestyle changes you make are supposed to be both healthy and pleasurable, why torture yourself?

Chances are, as your taste buds adapt to a new style of eating, cheesecake (or whatever your downfall is) will loosen its grip on you and won't taste as good as it once did. Barring that, look for a recipe for a low-fat, low-sugar version of your favorite treat, and indulge in small portions on occasion. Or, cut off a small piece for yourself and give away the rest so that you won't be tempted to eat more. You'll be surprised to discover that just knowing it's all right to allow yourself a treat now and then can make it easier to say no.

ACCENTUATE THE POSITIVE

Does this happen to you? You start your day by stepping on the scale and, as the needle rises, you think, "I'll never be able to lose this extra weight." Maybe you decide to skip your morning walk because "it won't work anyway." At breakfast, you're so down that you top off your cereal with a doughnut and a glass of chocolate milk because, you think to yourself, "I've already blown my diet anyway. What does it matter."

The scenario isn't uncommon, but it is unhealthy. Negative thoughts and attitudes like these can sabotage your self-esteem and your weight program. After all, you might reason, why plan healthy meals and make a habit of exercising if defeat is certain?

The endless stream of thoughts running through your head every day is called self-talk. Often critical and negative, self-talk can discourage and weaken you to the point of despair. You think: "I'm too fat." "I don't have any willpower." "The weight is coming off too slowly. There must be something wrong with me."

On the other end of the spectrum is positive self-talk, which can be a powerful tool for building self-confidence, correcting bad habits, focusing attention and powering your exercise and eating routines. Positive self-talk is motivating and encouraging — the basis for many a successful life change. You're using positive self-talk when you bike up that steep hill, repeating all the while, "You can do it! You can do it!"

With a little practice, you can turn your negative self-talk into positive self-talk. Throughout the day, stop and evaluate what you're thinking. Question any thoughts that you feel are upsetting, and then practice turning negative thoughts into positive statements. For instance,

Positive thinking and healthy eating

Put the power of positive thinking into your new healthy diet. Rather than focusing on what you can't eat, focus on what you can. Think about what new tastes you can discover that will enhance your health. If, for example, you've never been much of a fruit eater, experiment with adding different fruits to your menus. Add blueberries to your cereal in the morning — try frozen varieties if fresh blueberries aren't available. Toss some mandarin orange slices and raisins into a salad.

Flip through cookbooks and cooking magazines devoted to healthy cooking. By experimenting with new foods and new combinations, not only are you bound to find some tastes you can enjoy, thereby increasing your eating pleasure, but you'll also increase the variety of nutritious foods in your eating plan. Eventually, your taste buds will adjust to your new style of eating. You'll like foods you never thought you would, and you may find some of your old favorites less appealing.

Try getting into the habit of asking yourself, "Will what I'm about to put in my mouth contribute to my good health or simply add calories?" If it's just calories, then why eat it? Unless it's something you dearly love, skip it. If you dearly love it, try to have only a small amount. Your body will thank you.

instead of saying, "It will never work," say, "I'll give it a try." For more examples, see "Positive thinking and healthy eating" on page 80.

Some people find that they need outside help to change their negative thoughts into positive affirmations and to rid themselves of self-defeating attitudes and beliefs. What's called cognitive behavior therapy may help you do this.

Cognitive behavior therapy is based on the belief that much of what you are is what you think — that how you feel is a result of how you think about yourself and your life circumstances. If you're like many people, you allow your feelings to control your judgment ("I feel fat and ugly, so I must be fat and ugly"). You also magnify negative aspects of a situation while filtering out positive ones ("I've lost 5 pounds — but it's only 5 pounds, and I'll probably gain it back anyway").

With cognitive behavior therapy, a licensed therapist helps you replace these negative thoughts with more positive, realistic perceptions. Once you've learned new ways to view the events that make up your day, you're better able to cope with them in a positive manner.

BUILDING SELF-CONFIDENCE AND SELF-ESTEEM

Positive self-esteem and high self-confidence are essential to a successful weight program. When you're self-confident, you walk with your head held high knowing that your strengths and talents don't rely on your weight. You feel that you're an important and valuable person regardless of your size.

Why is this important to your weight program? Because it's that same attitude that will help you to decide, "I can do this," even when you step on the scale and the numbers climb disappointingly higher than the numbers from the week before. That's why it's important to have a healthy, positive view about yourself.

How do you build self-esteem?

- Practice positive self-talk, as described in this chapter.
- Make three lists: (1) things you do well, (2) why others like you and (3) things you like about yourself.
- Share your feelings. Talk with friends about your ups and downs.
- Keep a daily journal. Each day write about something you've accomplished, something you're looking forward to, and at least one thing you genuinely enjoyed that day.
- Join a professionally led support group or meet with a licensed therapist if you feel it would be helpful.
- Stay social. Interacting and socializing with others will give you a sense of belonging, which can build self-esteem.
- Set realistic expectations. Expectations that are too high can make you feel like a failure. Realistic expectations, on the other hand, help give you a sense of accomplishment.
- Celebrate. Take time to congratulate yourself when you succeed.

Maintaining self-esteem at any weight

If your weight is holding you back from building self-esteem and feeling good about yourself, keep these three thoughts in mind:

- Realize that you're an important, valuable person who can contribute to your community and to others — even if you stay at your current weight.
- Live your life now. Don't wait until you lose weight to try new things or do things you've always wanted to do. Buy nice clothes, go on vacations, go out with friends.
- Expand your goals beyond weight loss. Focus on other potential benefits as you work to lose weight, such as improving your cholesterol and blood pressure numbers.

- Change your perspective. Think about the things you do well instead of focusing on what you're not able to do.
- Don't hide behind oversized, drab clothing. Dress in clothing that makes you feel good about yourself.
- Do nice things for other people. Volunteer, take a meal to a sick friend, greet a stranger.
- Spend time with positive, supportive, life-affirming people.
- Don't expect perfection.

BUILDING SUPPORT NETWORKS

Think back to important life changes that you've made. Perhaps you've gotten married, changed jobs, moved to a new town, had a baby or lost a loved one. In each of these situations, you've probably leaned on the support of other people, which likely made a significant difference as you adjusted to your new situation.

Launching a healthy weight program is another time of great change in your life.

Getting support for your efforts, whether through a friend, a trained professional or a group of fellow travelers on this same path, can ultimately mean the difference between your success and failure.

Support can be emotional — a shoulder to lean on when you're discouraged. And it can be practical — someone to watch the kids while you exercise. It can provide the encouragement you need to get out and exercise on days when your favorite TV show seems like a better option.

In fact, one study found that people who had the support of friends were less likely to drop out of a weight-control program and more likely to maintain their weight loss over a six-month period than were people without such support.

Some people fare better with professional support, such as from a dietitian or personal trainer. Others like the personal support they get from friends and family members. Some combine professional and personal support.

For some, a professionally led group can be helpful. If you do join a group, keep in mind that what you'll get out of it will be in proportion to what you put into it. If you participate rather than just listen, you're more likely to reap the rewards of the group, which include encouragement and empathy.

If you're someone who likes to work alone and doesn't want to ask for anyone's help, that's OK. Do whatever works for you, but keep in mind that different approaches fit different needs.

CHALLENGING YOUR ASSUMPTIONS

We often unconsciously work to keep things exactly the same in our lives. If you disturb the balance, such as by losing weight, your body may try to right itself by returning to business as usual. This is why many people regain the weight they lost and return to the behaviors that caused them to be overweight in the first place. How can you avoid this? Try to create a new equilibrium.

The way to do that, according to one theory, is to challenge your big assumptions. Those are the things you think of as truth but are really just assumptions that you make. For example, say you're convinced that you're destined to be overweight because you were born into an overweight family, or, since you've never been athletic, you couldn't possibly stay with an exercise program. Those are assumptions, not truths. You have to recognize assumptions and examine them.

Here's a way to examine assumptions:

- Identify one of your big assumptions about weight.
- Analyze this assumption. How does it affect your behavior? How long has it been around? Where did it come from?
- Spend time thinking about how this assumption serves you. What does or doesn't happen when you accept it as gospel? What might happen if you view it as merely an assumption?
- Test the assumption in safe ways.

When challenging an assumption, take it gradually, in small steps. Listen to yourself as you go. What are your thoughts and feelings as you discover that your assumption isn't the truth? Are you relieved? Scared? Anxious? Talk these feelings over with a friend or a licensed counselor, if you feel you need to. Or write about them in a journal. There are wonderful benefits to achieving and maintaining a healthy weight. There are also potential drawbacks.

If you're deeply bothered by a change in your life resulting from weight loss, consider talking to a licensed counselor who specializes in weight-related issues. Remember, every problem has a solution.

PART III
Maintaining a weight program

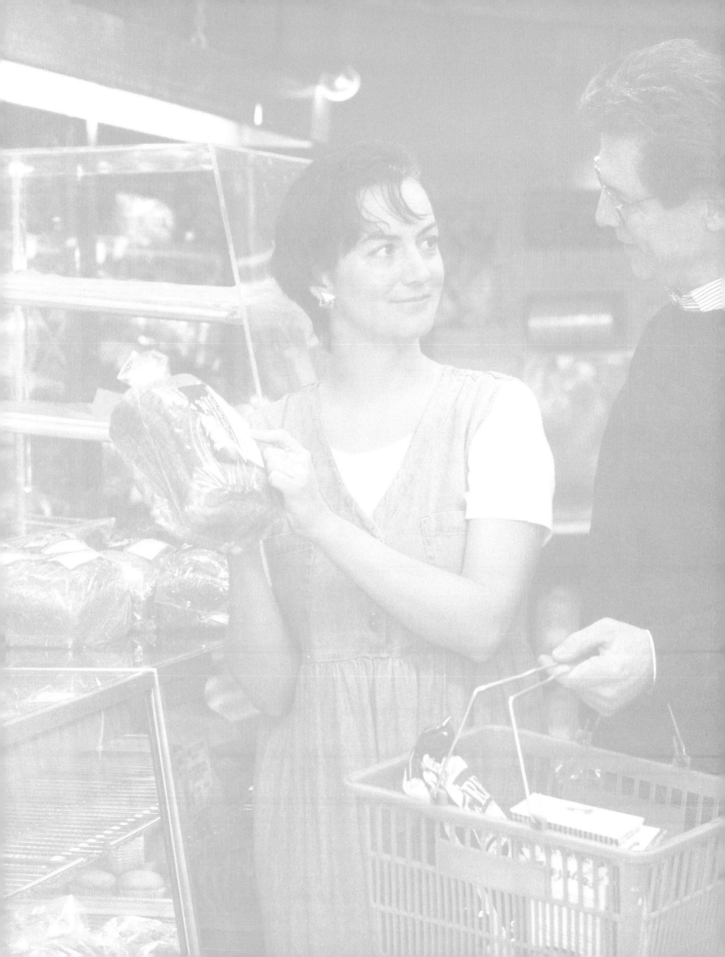

CHAPTER 9

Taking control of meal planning

If you follow the dietary approach promoted by the Mayo Clinic Healthy Weight Program, you'll benefit from a balanced diet and moderate portions, you won't go hungry, and you'll be working toward a healthy weight. If you remain physically active as well, you'll be better equipped to keep excess weight off.

As the healthy behavior changes that you make become routine for your diet and activity level, your health will steadily improve. This lifestyle approach works better than following a fad diet to lose weight, only to have the weight return once you go off the diet. The principles of Healthy Weight Program are the kind that everyone can follow, whether they need to lose weight or not.

CREATING WEEKLY MENUS

This book provides you with weekly menus to help you develop a healthier approach to eating. There will come a time when you'll want to be responsible for planning your own menus. In addition, as you become comfortable with your eating plan, you may be interested in trying new foods and cooking techniques. And that's good. This is a time to experiment and be adventurous.

If you're worried about being able to select and prepare healthy meals on your own, don't be. It's not difficult to integrate the Mayo Clinic Healthy Weight Pyramid into your daily diet and adjust it to suit your tastes. To plan menus, you just need to keep the basic principles in mind. In fact, you may already be familiar with and regularly using these principles in your kitchen. Fine-tuning is all that's required to get you started.

Know your daily calorie goal

As you plan meals for the day or the week, it's vital to know approximately how many calories you should eat each day (see Chapter 5). This may require an occasional reassessment or adjustment of your eating behaviors. If you're trying to lose weight, a good daily calorie goal for most women is 1,200 calories, and for most men, 1,400.

When you know your calorie goal, the daily serving recommendations for each food group will guide your menu decisions. It's also important to be familiar with serving sizes in each of the food groups. Try to include at least one serving from most food groups at each meal.

Plan by the week

It's more efficient to plan your meals for an entire week, especially if you shop for groceries on a weekly basis. That way, you'll know whether or not you have all of the ingredients on hand before you start preparing a meal.

As you work on planning your meals for the week, don't get hung up on hitting exact servings totals each day. It's easier to plan in terms of longer time periods. If on Monday, for example, you don't reach your fruits target, add an extra serving or two on Tuesday. Boost your weekly greens and whole-grain totals by making some lunches and dinners vegetarian — a strategy that will also help you incorporate healthy protein sources, such as legumes and low-fat dairy products.

Make pleasure a priority

Some of your planning efforts may seem like number crunching. You're working hard to make sure that you have the right foods and the right number of servings at each meal. But don't forget that good food is one of life's pleasures. Take advantage of flavors, colors and textures to create enticing dishes. A varied selection of foods helps delight the senses.

Adapt your menus to the seasons

Although it's possible to find bell peppers in January and summer squash in March, they may not be as fresh as you'd like and they may be more expensive. Whenever you can, look for recently harvested produce — asparagus, peas, and cherries in the spring, peaches, sweet corn, and tomatoes in midsummer, and apples, pears, and beets in the fall. This way you'll promote a varied diet with the freshest foods available.

In the spring, summer and early fall months, you can find farmers' markets in many urban areas. These markets provide an opportunity to purchase local produce, which tends to be the freshest around.

Customize your menus

Once you're comfortable with the principles of the Healthy Weight Program, you may want to explore other options for variety. For example, if you enjoy Asian cuisine, you may want to create menus that emphasize rice and noodles. You can achieve this by adding two carbohydrates servings and subtracting one protein and dairy serving and one fats serving. Some people prefer a Mediterranean-style diet that includes more servings of monounsaturated fats such as olive oil, nuts and avocado. In this case, you can add three fats servings and subtract one carbohydrates and one protein and dairy serving.

When switching servings from one group to another, keep in mind that serving totals from either the carbohydrates group or the protein and dairy group shouldn't drop below three each.

Be adventurous

Discovering new foods and flavors is part of the joy of cooking and eating, so don't be afraid to explore unfamiliar cuisines. Some of the world's most intriguing ingredients — quinoa, edamame, bok choy, bulgur — are as healthy as they are delicious. Bear in mind that the broadest range of health benefits comes from menus that feature a wide variety of nutritious foods.

Don't forget convenience foods

A healthy meal doesn't have to be complicated or time-consuming to prepare — especially if you have a busy day ahead. When meal planning, consider convenience foods for those days when there's little time to fix meals.

For example, plan at least one meal per week around a favorite convenience food, such as a frozen entree or a side dish. Just remember to be selective about which convenience foods you choose by reading the nutrition labels. Don't choose based on calories alone. Also look for items that are low in fat and that aren't loaded with sodium. Sodium is often used to help preserve food, but too much sodium isn't good for your health. Among other things, it can increase your risk of high blood pressure or make the condition harder to control.

Several brands of frozen entrees offer healthy versions of the following foods:

- Chicken chow mein with rice
- Salisbury steak
- Shrimp primavera
- Vegetarian chili
- Filet of fish Florentine
- Chicken cacciatore

You might also find it helpful to keep on hand convenient versions of foods such as pasta dishes and instant brown rice. Look for those that are lowest in fat and calories. You may need to alter the basic recipe on the package. Use the skim version when a recipe calls for milk and omit the margarine.

Look for shortcuts

Another way to help simplify meal preparation and save time is to purchase precut vegetables and fruits, precooked meats, shredded low-fat cheeses and packaged salads. Frozen or canned vegetables and fruits also may come in handy for some

Dietary don'ts

This chapter has provided you with plenty of nutritional do's. You may be surprised by some of the don'ts:

- Don't starve yourself. Try to eat regular meals. If you're hungry between meals, eat. Select most foods from the base of the pyramid — vegetables and fruits.
- Don't try to be perfect. You can learn from your mistakes.
- Don't let the occasional setbacks weaken your commitment to lose weight — expect them and know you can get past them.
- Don't be on a timeline. Changing lifelong behaviors is a gradual process and doesn't happen overnight.
- Don't give up — you can do it! Persistence is what carries you through difficult times.

dishes. Rinse the canned vegetables with water to help remove the sodium used in processing. To cut down on calories, buy fruit that's canned in its own juices rather than in syrup.

Be flexible

Remember that every food you eat doesn't have to be an excellent source of nutrients. Nor is it out of the question to eat high-fat, high-calorie foods on occasion. The main thing is that you choose foods that promote good health more often than those that don't.

BEGIN WITH THE BASICS

Vegetables and fruits should form the basis of your diet, so you might build your daily menus on which vegetables and fruits you're planning to eat.

To make sure that you get enough fruit, aim to include at least one serving at breakfast, lunch and dinner. To make sure that you get plenty of vegetables each day, plan lunches and dinners that incorporate two or three servings each, such as a salad or a vegetable soup. Another way to pack in the vegetables is to replace some or all of the meat in casseroles or pasta dishes with vegetables.

Getting enough servings is actually easier than it may sound, because many dishes contain more than one serving and the serving sizes are relatively small. Also keep in mind that vegetables and fruit make excellent snacks.

GO FOR THE GOOD FAT

Most healthy eating plans, including the Mayo Clinic Healthy Weight Program, recommend that you limit the amount of fat you consume each day, especially saturated fat and trans fats. Saturated fat is found in animal products, such as meat,

Is eating sugar unhealthy?

Sugar isn't necessarily bad, but most sugars provide calories and little nutritional value. Sugars are simple carbohydrates. Sources include table sugar (sucrose), fruits and juices (fructose), and milk and milk products (lactose). Natural sources of sugar are usually better for you than foods with lots of added, refined sugar. Refined sugar has a high energy density.

Current U. S. Department of Agriculture Dietary Guidelines for Americans offer the following recommendations:

- Limit your intake of beverages and foods that have simple sugars added during processing — not foods such as fruit and milk, which have natural sugar in them. Don't let soft drinks or other sweets crowd out other foods needed for health, such as water or low-fat milk and milk products.

- Check the food label before you buy. The ingredients list tells you what's in the food, including any sugar that has been added. Ingredients are listed in descending order by weight. In addition to the word *sugar* on the labels of many products, look for these lesser-known ingredients, which are actually forms of simple sugar: corn syrup or sweetener, dextrose, high-fructose corn syrup and maltose. A food is likely to be high in added sugar content if these ingredients appear first or second in the ingredients list.

butter and whole milk. Trans fats, also referred to as partially hydrogenated vegetable oils, are often used in the preparation of processed foods.

But there is such a thing as good fat. Unlike saturated fat, which can clog your arteries and increase your risk of heart disease, one type of fat — called omega-3 fatty acid — appears to have a beneficial effect. Omega 3s are thought to lower your triglyceride level (triglycerides are a type of blood fat) and improve your "good" (high-density lipoprotein or HDL) cholesterol level.

Foods containing omega-3 fatty acids are part of a healthy diet, but the typical American diet includes few of them. The best sources of omega 3s are flaxseed and fatty, cold-water fish, such as salmon, mackerel, herring, bass, swordfish, tuna and trout. Other foods containing this type of fat, but in lesser amounts, include walnuts, soybeans and cooking oils made from flaxseed, soybeans and canola.

This is an important reason why you'll see fish listed often in the Healthy Weight Program. In addition to being a source of protein, it provides "good" fat.

Health experts generally recommend eating fish — baked, broiled or grilled, but not fried — twice a week. (The Food and Drug Administration advises, however, that pregnant women, nursing mothers and children not eat king mackerel or swordfish because these fish contain higher amounts of mercury.) As you're planning your weekly menus, don't forget about including fish.

Adapting recipes

This book provides a number of recipes to help you eat better. These recipes are a starting point toward a healthier lifestyle. As you become more comfortable with the changes in your diet, you'll likely want to experiment with new foods and recipes.

Just because you're eating healthier doesn't mean that you can't enjoy your favorite foods on occasion. You can do this by making some traditional dishes more nutritious. Chances are, you can reduce the calories and fat without greatly affecting the taste (see the example on page 279). Here are some common healthy substitutions:

If the recipe calls for	Try substituting
■ Butter ■ Margarine ■ Shortening ■ Oil	■ Low-fat vegetable broth, for frying. ■ For baking, replace half of the butter, shortening or oil with the same amount of applesauce, prune puree or commercial fat substitute. To avoid dense, soggy baked goods, don't substitute oil for butter or shortening, and don't substitute diet, whipped or tub-style margarine for regular margarine.
Whole milk	1 percent or skim milk
Evaporated whole milk	Evaporated skim milk
Eggs	Egg substitute. A half cup generally equals two eggs. You can use two egg whites for each whole egg in most recipes, too.
Sour cream	Fat-free plain yogurt or low-fat sour cream. Fat-free sour cream isn't intended for baking.
Cream cheese	Light cream cheese or low-fat cottage cheese pureed until smooth. Fat-free cream cheese isn't intended for baking.
Chocolate	Less chocolate, but in smaller pieces for greater dispersal. In some recipes, substitute cocoa and oil or corn syrup. One square of unsweetened chocolate equals 3 tbsp. of cocoa and 1 tbsp. oil. One square of semisweet chocolate equals 3 tbsp. of cocoa and 1 tbsp. corn syrup.
Sugar	In most baked goods you can reduce the amount of sugar by one-half without affecting the food's texture or taste. Because sugar increases moisture in baked goods, make sure you use $1/4$ cup of sugar, honey or molasses for every cup of flour.
Flour	Whole-grain flour. Whole-grain flour can be substituted for regular flour in many recipes, such as bread or muffins. Whole-grain flour is higher in fiber than regular flour.

REMEMBER THOSE LEGUMES

Something else to keep in mind as you do your weekly planning is to include legumes in your menus. The term *legume* refers to a large family of plants whose seeds develop inside pods and are usually dried for ease of storage.

Because legumes are high in protein, these plant foods make an excellent substitute for animal sources of protein such as meat and dairy products. Legumes are also versatile and inexpensive.

Common types of legumes include:

- White and navy beans
- Lima beans
- Pinto and black beans
- Black-eyed peas
- Split peas
- Brown and red lentils
- Chickpeas (garbanzos)

There are many ways that you can incorporate legumes into everyday meals. Here are just a few suggestions:

- Feature beans, peas or lentils in soups, stews or casseroles.
- Add chickpeas or black beans to salads.
- Use pureed beans as a base for healthy dips and spreads.

DON'T FORGET WHOLE GRAINS

Grains are the seeds of plants. When left whole, they include the endosperm, germ and bran, all of which contain beneficial nutrients that your body needs. Although vitamins and minerals are often added back into refined grains after the milling process, they don't pack the nutritional wallop that whole grains do.

Whole grains are an important part of a healthy diet because they're relatively low in fat and high in fiber. Foods high in fiber help fill you up — you eat less because your hunger is satisfied sooner. In addition, fiber has many health benefits. It promotes healthy digestion and it may lower your risk of cardiovascular disease, diabetes and cancer.

When planning your menus, try to include whole-grain products. Some examples include oatmeal, brown rice, wild rice, whole-gain bread, whole-wheat pasta, bulgar and hulled barley.

GET YOUR CALCIUM

Calcium is a mineral important for strong teeth and bones and for muscle and nerve function. Sufficient amounts of calcium in your diet greatly reduces your risk of osteoporosis. The recommended daily intake of calcium is 1,000 to 1,200 milligrams (mg) for adults. Unfortunately, many adults don't consume enough calcium. If you're trying to lose weight, you may need to monitor calcium intake because of reduced calorie consumption.

To help reach your calcium goal, consider eating more low-fat dairy products and dark-green vegetables such as broccoli. Some cereals, breads and juices may contain added calcium. You may also consider taking a daily calcium supplement.

Understanding nutrition labels

The Nutrition Facts food label is a great tool to help you seek out foods that are healthy. At first glance, the numbers and percentages on the label may look intimidating. But as you become more familiar with its format, you'll find that the label informs you about the contents of a product and helps you compare the nutritional qualities of similar products.

Serving size. Serving size information is based on the amount of this particular food people typically eat. It defines the amount for which the rest of nutrition information on the label applies. Serving sizes are based on standard household measurements, such as cups, ounces and pieces. Similar foods usually have similar serving sizes.

Calories. The calories listed relate to one serving of this particular food. In this example, there are 130 calories in six wafers. So as you achieve or maintain a healthy weight, be mindful of calorie options when comparing like products. This label also reveals how many calories in one serving come from fat. In this example, 40 of the 130 calories come from fat.

Nutrients. Food companies must list, at the minimum, the amounts of fat, total fat, saturated fat, cholesterol, sodium, total carbohydrate, dietary fiber, sugars, protein, vitamins A and C, calcium and iron that are contained in one serving of a product. Too much or too little of these nutrients can have an impact on your health. Some labels also display trans fat, but this information isn't required until January 1, 2006.

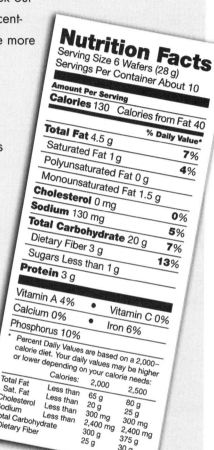

- Limit these nutrients: Total fat, saturated fat, trans fat, cholesterol and sodium.
- Get plenty of these nutrients: Dietary fiber, vitamin A, vitamin C, calcium and iron.

Percent Daily Value. The Daily Value numbers (%DV) on a Nutrition Facts label tell you how much of the daily recommended amounts of nutrients are contained in one serving of this food. These percentages are based on a 2,000-calories-a-day diet. For example, the label pictured here indicates that the 4.5 grams of total fat in one serving is 7 percent of all fat that an average person should consume in a day. That means there's 93 percent remaining total fat for the day. You may consume more or less than 2,000 calories a day, but you can still use the %DV as a frame of reference.

Label lingo

It can be confusing when you see terms such as reduced fat and low fat on food labels because no definition or explanation is provided. Is reduced fat the same thing as low fat?

The Food and Drug Administration (FDA) defines and regulates the use of terms involving nutrient content. Manufacturers can use these terms to draw your attention to foods that are high or low in various nutrients. Here's what some common terms mean:

Food label claim	What it means	Related terms	Specific examples
Free	Product is absolutely free of the nutrient in question, or if the nutrient is in the food, the amount must be insignificant.	■ Without ■ Negligible source of ■ Dietarily insignificant source of ■ No, zero, non	■ Fat-free: 0.5 grams (g) or less ■ Cholesterol-free: 2 milligrams (mg) or less ■ Sodium-free: 5 mg or less ■ Sugar-free: 0.5 g or less
Light	■ Must have half the fat or one-third fewer calories than the regular product. ■ Must have at least 50 percent less sodium than the regular product and be low in calories and fat.	■ Lite	■ Light sour cream ■ Light in sodium
Low	Meets the definition of "low" if food can be eaten frequently without exceeding dietary guidelines for: fat, saturated fat, cholesterol, sodium or calories.	■ Little ■ Few ■ Contains a small amount of ■ Low source of	■ Low fat: 3 g or less ■ Low in saturated fat: 1 g or less ■ Low in sodium: 140 mg or less ■ Very low sodium: 35 mg or less ■ Low calorie: 40 calories or less ■ Low cholesterol: 20 mg or less and 2 g or less of saturated fat
Reduced	Food must contain at least 25 percent less of a nutrient or calories than the regular product.	■ Less ■ Fewer	■ Reduced sodium ■ Reduced fat ■ Fewer calories

Adapted from the Food and Drug Administration, Food Labeling Guide, 1999

SAVVY SHOPPING STRATEGIES

To eat healthy, you don't have to drastically change the way you shop. Some simple steps you can take will help make the shopping trip successful.

Step 1: Plan ahead
Decide how many major meals are involved with this shopping trip. Then, consider the number of food items you'll need for breakfasts, lunches and snacks. Take an inventory of your staples.

Step 2: Make a shopping list
A list will make your shopping trip more efficient and help you avoid impulse purchases. Base your list on the menus from this book or those that you develop on your own. Add to the list one indulgence — perhaps a favorite dessert or a new convenience item. Try to stick only to what's on your list, but don't let your list prevent you from looking for or trying new healthy foods.

Step 3: Buy fresh
Fresh foods are generally better than canned or other ready-to-eat foods because they have more flavor and color and because they don't contain added ingredients. When you can, purchase fresh food.

Step 4: Shop the perimeter
Have you ever noticed how the freshest and healthiest foods tend to be around the perimeter of a grocery store? Picture

Cookbook shopping
If you find yourself in a cooking rut, look for a little inspiration. Cookbooks are available that suit almost every need, including eating healthy. To find quality recipes, look for the following in a cookbook:

- General information on nutrition and healthy eating. Does the cookbook devote several pages or a chapter to the principles of eating healthy?
- Nutritional analysis. Does the cookbook provide information on nutrients, such as calories, fats, carbohydrates, protein, sodium and fiber, per serving? Do the recipes closely follow recognized nutritional guidelines?
- Healthy ingredients. Do the recipes emphasize plant foods — vegetables, fruits, grains, legumes — and de-emphasize foods of animal origin?
- Practical advice. Are the recipes easy to make and the ingredients easy to find? Is the information well organized and easy to understand?
- Reputable author. Is the cookbook written, authored or endorsed by an established health care organization or dietary professional?

In addition, make sure the cookbook appeals to your tastes and matches your lifestyle. For example, if you don't have time to cook, find a cookbook that emphasizes easy, nutritious meals. Magazines are another source of new recipes. Look those that offer a nutritional analysis of their recipes.

Handling food safely

Here are tips for the safe handling of food:

- Plan ahead. Thaw meats and other frozen foods slowly in the refrigerator, not on a counter-top where it can attract bacteria.
- When shopping, don't buy food in cans or jars with dented or bulging lids.
- Before preparing food, wash your hands with soap and water. Rinse produce thoroughly or peel off the skin or outer leaves. Launder dishcloths and kitchen towels frequently.
- Don't mix raw meat with fresh produce during meal preparation. Wash knives and cutting surfaces frequently, especially after handling raw meat and before preparing other foods to be eaten. You may wish to use separate, even color-coded, cutting surfaces for different types of foods.
- When cooking meat, use a meat thermometer. Cook red meat to an internal temperature of 160 F, poultry to 180 F. Cook fish until it flakes easily with a fork. Cook eggs until the yolks are firm and no longer runny.
- When storing food, always check expiration dates. Use fresh red meats within three to five days after purchase or freeze them immediately. Use fresh poultry, fish and ground meat within one to two days or freeze them immediately. Refrigerate or freeze leftovers within two hours of serving.

the store in your mind and take a tour around the outer sections — can you visualize the produce department, meat and seafood counter and dairy case? While there are good and necessary choices in the middle aisles of the store, such as pastas, grains and beans, many of your healthiest selections will likely come from the store's perimeter.

Step 5: Don't shop on an empty stomach

When you're hungry, it's hard to resist the bright packaging and enticing smells of many snack items, which are often high in fat, calories and sodium.

To reduce the temptation, shop after you've eaten a good meal. Sometimes, though, that just isn't possible. If you find yourself shopping when you're hungry, buy a piece of fresh fruit or another healthy item to munch on while you're at the store.

Step 6: Read food labels

Since May 1994, packaged goods sold in the United States have carried the Nutrition Facts label (see the sidebar, "Understanding nutrition labels," on page 93). This panel is an at-a-glance method for verifying how a food fits into a typical weight-control plan.

Each label contains information pertaining to serving size, calories, nutrients and percent daily values. This information can inform you about foods that are healthy, and warn you of those that aren't so healthy — often those that are highly processed or refined. Routinely checking food labels helps you compare the nutritional qualities of similar products.

KEEP IT SIMPLE

The menus you plan should reflect your tastes, abilities and lifestyle. Base your food decisions on the principles of the Mayo Clinic Healthy Weight Pyramid and include lots of vegetables, fruits and whole grains in meals.

If you make changes to your diet that are too drastic or too complicated, they're not likely to pass the test of time. So try to keep things simple. Focus on recipes that can be prepared relatively easily within your daily routine — meals that are practical, healthy, low in calories and satisfying. Soon your new eating behaviors will become second nature and making a trip to the grocery store won't require more than a moment's thought.

CHAPTER 10

Expanding your exercise program

Physical fitness, like healthy eating, is a lifetime pursuit. Because you have to eat every day, you also need to stay physically active to balance your calorie intake. Fitting more activity into your daily routine and taking regular walks are great ways to do that. Adding structured exercise gives you even greater control of your weight-control program.

Just as your diet benefits from a variety of foods, your body benefits from a variety of activities. Aerobic exercise such as walking makes your heart and lungs work more efficiently. But this is just one element of an optimal fitness program. Strength training builds stronger muscles, which stabilize and protect your joints and make daily activities easier. Flexibil-

ity or stretching exercises help extend the range that you can bend and stretch your joints, muscles and ligaments.

This chapter helps you increase and expand your activities by adding strength training and stretching exercises to your workouts. It helps determine how much exercise you'll need and provides tips on staying with a program. Stepping up the intensity doesn't mean you have to become a superathlete. It's not necessary to work out for hours at a time, do strenuous exercise or join an expensive gym. To become fit and lose weight, however, you do need to be consistent and committed to exercise. Maintaining an exercise program is one of the best predictors of long-term weight control.

HOW MUCH EXERCISE DO YOU NEED?

If your goal is to lose weight, you're more likely to succeed if you can increase the duration, frequency and intensity of your regular workouts. Exercising longer, more often and harder burns a greater number of calories. However, this increase needs to be balanced with other aspects of your lifestyle so that your exercise program is realistic, enjoyable and sustainable.

You've probably heard different recommendations about how much exercise is enough. One common guideline for fitness, supported by the U.S. Surgeon General, is to get 30 minutes of moderately intense physical activity on most days of the week.

But researchers have concluded that the amount of exercise you need for successful, long-term weight control may be more than what's required for improved fitness. The Institute of Medicine (IOM) now recommends that adults spend at least 60 minutes in moderately intense physical activity every day of the week. This recommendation reflects the fact that people in the United States are consuming more calories and getting heavier.

If you've been inactive or just starting to add more exercise, increase your activity level gradually. Begin with 10 or 15 minutes at a time and add one to five minutes to your workout until you can exercise for 45 to 60 minutes at a session.

The frequency of exercise is just as important as the duration. If you're just starting an exercise program, try working out three days a week on nonconsecutive days. Over several weeks, increase your sessions to five or six times weekly.

Another way to increase the demands of your workout is to add to the intensity of your exercise. You can gradually increase the intensity of activities you're already doing, based on the Borg exertion scale (see page 60). Or you can switch to higher-intensity activities — such as jogging or playing tennis instead of walking.

You can meet the IOM's guidelines for moderately intense activity by walking at three to four miles an hour for 60 minutes each day. Or you can use more intense activity, such as jogging for 20 to 30 minutes on most days of the week.

Many people find it hard to reserve even half an hour a day for exercise. You don't have to do it all at once. Try shorter sessions of activity, such as three 20-minute walks throughout the day. The bottom line is to aim for 60 minutes of accumulated activity — including both regular exercise and lifestyle activity — on most days of the week.

BUILDING A PROGRAM

Combine an active lifestyle with a regular exercise program and you can't go wrong. A balanced program that includes aerobic activities, strength training and stretching can improve your levels of physical fitness, muscular strength, endurance, balance and flexibility.

A typical workout might include the following routine:

- five minutes of warm-up
- 30 to 60 minutes of aerobic activity
- 20 to 30 minutes of strength exercises
- five to 10 minutes of cooling down and stretching

This routine isn't inflexible. Create a routine that fits your schedule and your interests. Maybe you can walk for an hour on most days of the week and do strength exercises for 20 minutes three times a week. It's always important to warm up before each exercise session, no matter how short, and cool down afterward.

Once you're in the habit of exercising, keeping a routine won't feel like such a hassle. You may look forward to the break from other obligations. And remember, you don't have to do your daily exercises all at one time.

Schedule time for rest in your routine. Your body may need time to physically recover. Alternate between low-intensity and higher-intensity exercise from day to day. For example, if you jog one day, do easy cycling or gardening on the next day. Take a break at least one day a week from your formal exercise program — but continue your active lifestyle.

How intense is your exercise?

Intensity reflects how hard you're working when you exercise. When you do an activity faster or harder, you add to its intensity. Walking is usually a light to moderately intense activity, while jogging and running can be vigorous.

Chapter 6 describes one way to gauge exercise intensity by using the Borg ratings of perceived exertion scale (see page 60). To receive aerobic benefits, you should exercise at a moderate intensity, which is in a range between 12 and 14 on the Borg exertion scale.

Another simple tool for assessing exercise intensity is the talk test. While exercising at a moderately intense level, you should be breathing harder, developing a light sweat and feeling some strain on your muscles, but you should still be able to speak in brief sentences.

You can also use your target heart rate (THR) to gauge the intensity of an activity. Your THR is between 60 percent and 85 percent of your maximum heart rate (MHR). To estimate your MHR, subtract your age from 220. For example, if you're 62, your MHR is approximately 158 beats a minute. Then, calculate the lower and upper limits of your THR by multiplying your MHR by 60 percent and 85 percent:

- 0.60 x 158 = 95 beats a minute (the approximate lower limit of your THR)
- 0.85 x 158 = 134 beats a minute (the approximate upper limit of your THR)

So, if your age is 62, maintaining a heart rate between 95 and 134 beats a minute is a good estimate of moderately intense exercise. While exercising, place two fingers on the inside edge of your wrist and press gently to feel your pulse. Count your pulse for 10 seconds and multiply that number by 6 to determine your heart rate in beats a minute.

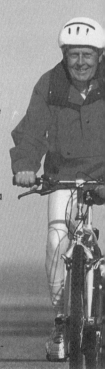

Staying with a program

About half the people who start an exercise program will drop out within six months. Some stop when they get bored or think the results come too slowly. Others overdo exercise at the start of their programs and are quickly discouraged by the pain and stiffness they feel later.

Even if you've never stuck to an exercise program before, you can do it now. The following tips may help you stay involved and motivated:

Be patient. It's better to progress slowly than to push too hard and be forced to abandon your program because of pain or injury. Improvements to your fitness and health may not develop overnight, but you'll notice a difference within about a month. It generally takes about three months for exercise to become routine. If you can stay with your program for that long, you're more likely to continue it.

Make it fun. Boredom is a major reason why people stop exercising. You're more likely to stay with your program if you choose activities you enjoy.

- Listen to music, watch television or read while you work out.
- Work out with a friend or in a group.
- Join an exercise club or fitness class.
- Get a new piece of equipment, such as a pedometer, which measures the number of steps you take each day.

Include variety. Alternating between different activities (cross-training) reduces your chance of injury from overusing a muscle or joint. It also keeps you interested. For aerobic exercise, you might walk one day, bicycle the next and swim later in the week. On days when the weather is pleasant, do your stretching exercises outside. Don't be afraid to try a new activity or join a health club.

Suit your personality and lifestyle. Do you like to exercise alone or in groups? If you prefer solitude, you may enjoy walking or biking. If group activities appeal to you, consider enrolling in a dance class or joining a bowling league.

Plan exercise for a time of day that suits you. For example, if you're a morning person, exercise before you begin the rest of the day's activities. Make exercise convenient. Even if you prefer to exercise outdoors, you can still plan indoor activities in case of bad weather.

Get support. Encouragement from family and friends can be motivating. Studies show that social support helps people stay with an exercise program. Working out with a partner helps you get out the door on days when you're not inspired.

Track your progress. An exercise diary shows what you've accomplished and helps you set goals for the future. After each workout, record the date, intensity and duration of your exercise, and your mood. These entries are more in-depth and personal than in an activity record (see pages 212-221). Seeing your progress in writing can be a powerful motivator.

Reward yourself. Work on developing an internal sense of reward based on feelings of accomplishment, self-esteem and self-control. After each exercise session, take a few minutes to sit down and relax.

It's only temporary

Everyone's been there. Work gets extra busy, you take a vacation or get sick, and all your good exercise intentions fly out the window. How do you get back to your routine? Try these tips:

- Don't be too critical. Consider every lapse as a learning experience. Remind yourself it's a temporary break and not a catastrophe.

- Be realistic. Do you think you can exercise two hours a day 365 days a year? If this is your goal, you're setting yourself up to fail.

- Continually plan. Always be thinking of ways to incorporate short periods of physical activity in your day even if you have an upcoming trip or your workload increases.

- Make it a priority. Exercise is just as important as anything else you do during the day.

- If you're losing interest in your exercise program, take a few days off to refresh yourself. Think of something new you can do to keep yourself interested.

- Get going. Do some kind, any kind, of physical activity today.

Savor the good feelings that exercise gives you, and reflect on what goals you've just accomplished.

External rewards can also help keep you motivated. When you reach a longer-range goal, treat yourself to a new CD, a massage or tickets to a sporting event.

Allow yourself breathing room. Be flexible with your schedule. If you're tired, feel a cold coming on or have a hectic day, don't force yourself to work out. Take the day off, and continue your program when you're feeling better.

Expect lapses. A brief period of time when you can't exercise isn't a disaster. Just get going again. See also pages 292-301 in the Healthy Weight Program.

STRENGTH TRAINING

When it comes to physical fitness and weight control, investing in a set of weights or resistance bands may pay dividends as great as those gained with a pair of walking shoes. Strength training, also referred to as resistance training or weight lifting, builds the strength and endurance of your muscles. The stronger your muscles are, the easier your daily tasks become and the longer you can work before getting tired.

Strength training reduces body fat and increases lean muscle mass. That doesn't mean you'll bulk up. You may actually look thinner because your muscles are better toned. Increased lean muscle mass will provide you with a bigger "engine" to burn calories. The more muscle mass your body has, the more efficiently it burns calories, even when you're at rest.

Strength training also helps:

- Increase your strength and stability, making it easier to move and lift things.
- Maintain your balance and coordination. This helps reduce the risk of falls.
- Maintain and increase your bone mineral density and decrease your risk of osteoporosis. When bone is stressed appropriately through muscle movement, it gets stronger.
- Reduce your risk of injury. Strong muscles protect your joints and lower back from injury during aerobic exercise and normal daily activities.
- Boost your self-confidence and self-image. Studies indicate that people who participate in strength training feel better about themselves.

Strength training is especially important as you get older. Muscle mass diminishes with age — your muscles shrink if you don't use them. Each year between the ages of 30 and 70, you lose about 1 percent of your muscle strength, primarily through inactivity. That means you could be 40 percent weaker at age 70 than you were at 30. If you don't replace that loss, you might be increasing the percentage of your body weight that is fat.

Strength training helps preserve your muscle mass. And studies involving middle-age to older men and women found that resistance training had the added benefit of reducing their risk of cardiovascular disease, cancer and diabetes.

It's never too late to start, no matter what your age. In one study of people over age 50, several months of strength training reversed two decades' worth of lost muscle mass. Even frail people over age 90 were able to regain some muscle mass with resistance exercises. These gains translated to improvements in their ability to get out of chairs, climb stairs and walk without falling.

You can benefit from strength training with just two sessions a week. If you work all major muscle groups, each session may last 20 to 30 minutes.

Getting started

Strength training involves working your muscles against some form of resistance. When your muscles push or pull against a force such as gravity or a weight, they grow stronger. Strength training is typically done with free weights or weight machines. You can also exercise using the weight of your own body as the resistance or with equipment such as resistance bands and stability balls.

Free weights — dumbbells and barbells — are freestanding weights that you lift. Dumbbells are small hand-held weights and barbells are long bars with weights attached at each end. Weight machines come in a variety of forms and typically work different parts of your body. If you don't have access to free weights or machines, try adapting two empty 1-gallon milk containers. Pour a little bit of water into each to add weight. Increase the weight by simply adding more water.

Body composition and weight

After you add strength training to your exercise routine, you may notice the numbers on the scale creeping up a bit. Strength training builds lean muscle tissue, and muscle weighs more than fat because it's denser. So you might weigh a little more, but you'll look leaner. In the long run, your added muscle will burn more calories, which will help with weight loss.

The amount of your body's fat tissue and lean tissue (muscles, bones and organs) is known as body composition. Because body composition reflects the specific amounts of fat and lean tissue, it's often a better indicator of your overall health than body weight is. Your body composition is based not on how much you weigh, but on how much of your weight is fat and how much is lean. Excessive body fat is unhealthy.

Your bathroom scale doesn't tell you how much of your weight is fat. And a well-muscled person with relatively little body fat may be designated as overweight on the standard weight charts, while a thin person with poor muscle development and relatively more fat may be designated as healthy. For most people, however, the BMI is an effective tool for determining whether or not they're overweight (see page 18).

The best way to achieve a healthy body composition is to burn calories through regular aerobic exercise while using strength exercises to build lean tissue.

Not all strength training is done with weights. Exercises that use your own body weight to create resistance include push-ups against a wall, chair dips, lunges and standing squats.

Regardless of the method you choose, begin strength training slowly. If you start with too much resistance or too many repetitions, you may damage muscles and joints. A single set of 12 repetitions (reps) can build muscle just as effectively as doing multiple sets. Start with a weight you can lift comfortably eight times and build up to 12 repetitions. The weight should be heavy enough so that the last three to four repetitions are difficult to complete. After you can easily do 12 repetitions, you may increase the weight.

If you're a beginner, you may find that you're able to lift only 1 or 2 pounds in a set. That's OK. The weight should be heavy enough to tire your muscles but not cause pain. As your body gets accustomed to strength exercise, you'll be able to do a set using a heavier weight.

Before each session, take a five- to 10-minute walk to warm up your muscles. When doing the exercises, try to work all of your major muscle groups, including the legs, abdomen, chest, back, shoulders and arms. Try to work opposing muscles equally for balance.

You can work your whole body during each session, or you can focus on your upper body during one session and your lower body during the next. Take at least one day off before working the same muscle group again to allow time for recovery.

If you're new to strength training, consider finding a certified professional to teach you the proper technique. Or look for a class offered through a community education program.

Guidelines for strength training include:

- Complete all movements slowly and with control. If you're unable to maintain good form and posture, decrease the weight or number of repetitions.
- Breathe normally and freely, exhaling as you lift a weight and inhaling as you lower it. Don't hold your breath.
- Stop exercising immediately at the moment you feel any pain.
- Stretch your muscles before and after your workout. When stretching beforehand, warm up first with walking.
- Work at a somewhat hard intensity when strength training — 12 to 16 on the Borg scale (see page 60). You should feel a sense of strain (not pain) in your muscles and develop a light sweat.
- It's normal to experience mild muscle soreness for a few days after starting strength training.

STRETCHING AND FLEXIBILITY

Flexibility is the ability to move your joints through a range of motions. This applies to the vertebrae in your back as well as the joints of your fingers, wrists, elbows, shoulders, hips, knees and ankles. The ability to bend and move your joints requires that the muscles around the joints be stretched regularly.

Some people are naturally more flexible than others due to their genetic makeup. Flexibility is also influenced by gender, age and physical activity. Stiffness that's often attributed to aging is more often caused by inactivity. Flexibility is a use-it-or-lose-it function — the less active you are, the less flexible you're likely to be.

No matter what your starting level for exercise, you can improve your flexibility. Regular exercise and stretching can reverse stiffness. Flexing your muscles and moving your joints through their full range of motion prevents your muscles from tightening.

Regular, careful stretching brings:

- **Increased flexibility.** Flexible muscles allow greater freedom of movement and can make daily tasks, such as lifting packages, bending to tie your shoe or hurrying to catch a bus, less tiring.
- **Improved circulation.** Stretching increases blood flow to your muscles, literally warming them up. Blood flowing to your muscles brings nourishment and gets rid of waste byproducts in the muscle tissue. Improved circulation can help shorten your recovery time if you've had any muscle injuries.
- **Better posture.** Frequent stretching helps keep your muscles from getting tight and helps maintain good posture.
- **Stress relief and relaxation.** Stretching releases muscle tension and soreness and allows you to feel more relaxed physically and mentally.

- **Enhanced coordination and balance.** Maintaining a full range of motion in your joints keeps you in better balance. Especially as you get older, coordination and balance will help keep you less prone to falls.
- **Reduced risk of injury.** Stretching prepares your muscles for activity and helps protect you from injuries to your muscles or tendons.

Getting started

Stretching improves the flexibility of your muscles by lengthening muscle tissues and training your muscles to relax. Flexibility also helps improve posture, relieve pain and improve performance.

Stretching can be done in a number of ways. If you have a tight muscle, it may be beneficial to stretch before exercise. But stretching, especially before exercise, isn't always necessary. Recent research has questioned whether pre-exercise stretching actually reduces the risk of injury. In addition, some research suggests that traditional stretching — holding a muscle in a stretched position for 30 to 60 seconds — before high-intensity exercise may actually impair your performance.

Some fitness experts recommend simply warming up before exercise, using the same muscles you'll be using during your workout. For example, brisk walking is a way to warm up before more intense aerobic activity. Some stretching during cooldown after exercise is still recommended.

Although a regular stretching program is the easiest way to increase flexibility,

activities such as swimming, low-intensity cycling, walking, dance, yoga and tai chi also may be effective.

In addition to stretching the major muscle groups, your basic stretches should focus on muscles and joints that you routinely use at work or play. For example, if you frequently play golf or racquet sports, be sure to stretch your shoulder muscles. If you walk or run, stretch your calf muscles, hamstrings and quadriceps.

No matter what activities you do, keep your torso flexible by stretching your back and chest muscles. A healthy spine is crucial to every activity, so you'll want to keep it limber and strong.

Stretching technique is fairly simple and easy to learn. Follow these guidelines:

- Warm up first. Stretching muscles when they're cold may increase your risk of injury. Warm up by walking and gently pumping your arms, or exercise at low intensity for five minutes.
- Always stretch slowly and gently.
- Hold your stretches for at least 30 seconds and up to 60 seconds for a particularly tight muscle. That can seem like a long time, so wear a watch to make sure you're holding the stretch long enough.
- Don't bounce. Bouncing as you stretch can lead to muscle injuries.
- Stretch until you feel mild tension or noticeable pull in your muscle. If a stretch hurts, you've gone too far — ease up. As you hold each stretch, try to relax the muscle being stretched.
- Relax and breathe freely. Don't hold your breath while stretching.

CHOOSING WORKOUT SPACE

As you develop your regular exercise program, consider investing in a health club membership or in fitness equipment. Of course, it's possible to exercise with little or no equipment and without spending a lot of money. For example, you can do strength and flexibility exercises at home and get your aerobic workouts from walking or jogging.

There are distinct advantages to either a health club or home gym. For one, it may keep you motivated to stay with your exercise program. But before paying membership fees or spending money on a fitness machine, think about your weight goals, fitness goals, budget, space, preferences and personality.

Health clubs

When you join a health club or gym, a wealth of resources and expertise is at your fingertips. Clubs offer a greater variety of equipment than you could afford to buy on your own. Clubs also have fitness professionals to field questions, help plan exercise programs and teach proper technique for various exercises.

Health clubs also may have features such as a swimming pool, running track, sauna and racquetball court. Many clubs offer a variety of fitness classes. A health club is a good option if you enjoy group activities or are motivated by the social aspects of exercise. You may also be more motivated to work out if you've paid a hefty fee to do so.

Here's what you can expect from a health club:

- **Fitness at your level.** If you're just starting a program, look for a health club geared for beginners. Advanced classes and experienced members, though, can be an incentive as you learn.
- **Certified staff members.** Instructors should be certified by a nationally recognized organization, such as the American Council on Exercise, the American College of Sports Medicine, or the National Strength and Conditioning Association.
- **Friendly employees.** Do staffers smile and greet you? Do they offer encouragement? Do they show interest in helping you attain your goals?
- **Clean, safe environment.** Are the equipment and floors clean? Are staff members certified to give first aid and cardiopulmonary resuscitation (CPR)?
- **Comfortable atmosphere.** Not all health clubs are filled with hard bodies. Take a look around the center. Will you want to visit regularly?
- **Updated equipment.** Does the facility have equipment you want to use? Is it fairly new and in good condition?

Choose a club that's not too far from your home or workplace and has hours that are convenient for you. Try to visit a few facilities to comparison shop. Many clubs allow you to work out a time or two for free before you join. Take advantage of trial opportunities. Meet with a staff member, learn what services are available and take a tour.

Yoga, Pilates and tai chi: Working body and mind

If you want to try an activity that combines more than one type of exercise — and is relaxing and refreshing to boot — consider taking a class in yoga, Pilates or tai chi. These three disciplines have very different origins and techniques. But they all emphasize the mind-body connection and are relaxing ways to increase your flexibility, strength and balance.

Yoga

This system of breathing and poses (postures) has been around for thousands of years. Yoga promotes flexibility, strength, endurance and balance. It can be as vigorous or as gentle as you choose, and its techniques for stretching and strengthening the body can be practiced by people of all ages and abilities. Many of the yoga classes offered in the United States teach hatha yoga. This style combines gentle breathing exercises with slow stretches and movement through a series of postures (asanas). Yoga classes are offered at many places, including yoga schools and centers, health clubs, community and senior centers, and churches.

Pilates

This low-impact system of exercises originates from dance and ballet. Designed to strengthen your core muscles — lower back, hips, abdomen and buttocks — Pilates exercises also improve flexibility, strength and posture. In Pilates, you perform a set of controlled stretches and movements, focusing on each muscle group both physically and mentally. Although some Pilates exercises are done on machines, many programs offer floor-work classes. Classes by certified Pilates instructors are offered at health clubs and community centers.

Tai chi

This ancient form of martial arts involves gentle, circular movements combined with deep breathing. The poses are performed slowly and gracefully, with smooth transitions between them. Tai chi helps strengthen muscles, improve flexibility and reduce stress. It also helps you maintain and improve your balance. Classes with qualified instructors are found at martial arts schools, health clubs and community centers.

Making a home gym

Working out at home has its advantages, too. It's less expensive, and you don't have to drive back and forth to a gym. You don't have to wait in line to use exercise machines. You can work out whenever you want and in privacy.

But if you plan to exercise at home, you'll need to be highly motivated to ignore the inevitable distractions that come along, such as housework, ringing phones and drop-by visitors. You may have to be creative to keep home workouts from getting boring.

Before buying home fitness equipment, consider your needs and your personality. If you've already made exercise a habit, then you're ahead of the game. But if your good intentions of getting to the gym often fizzle, chances are that you won't work out at home, either — and before long, you'll be selling that expensive treadmill at your next garage sale.

What type of equipment you invest in should be determined by your fitness goals, budget and space. Dedicating a specific place in your home for exercise will help you be successful. You also want the equipment to be easily accessible. An inexpensive way to start is with a good pair of shoes, appropriate free weights and an exercise mat. Other inexpensive options include resistance bands, fitness balls, fitness videos and jump ropes. After that, your choices of equipment will depend on what you like to do. If your favorite activity is walking, a treadmill may be a good investment.

A REWARDING HABIT

Starting an exercise program is an achievement in itself. As soon as you take that first walk or lift that first weight, you're one step closer to your fitness and weight goals. And the progress you make is as important, if not more so, than reaching the goals themselves.

Many people who start an exercise program are amazed to find that the activity they've been dreading for all these years is actually pleasant and rewarding. After you've been active for a while, you may find that you're stronger and more fit, and you look and feel better. That's a transformation worth savoring!

CHAPTER 11

Staying
motivated

I t's the million-dollar question. How do you maintain a lifelong commitment to weight control? If this question had an easy answer, nearly everyone would be at a healthy weight.

The truth is, maintaining a healthy weight is challenging. Even if you're committed for the long haul for all of the right reasons, your resolve will be tested time and again. You might hit a plateau where you'll see no results for weeks, or be faced with a life crisis that puts weight loss on the back burner. You may find that old habits die hard, and negative attitudes undermine your effort.

This chapter can help you overcome these challenges and help you maintain a healthy weight for a lifetime. You'll learn how to turn problems into opportunities for change and to reward yourself for what you've accomplished.

BUMPS IN THE ROAD

Even with a good plan and the best of intentions, you'll run into roadblocks on your path. How you respond to these obstacles can be the difference between success and failure. Following are common problems you may experience:

Plateaus

There's no greater reward for your effort than to step on the scale and see that you've lost weight. But what happens when the indicator on the scale doesn't change from week to week? Even if you're eating a healthy, low-calorie diet and exercising regularly — by all accounts, doing everything right — the results aren't showing up. Or you may see results for the first few weeks, then hit a plateau. Days may go by, even weeks, when your weight remains unchanged.

Before you get discouraged, understand that long-term results don't always show up right away. Try not to become too self-critical, and above all, don't give up! Stick with the program.

If your program has stalled for weeks, make sure you're on track with weight-loss basics. Consider one of the strategies described on page 158 of the Action Guide. Or try one of these suggestions:

- Assess your food and activity records. Make sure you haven't loosened the rules, letting yourself get by with larger portions or less exercise.
- Focus on three- to four-week trends in weight loss instead of daily fluctuations. You may find that, although progress is not evident immediately, you're nevertheless losing weight.
- If you've hit a plateau, reassess your program. Is it possible that you've accomplished about as much as you can with the goals you've set? You may need to adjust or change your focus.
- Remain positive. Remember that results aren't measured in pounds alone.
- Be willing to try new alternatives. Look for inspiration from the experiences of others trying to lose weight.

Lapse and relapse

Rare is the person who doesn't experience a lapse from time to time. Whether it's sneaking dessert after an already decadent meal or missing a daily walk, lapses are bound to happen. The danger occurs when lapses turn into relapses.

What's the difference? A lapse occurs when you revert to old behaviors once or twice. It's temporary, common and a sign that you need to get back in control.

A relapse is more serious. After several lapses have occurred in a short span of time, you're at risk of completely reverting back to your old behavior. You panic, afraid that you'll undo all your good effort. You may give up and say, "I guess I just can't do it."

Calm down. Remember that lapses are normal, temporary and can be anticipated. Know that, no matter how dedicated people are, they all make mistakes. Assess your situation and see the lapse for what it is. Use the experience as an opportunity to strengthen your resolve (see also pages 292-301 in the Healthy Weight Program).

Consider these tips for getting back on track when you experience a lapse:

- Don't let negative thoughts take over. Remember that mistakes happen and that each day is a chance to start anew.
- Clearly identify the problem, then create a list of possible solutions. Pick a solution to try. If it works, then you've got yourself a plan for preventing another lapse. If it doesn't work, try the next solution and go through the same process until you find one that works.

- Get support. Talk to your spouse, friend or a professional counselor.
- Work out your guilt and frustration with exercise. Take a walk or go for a swim. Keep the exercise upbeat. Never use exercise as punishment for a lapse.
- Recommit to your goals. Review them and make sure they're still realistic.

What if you do relapse? Although relapses are disappointing, they can help you learn that your goals may be unrealistic, that you have high-risk situations, or that certain strategies don't work for you.

Above all, realize that you're not a failure. Reverting to old behaviors doesn't mean that all hope is lost. It just means that you need to recharge your motivation, recommit to your program and return to healthy behaviors.

Stress

Everything is going along well until something happens that throws a wrench in your progress toward a healthy weight. A family member has a major illness. You get a promotion. The holidays arrive in all their cookie-covered glory.

When stressful situations occur, your natural response may be to turn to food for comfort. You may lose focus on your exercise routine. Unfortunately, these solutions to stress just create more havoc in your life.

You can avoid this scenario by finding better ways to deal with stress. Go for a walk, listen to music or call a friend. Remind yourself every day that you *will* return to your regular routine, and you *will* continue to lose weight.

Getting friends and family on board

It's difficult to lose weight alone — but it's even more challenging when those closest to you aren't supportive. Whether it's a spouse who's doesn't want to share your experience, a mother who insists that you eat her famous dessert or friends who beg you to skip a workout to go out for pizza, handling these relationships can make the road ahead difficult. Help turn the tables in your favor with these suggestions:

- Call on your weight-loss partners or a professionally led support group. They can help you counteract the temptations or negative messages you're getting from others.
- Support yourself. Remind yourself everyday why you're changing your behaviors. Post positive messages where you'll see them several times a day.
- It's not uncommon for a spouse or companion to fear you're going to leave after losing weight. Remind your loved one that while you're changing your lifestyle, you're not changing the feelings you have for him or her. After all, the focus of the Healthy Weight Program is on your better health, not on your appearance.
- Ask for support. Tell family and friends that you'd appreciate their help and give them specific ways that they can assist you.

Coexisting mood conditions

Clinical disorders such as depression and anxiety can put a halt to your weight program. There's a clear link between obesity and depression. So, if you show signs of a mood disorder, such as sleeping more than usual or feeling down a lot of the time, it's a good idea to seek professional help. Talk to your doctor about your symptoms and treatment options. Generally, weight loss is easier once treatment for the mood disorder is underway.

BREAKING BEHAVIOR CHAINS

It's happened to everyone. You've had a healthy day — biked to work, eaten fresh fruit at breakfast and taken a 15-minute walk during your lunch break. Then a midafternoon craving sends you sprinting for the vending machine. Three minutes later, you're back at your desk with an extra-large candy bar in hand.

What happened? Maybe you were tired, or you didn't eat enough at lunch. Whatever the reason, you let a craving get the best of you. Now you feel guilty, frustrated and angry with yourself — feelings that may send you back to the vending machine. Where do you go from here?

Imagine this chain of events as a series of separate but interconnected behaviors. Try to separate this chain into discrete parts. Examining each link of the chain can lead to possible solutions and help you control poor decision-making that can lead to overeating. Take the example of a woman named Laura, who feels guilty after eating cookies but continues to eat more. Here's her chain of behavior:

- Agrees to bring cookies instead of a salad to a friend's potluck dinner.
- Buys the cookies two days beforehand.
- Works late and misses her lunch.
- Arrives home very hungry.
- Thinks, "I'll eat one cookie, then go to the grocery store."
- Takes the box of cookies to the den.
- Eats cookies while watching television and reading her mail.
- Eats rapidly and without awareness.
- Feels guilty and like a failure.
- Eats more.
- Quits her weight program.

At every link, Laura could have done something to break the chain of events. She could have agreed to bring a salad or a dessert she doesn't crave. She could have waited until the day of the party to buy the cookies. Knowing that missing lunch is a high-risk situation for out-of-control eating, she could have planned an evening meal in advance. She could have taken one or two cookies into the den, not the entire box. Finally, she could tell herself that this was a lapse and start again.

You can do the same with your behavior chains. Try interrupting a chain at the earliest link. If a midafternoon craving regularly strikes, you may break the chain by stocking your office desk with healthy snacks. Or maybe you can plan a healthy dinner before leaving for work. Self-control is easier to exercise than willpower. Don't lead yourself into temptation.

Below are four different approaches to help break a behavior chain. Find one that works for you. If one approach isn't successful, try something else. Different approaches may work on different days.

ABC approach

Heading off problems before they develop can be effective in changing your behavior. This is sometimes called the ABC method: *A* stands for antecedent, *B* for behavior and *C* for consequence. Most behaviors have a cause or antecedent. And behaviors lead to consequences.

Generally, people are more aware of the consequences of a behavior because these often demand their immediate attention. By addressing antecedents first, you may avert behaviors before they start and thus not have to deal with any consequences.

For example, keeping a tub of ice cream in the freezer (antecedent) may cause you to sneak spoonfuls throughout the day (behavior), ultimately causing you feelings of guilt and disrupting your weight program (consequence). Using the ABC approach, you might decide to keep ice cream out of your house entirely. This addresses the antecedent and helps you maintain your weight-control program.

Distraction approach

Imagine that ever since you were a child, you've enjoyed a bowl of ice cream before going to bed. So now, when you get ready for bed each night, the carton you've hidden in the back of the freezer starts calling your name. Focus on turning your attention away from your craving. For instance, you might read, listen to music, write a letter or switch on the television. Whatever your solution, the key is to find something that keeps your attention until the craving passes. You'll find that cravings are short-lived when your mind is occupied with something else.

Confrontation approach

This approach involves facing the negative consequences of your behavior head-on. For example, if you're craving ice cream, think about the unneccesary calories and fat you'll be consuming. Think about how tired and sluggish you'll feel afterward. Think about how overeating will impact your health. Remind yourself that this isn't what you want to do with your life. What you want is to improve your health and feel better about yourself.

Shaping approach

Shaping encourages you to change your behavior gradually, one step at a time. For instance, instead of cutting ice cream out of your diet entirely, you eat a smaller bowl every night. Then you eliminate one evening snack completely — deciding, for example, to not eat ice cream on Mondays. In time, you'll be able to scale back to a small bowl of ice cream once a week. That's a nice compromise.

Making gradual changes over time is less intimidating than changing your life in a single day. As you succeed with step-by-step changes, your confidence will grow and will fuel further successes.

ADJUSTING YOUR ATTITUDE

Maintaining a successful weight program requires more than adjusting your behaviors. The attitudes you have about yourself and about your body also affect your success. Below are five common problems that you may encounter, along with strategies for overcoming them.

Negative self-talk

As you learned in Chapter 8, self-talk — the internal dialog you have with yourself each day — influences your actions. When that self-talk is negative, it can wreak havoc on your self-esteem and stall your progress. After all, if you convince yourself that you'll never lose weight, it seems reasonable to say to yourself, "Why even try in the first place?"

Remove yourself from this self-defeating behavior by replacing negative self-talk with positive self-talk. Chapter 8 outlines strategies for doing just this.

Negative attitude

Negative attitudes and beliefs can be as destructive as negative self-talk. For instance, you may believe that you can't go to the gym because people will stare and make fun of your body. Or maybe you credit a special diet for your initial success instead of your own abilities and hard work. Such perceptions can sabotage your ability to lose weight.

Fight back by identifying your negative attitudes. Write them down and think of alternative attitudes to counteract them.

Motivation methods

Motivation comes in many forms. Here are ways to keep your weight program on track:

- Set goals. Write them down and post them where you can see them.
- Keep track of your progress. Record exercise times, pounds lost, milestones met, and improvements in health.
- Put it in writing. Make a contract with yourself and post it where you can see it.
- Create a support team. Tell friends and family about your progress, ask your spouse to help cheer you on and make time to exercise with friends.
- Reward yourself with something that matters to you every time you reach a goal.
- Set a regular time for your physical activity so that it becomes habit.
- Develop positive self-statements or affirmations. Repeat them to yourself daily or type them and post them where you'll see them regularly. An example is, "I'm getting stronger and better every day," or that old standby, "Every day in every way, I'm getting better and better."
- Cut yourself some slack. For instance, when it comes to your exercise program, remember that you're not in boot camp. It's OK to take a day off now and then when you need it. The more responsibility you take for your weight program, the more you'll make it your choice and the less likely you are to rebel against it.

Consider these examples:

- *Negative attitude:* "Exercise is painful and boring."
  New attitude: "I like being physically active. I'll call a friend to go walking and enjoy the beautiful day."
- *Negative attitude:* "I'm only losing weight because this program works. Once it's over, I'll regain the weight."
  New attitude: "I'm making this happen by making positive choices. My success will continue even when my program ends because I'm committed to changing my lifestyle for a lifetime."

Unrealistic dreams

Sometimes, you may imagine that losing weight will cure all your problems. But you know this is just a dream.

Be realistic about what weight loss will do for you. Yes, you'll probably be healthier. And yes, you'll likely have more energy and higher self-esteem. But losing weight doesn't guarantee a better social life or a more satisfying job.

Your life will likely change with weight loss, but slowly — and maybe not in the ways that you imagine. Try to counteract idealistic dreaming with these strategies:

- **Set realistic expectations.** Recognize your unrealistic dreams, then counter them with more rational goals.
- **Set short-term goals.** Instead of focusing on how happy you'll be after reaching your ultimate weight goal, focus on what you want to accomplish this week. This gives you the opportunity to celebrate successes every week.

- **Celebrate changed behaviors.** Don't just reward yourself for pounds lost. You're working hard, and there are other achievements to be excited about.

Inflexibility

Words such as "always," "must" and "never" add undue pressure to your program. For instance, you decide that you'll "never eat chocolate again." You demand, "I must walk two miles every day."

Why be so tough on yourself? After all, to "never" or "always" do anything is a lot to ask and may be a path to guilt-ridden lapses. Your urgency doesn't allow you to be flexible, and everyone makes mistakes. Besides, if you beat yourself up over one momentary slip, it's easy to overlook the progress you're making.

Denying yourself something, such as chocolate, is a sure way to fuel a craving. When you finally break down, you're as apt to buy two candy bars as you are one. Once you've broken your rule, you allow yourself to have chocolate ice cream before dinner or chocolate cake before bed. Suddenly, your eat-no-chocolate rule has made you feel like a failure.

The sensible approach is to plan for a treat now and then but do so in appropriate situations. For example, when you're out to dinner with friends but not when you're alone or feeling sad.

All-or-nothing thinking

All-or-nothing thinking causes you to see a situation as either all good or all bad. For instance, you may think, "If I succeed

Staying the course

You may think that once you've achieved a healthy weight, your work is done. Sorry, but that's the diet mentality talking. It goes back to the idea that you go on a diet to lose weight, and once you lose the weight, you go off the diet. That kind of thinking leads to regaining weight. Been there, done that. Not going there again.

This time you're going to hold on to your hard-won victory. Maintaining your weight follows the same principles as losing it. Because you've made lifestyle changes, you can continue them indefinitely. Instead of going off a diet, it's best to stay on the path you're on to maintain your weight. Whatever you used to help you lose weight, you'll need again to keep it off.

That's why we've stressed the need for lifestyle changes. That's why it's so important to make changes that you can live with permanently. You're already doing what you need to do. You're making healthy food choices and moving your body every day. You look good. You feel good. You're justifiably proud of yourself. Just keep on keeping on.

my calorie count today, I'm back to being overweight," or "If I eat ice cream, I've blown the program." In short, what you feel is, "If I'm not perfect, I'm a failure."

Few things about weight loss are all or nothing. The truth is that one setback doesn't mean you're a failure. If you let yourself believe this, you're likely to suffer guilt and depression and take a serious blow to your self-esteem. And as the problem snowballs, you'll be tempted to handle those feelings with comfort food.

Counteract all-or-nothing thinking with moderation. Tell yourself, for instance, that there are no "good" and "bad" foods, and that it's OK to have dessert once in a while. Or, instead of calling yourself a failure when you eat more than you planned or miss an exercise session, remind yourself that you can get back on track tomorrow. Be realistic in your assessment of your behaviors.

REWARD YOURSELF

When you reach goals, it's important to reward yourself. Giving yourself a pat on the back — whether a simple foot massage or a weekend getaway — will help you to stay with your weight program.

It starts with the realistic goals you've set. After all, if your goals are unattainable, you won't have anything to celebrate — and, worse, you'll feel bad about yourself. You can't expect to lose 30 pounds in your first month, but you can celebrate the pound you lost this week or the charity walk you participated in.

Don't get discouraged when you run into roadblocks. Instead, take time to appreciate even the smallest successes. Make a list of how you've succeeded in changing your eating and activity habits. Think about all the ways you feel better as a result of the weight you've lost. Then

25 years of weight loss

I'm not sure how much I weighed at my peak. I avoided scales. But I'm sure I was 215 pounds or more — too heavy for my 5-foot, 5-inch frame. I know I was a size 22.

That's history. For the past 25 years, I've weighed between 140 and 145 pounds. I made a lifetime commitment to lose weight and keep it off. I didn't like how I felt. Though I was only 26 years old, I felt old. I felt limited in my activities. I felt like I couldn't wear what I wanted to wear.

I put on my sweat suit. It was tight, and I didn't feel confident about exercising. But I was determined to run every day for a year. I never missed one of those 365 days. One thing I learned is you get kind of compulsive when you start something, and then you begin to balance out. Now, I exercise 30 to 45 minutes, five or six days a week. I started with jogging, but as I became healthier, I added other activities: tennis, racquetball, swimming. I run in one or two races a year partly because I like the T-shirts I get. They're a symbol of victory to me. I'm going to make them into a quilt someday.

Exercise is what helps me most because it's a victory that's contagious. For me, victory in exercising leads to victory in diet. If I go through a hard time where I overeat, or if it's Christmas — when I choose to enjoy sweets — I can still exercise. And if my weight hits 152 or 153 — I prefer to measure with my tight jeans instead of scales — I start a food diary to get back on track.

Besides helping me keep tabs on what I eat, the food journal has helped me identify my vulnerable eating times. One of those times is what I called the 5 o'clock frenzy. I'd rush home from work, hungry and worn out. I'd start cooking and eat while I cooked. But I learned that I could take the edge off being hungry by taking an apple or a bag of carrots to work, and then snacking on them during the drive home.

As I get older, it's harder to keep the weight off. I added lifting weights about three or four years ago. I spend only about 15 minutes, three times a week. I do it mostly to maintain my weight loss, but I also need it for my osteoporosis prevention and because women lose their muscle mass big time as they grow older.

I have to be honest, every day takes a new commitment. I'm moving into another house right now, so I'm tired. But I know I need to do 30 to 45 minutes of my cross-country ski machine and treadmill, which are my main exercises during the winter.

I look in the mirror and still can't believe what I see — even after 25 years. I still have the mental image that I'm overweight. Those memories stay in your head a long time. But the reality is the picture I see in the mirror, and the record of good health.

Faye
Byron, Minnesota

reward yourself every week or day, for instance, for simply staying on track. This is an accomplishment in itself.

Finally, spend time looking at the big picture. This means that you shouldn't rely only on your bathroom scale when it comes to measuring success. The scale won't reveal all the factors that really count. Are you more active? Do you have more energy? Have you gained muscle? Has your blood pressure improved?

Losing weight isn't just about appearances. Reward yourself for all the positive changes you've made in your life — even when they aren't reflected on the scale.

AND FINALLY ...

You may have already heard the statistic about the likelihood of keeping weight off permanently — 95 percent of those who lose weight regain it within five years. However, this statistic doesn't mean you're doomed to failure.

According to a study from the National Weight Control Registry (NWCR), success with lifetime weight control is possible. In fact, the study followed 629 women and 155 men who had been overweight for years. They lost an average of 66 pounds each. And although they did gain some weight back, they kept a minimum of 30 pounds off for at least five years. Most of them did it through a combination of exercise and restricting fat and calories. They did it by making the lifestyle changes we're recommending to you. A big surprise of the study was that 42 percent of the participants claimed that maintaining a healthy weight was easier than their intial weight loss.

The most heartening news is that 95 percent of the study participants were pleased with the overall results of their weight loss. They said it improved their overall quality of life, including their mood, their health and their self-confidence. The people of this NWCR study are living testimony that long-term weight loss can be achieved and that the benefits are many.

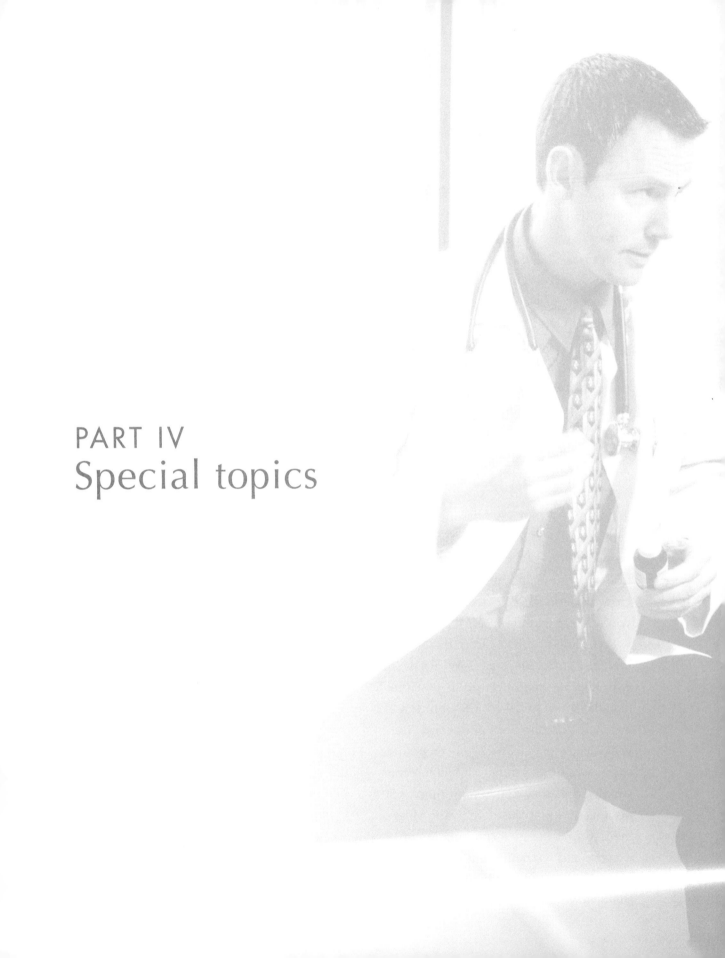

PART IV
Special topics

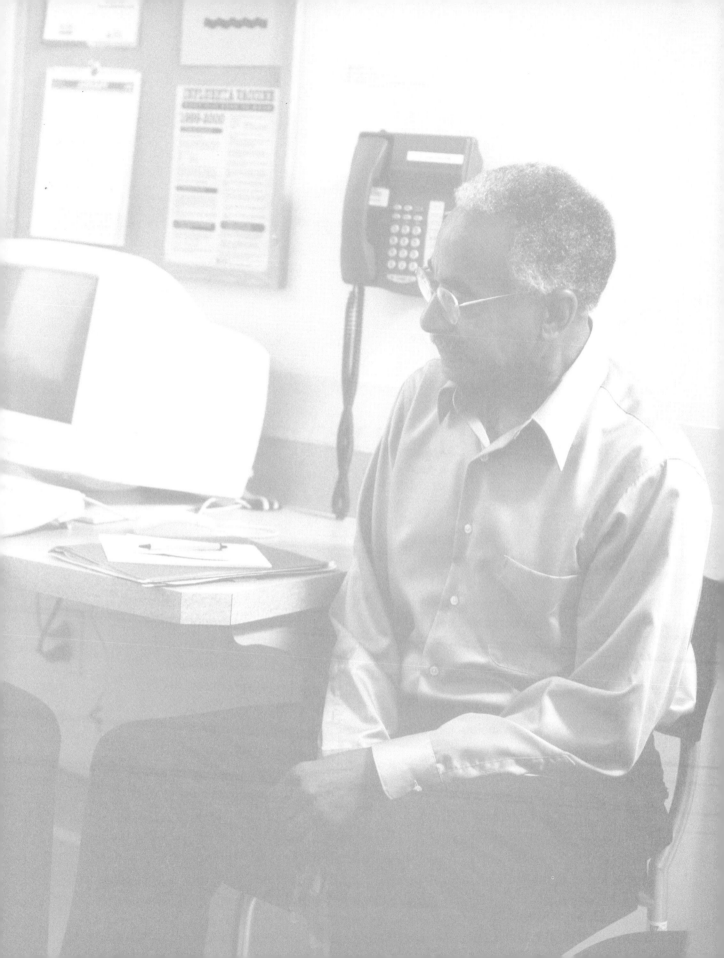

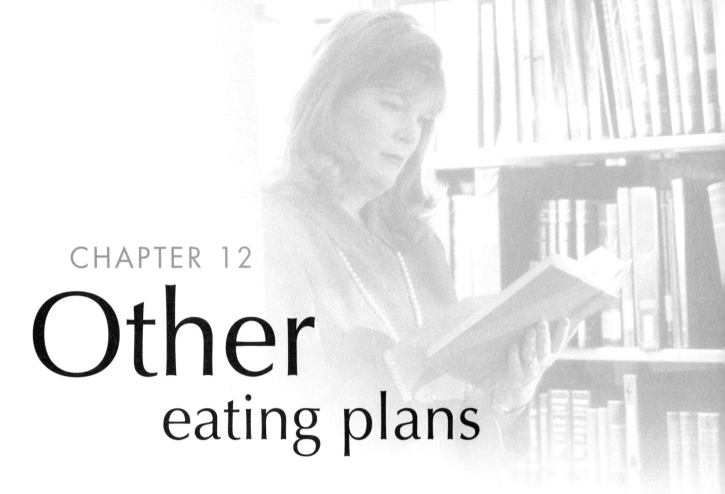

CHAPTER 12

Other
eating plans

If achieving a healthy weight were easy, there wouldn't be so many weight-loss programs and products out there. In fact, Americans spend billions of dollars a year on diet aids and services, ranging from diet soft drinks to health clubs, all in search of a magic bullet that helps them shed pounds quickly.

Unfortunately, people often find that specific diets are hard to sustain for long periods of time, in part because they get tired of avoiding certain foods, loading up on others or feeling hungry. As a result, whatever pounds they drop come right back after they go off the diet.

Maintaining a healthy weight requires long-term commitment. Even worthy diet plans fail when good intentions can't overcome a feeble dedication to making permanent lifestyle changes.

It's easy enough to lose weight quickly with most popular diets, often because they restrict your total calorie intake. A calorie is a calorie, no matter where it comes from or how it's consumed, and when you eat fewer calories than your body regularly burns, you're bound to lose some weight.

But most people underestimate the number of calories they eat by at least 10 percent to 20 percent — more if they're very overweight. You may think you're holding your calorie level to 1,500 a day, for example, when you're really consuming closer to 1,800 calories or more. People also misjudge the amount of physical activity they get daily, believing a walk from the car to the office will suffice for half the day's needed exertion. As a result, people get discouraged when they think they ought to be losing pounds and they're not losing weight at all.

Because responsibility for a weight program can seem overwhelming, some people feel more comfortable following a prescribed eating plan that offers instructions and promises desired results. Some structured diet plans require that you count fat grams or allot points to the foods you eat. Although these systems may not be the ultimate solution to your weight-loss quandary, they may help you see a direct relationship between what you put in your mouth and its eventual effects on your body. But will they also help you make long-term changes that result in a healthy, sustainable way of eating?

This chapter discusses some of the popular diets in circulation today.

VERY LOW-CALORIE DIETS

Very low-calorie diets (VLCDs) generally provide less than 800 calories a day and are typically administered under medical supervision. They may be prescribed as an intervention for obese people for whom nothing else has worked. VLCDs use commercially prepared formulas that replace all of your food for several weeks or months. These diets are usually combined with behavior modification, nutrition education, physical activity or drugs.

Assessing a diet plan

If you're considering a new weight-loss program, evaluate it by the following statements and see how the program holds up. If one or more of these statements apply, it should send up a red flag.

- Promises of a quick fix
- Dire warnings that, unless you use a certain product, terrible things will happen
- Claims that sound too good to be true
- Overly simplistic conclusions drawn from a complex study
- Advice based on a single study
- Dramatic statements that are refuted by reputable scientific organizations
- Advice given to help sell a product
- Opinions based on studies published without peer review
- Recommendations from studies that ignore differences among various individuals or groups

Based on information from the Food and Nutrition Science Alliance

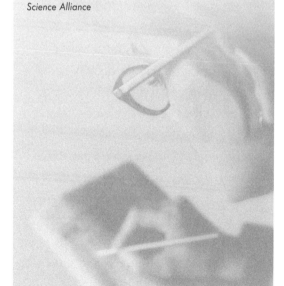

VLCDs can cause substantial weight loss in the first 12 weeks — usually about 3 to 5 pounds a week — and can improve conditions such as diabetes, high blood pressure and abnormal cholesterol levels. However, long-term weight control is difficult after stopping such a diet, particularly if you aren't practicing healthy eating habits or you're not being physical active on a regular basis.

If you're on or considering a VLCD, it's important to receive ongoing monitoring from a health care professional.

LOW-FAT DIETS

Eating foods that are low in fat is a logical strategy for losing weight. A gram of fat contains twice as many calories (nine calories per gram) as a gram of carbohydrate or of protein (four calories each). Current government guidelines recommend keeping dietary fat to no more than 35 percent of your total calories and limiting saturated fat to 10 percent or less.

Cutting down on high-fat foods can help you cut down on your daily calories and thus help you lose weight. So why don't low-fat diets always work? The truth is that even a low-fat diet can lead to weight gain when people ignore the total amount of calories they're eating and regularly exceed their daily calorie goals. Too many calories from any source, low-fat foods included, can add pounds.

It's also not a good idea to cut most or all fatty foods from your diet. This may deprive you of other necessary nutrients found in those foods. In addition, your body needs some dietary fat to help absorb certain essential vitamins, such as vitamins A, D, E and K.

Whatever percentage of your calories are from fat, choose fats that will promote your long-term health. Limit animal-based (saturated) fats and trans fats (hydrogenated oils). Instead, use plant-based (monounsaturated and polyunsaturated) fats. Monounsaturated fats are considered the most desirable. These are found in nuts (almonds, walnuts, hazelnuts, pecans and peanuts), olives, avocados, and olive, canola and nut oils.

Remember to eat a variety of healthy foods. If you're in the habit of eating processed, fat-free snacks, switch to eating whole foods instead. Include more vegetables, fruits, whole grains and plant-based proteins such as beans. These foods are low in calories and fat and provide essential vitamins and minerals not always found in processed foods.

Some people with heart disease go on very low-fat diets — 15 percent or less of total calories from fat. Such diets may help reverse the progression of heart disease, but they're usually undertaken under medical supervision and combined with a healthy eating plan, daily exercise and stress management techniques. If you're considering a very low-fat diet, check with your doctor first. He or she, and perhaps a registered dietitian, can help you weigh the pros and cons based on your personal health needs.

LOW-CARB DIETS

Another popular strategy for losing weight is to limit the amount of carbohydrates you eat. The theory behind this type of diet is that carbohydrates raise blood sugar levels, which cause an increase in your body's insulin production. Insulin drives blood sugar into your cells and prevents the breakdown of fat, thus it's considered a possible mechanism for weight gain.

Proponents of low-carb diets hypothesize that if this is the case, a decrease in carbs will result in lower blood sugar and insulin levels, leading to weight loss. By reducing the amount of carbs you're taking in, your body turns to stored carbohydrates (glycogen) for energy. When these reserves are exhausted, your body turns to the next source of energy, fat tissue, leading to further weight loss.

Some people do lose weight on low-carb diets, but the weight loss probably isn't related to blood sugar levels. More likely, it's related to three factors:

- **Loss of water weight.** When you initially decrease your carbohydrate intake, your body burns glycogen, releasing water and causing weight loss.
- **Decreased appetite.** Burning fat without carbohydrates creates byproducts called ketones that build up in your bloodstream (ketosis). When you're in a state of ketosis, you'll find that you have a decreased appetite.
- **Reduced calories.** Most low-carb diets reduce your overall calorie intake because they limit certain foods that contain carbohydrates, including grains such as bread and pasta, and sometimes vegetables and fruits.

Several different versions of the low-carb diet have become prominent.

Atkins diet

Robert Atkins, M.D., was a pioneering proponent of a high-protein, low-carbohydrate diet back in the 1970s when his *Dr. Atkins' Diet Revolution* hit the bookstores. His ideas went out of vogue with the low-fat craze in the '90s but have since been re-energized in another book, *Dr. Atkins' New Diet Revolution*.

The Atkins diet limits carbohydrates to 20 to 40 grams a day initially. Most grains, beans, fruits, breads, pastas and vegetables are excluded except for salad vegetables and small amounts of other foods. Generous amounts of meat, eggs, cheese, butter and cream are allowed.

A multicenter, controlled clinical trial compared an Atkins-type diet with a low-fat, low-calorie, high-carbohydrate diet over the course of a year in 63 obese men and women. In the first six months, the low-carb diet produced greater weight loss than did the low-fat diet, but at the end of the year, the weight loss in both groups was approximately the same. As with most diets, the dropout rate was high, around 40 percent for each group. The researchers concluded that more studies need to be done to determine the safety and effectiveness of a low-carb diet, particularly over the long run.

Zone diet

The Zone diet, created by Barry Sears, Ph.D., is a high-protein, low-carb diet intended to produce a metabolic state in which your body works at peak efficiency, leading to weight loss, increased energy, improved mental focus and decreased illness. You achieve this by maintaining a strict caloric ratio of 40 percent carbohydrates, 30 percent proteins and 30 percent fats (*Dietary Guidelines* recommend 45 percent to 65 percent carbohydrates, 10 percent to 35 percent proteins and 20 percent to 35 percent fats in your diet).

Like most diets that limit carbohydrates, the Zone diet is based, at least in part, on the idea that carbohydrate intake promotes the production of insulin. Maintaining appropriate levels of insulin and blood sugar, according to Dr. Sears, contributes to the balancing of hormone-like substances in your body called eicosanoids. The best way to enter "the Zone," claims Dr. Sears, is by preserving your eicosanoid balance.

However, there's little evidence that health and disease risk can be influenced by changing the eicosanoid level in your diet. People will lose weight if they follow the prescribed Zone diet because it's low in total calories and it emphasizes vegetables and fruits. A typical Zone diet consists of fewer than 1,000 calories a day.

Protein Power

The Protein Power plan also emphasizes decreased carbohydrate intake on the premise that carbohydrates promote elevated insulin levels. The plan involves three phases. In the first phase, carbohydrate intake is reduced to 30 grams a day until you reach your weight goals. In the next two phases, carbohydrate intake is gradually increased to an amount that allows you to maintain your new weight.

Despite the diet's name, the amount of protein recommended on this plan — 60 to 120 grams a day based on lean body mass and activity — is similar to the amount most people currently consume.

Does too much insulin cause weight gain?

Most low-carbohydrate diets are based on the theory that carbohydrate intake promotes insulin production in your body. Levels of insulin that are too high can lead to insulin resistance, in which your body doesn't respond to or can't use its own insulin. Insulin resistance is a prominent trait of type 2 diabetes.

The problem with the insulin-related weight gain theory is that its reasoning is somewhat backward. Excess total calories from all foods, not just from carbohydrates, leads to obesity, and obesity then leads to increased insulin levels and insulin resistance, not the other way around. Obesity, not excessive carbohydrate intake, is the basic predisposing factor for insulin resistance. This is particularly true of central or upper body obesity.

GYLCEMIC INDEX DIETS

The glycemic index ranks carbohydrate-containing foods based on their effects on blood sugar. For example, eating highly processed foods, such as bread made with refined flour, raises blood sugar higher and faster than does eating whole foods, such as an apple. This earns white bread a high glycemic-index rating and apples a low glycemic-index rating.

Similar to the theory behind low-carb diets, most diet plans involving the glycemic index say that rises in blood sugar lead to overproduction of insulin, leading to weight gain.

In addition, the rapid drop in your blood sugar level that follows eating high-glycemic-index foods can cause you to quickly feel hungry again — sooner than if you had eaten foods high in proteins and fats, nutrients that can increase your feeling of being full. Feeling hungry more often can make you eat more often.

The idea behind diets based on the glycemic index is that eating the right carbs — foods low on the glycemic index — can help you lose weight by lowering insulin production and regulating your appetite.

You may encounter problems with a diet that emphasizes only foods with a low glycemic-index rating. Many other factors influence your blood sugar level, including age and weight. People typically eat a combination of foods, which may affect blood sugar differently than does a single food. Food preparation and portion size also affect blood sugar levels.

Two diets loosely based on the glycemic index are the South Beach diet and Sugar Busters diet.

South Beach diet

Similar to the Protein Power plan, the South Beach diet has three phases. Phase I is very low in carbohydrates and high in protein and fat. This phase attempts to break you of your food cravings, decrease your appetite, and return your blood sugar and cholesterol levels to normal by focusing on low-glycemic-index foods and healthy fats. Phase II allows you to add in more of the right carbs, but total calories stay about the same — between 1,500 and 1,800 a day. You stay in Phase II until you reach your desired weight goals. Phase III is considered the maintenance phase in which you aren't on a diet anymore, but you follow the basic rules of eating the right carbs and the right fats to avoid swings in blood sugar and cholesterol. You can repeat Phase I at any time.

Sugar Busters

For all of the sugar Americans eat, the premise of the book *Sugar Busters! Cut Sugar to Trim Fat* may seem like a diet whose time has come. The authors state that sugar promotes the insulin production that, in large amounts, promotes weight gain. The plan recommends eliminating high glycemic-index foods. But the concept lumps in whole foods such as potatoes, corn and carrots with products filled with refined sugars such as cakes, candies and soft drinks. Author H.

Leighton Steward and his associates don't advocate the heavy fats of the Atkins diet, but the Sugar Busters diet still promotes its fair share of rich foods.

Cutting back on sugar is only one aspect of healthy dietary change. Without making any other nutritional alterations, and particularly when encouraging the intake of saturated fat and decreasing the intake of beneficial vegetables, this diet is unlikely to help you lose weight — or at least keep it off over the long term.

OTHER POPULAR DIETS

Many diet plans sound downright unbelievable. It's hard to believe that anyone would spend much time, for instance, eating only pineapple, corn and salad one day and prunes, strawberries and baked potatoes the next. Still, many similar weight-loss plans cause people to hope that a new food combination or nutritional revelation will help them lose those extra pounds once and for all. But are these diets safe?

As with most diets, you'll probably grow tired of them before they can do any real damage. But the potential for harm arises if you attempt any long-term commitment to these dietary disasters. Will you lose weight? If you're cutting calories, you'll probably drop pounds, but the chances are good you'll gain them back once you go off any unsustainable diet. What follows are a few of the more popular fad diets.

Grapefruit diet

Each of the many versions of this plan — even one erroneously called the Mayo Clinic diet — requires you to eat half a grapefruit before every meal to reap the benefits of the fruit's so-called fat-burning enzymes. Typically, calories are limited to fewer than 800 a day, although some versions require that you eat until you're full.

Grapefruit has no fat, is low in calories and sodium, and is packed with vitamin C. But the very low calories — and deficits in protein, fiber and several important vitamins and minerals — can make this diet dangerous in the long run.

Blood-type diet

The blood-type diet provides a very detailed list of foods that you should eat or avoid, depending on your blood type. Based on the book *Eat Right for Your Type*, by Peter D'Adamo, the premise is that each blood type has its own unique antigen marker that reacts in negative ways with certain foods. According to the book, individuals have varying levels of stomach acidity and digestive enzymes, which seem to correlate with blood type.

Although you may find it comforting to have a list of foods to eat or avoid, no scientific evidence supports the idea that diets should be based on blood type.

Cabbage soup diet

What could be simpler? Eat as much cabbage soup as you want for seven days, and you'll lose 10 to 15 pounds. Other foods, too, are prescribed during the

Visual Guide
to a Healthy Weight

Mayo Clinic Healthy Weight for EveryBody is a lifestyle program based on the fundamentals of the Mayo Clinic Healthy Weight Pyramid. It encourages smart decisions and healthy behaviors that can help you control your weight. The program isn't driven by unrealistic expectations or the latest fad. It's a common-sense approach to better health that focuses on a balanced diet, moderate food portions and daily physical activity. Your commitment to this program can reduce your risk of many diseases and conditions associated with being overweight and provide you with increased energy, added self-confidence and improved odds for living a long and healthy life.

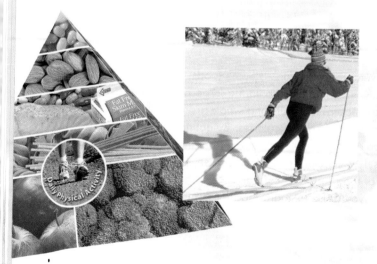
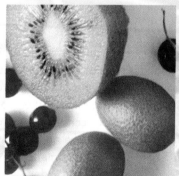
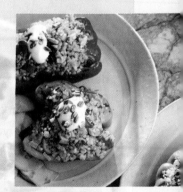

Hearty grain-filled peppers

SERVES: 6 • PREPARATION: 25 minutes • COOKING: 1 hour

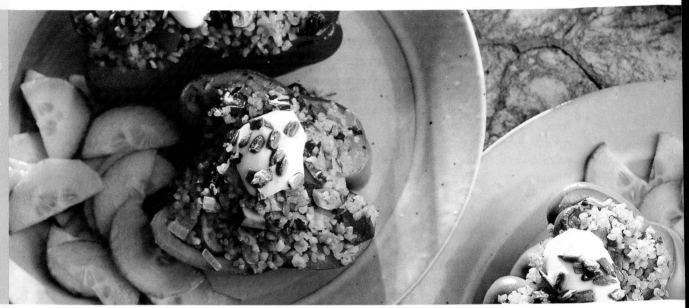

4 c. water

½ tsp. ground cinnamon

½ tsp. ground cumin

2 c. bulgur wheat

8 oz. white mushrooms, coarsely chopped

1½ c. diced fresh tomatoes or 14½ oz.
   canned diced tomatoes, drained

1 onion, finely chopped

2 garlic cloves, minced

½ c. chopped fresh flat-leaf
   (Italian) parsley

⅓ c. raisins

3 red bell peppers, halved, stemmed
   and seeded

3 green bell peppers, halved, stemmed
   and seeded

6 tbsp. plain fat-free yogurt

1 tbsp. sunflower seeds, toasted

1. In large saucepan, bring the water, cinnamon and cumin to a boil. Stir in the bulgur. When the water returns to a boil, reduce heat to low. Cover and simmer until the water is absorbed, about 15 minutes.

2. In large frying pan over medium heat, combine the mushrooms, tomatoes, onion, garlic and parsley. Cover and cook, stirring occasionally, until the vegetables are tender but not mushy, about 10 minutes. Stir the mushroom mixture and raisins into the cooked bulgur.

3. Preheat the oven to 400 F. Coat a shallow baking dish with nonstick cooking spray. Arrange the bell pepper halves in a single layer, cut side up, in the dish. Divide the bulgur mixture among the bell peppers, mounding slightly. Cover with aluminum foil and bake until the peppers are tender and the filling is heated through, about 45 minutes.

4. To serve, top each pepper half with ½ tbsp. of yogurt. Garnish with sunflower seeds.

This recipe is reprinted from *The Mayo Clinic* l *Williams-Sonoma Cookbook*, with permission of Weldon Owen, Inc.

Seared scallops with new potatoes and field greens

SERVES: 4 • PREPARATION: 45 minutes

Dressing

1 c. silken or soft tofu

1 tsp. lemon zest

1 tbsp. fresh lemon juice

1½ tsp. Dijon mustard

½ tsp. anchovy paste

1 clove garlic, minced

¼ tsp. salt

¼ tsp. freshly ground black pepper

2 tbsp. extra-virgin olive oil

Salad

1 lb. Yukon gold or red-skinned
new potatoes

1¼ lbs. sea scallops

¼ tsp. salt

¼ tsp. freshly ground black pepper

1 tbsp. olive oil

8 c. mixed field greens such as baby
lettuces, sorrel and tatsoi

6 tbsp. chopped fresh chives

2 tsp. cracked pepper

1. To make the dressing, in a blender or food processor, combine the tofu, lemon zest and juice, mustard, anchovy paste, garlic, salt and pepper. Process until smooth. With the motor running, slowly add the olive oil in a thin stream until emulsified. Cover and refrigerate until needed.

2. Put the potatoes in a saucepan, add water to cover and bring to a boil over high heat. Reduce the heat to medium and cook, uncovered, until the potatoes are tender, 15 to 20 minutes. Drain and let stand until just cool enough to handle. Cut each potato in half (or quarters, if the potatoes are large). In a bowl, toss the potatoes gently with half of the dressing. Set aside and keep warm.

3. Season the scallops with salt and ground pepper. In a large frying pan, heat the olive oil over medium-high heat. Place the scallops in the hot pan and sear on one side until golden, about 1 minute. Turn and cook on the other side until the scallops begin to turn opaque at the center, 1 to 2 minutes longer. Remove from the heat.

4. To serve, toss the greens with the remaining dressing and divide among individual plates. Scatter the potatoes and scallops over the greens. Sprinkle with chives and cracked pepper and serve.

This recipe is one of 150 recipes collected in *The New Mayo Clinic Cookbook*, published by Mayo Clinic Health Information and Oxmoor House and available in bookstores in the United States and Canada.

Jamaican barbecued pork tenderloin
SERVES: 4 • PREPARATION: 25 minutues • COOKING: 30 minutes

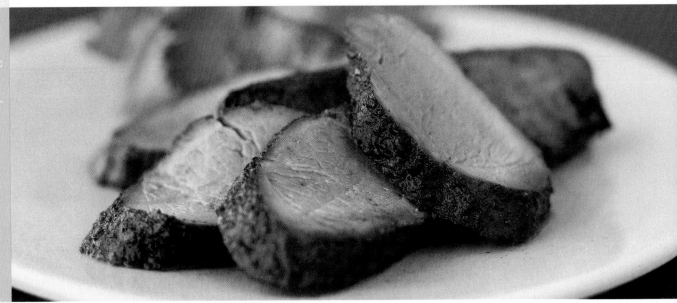

Visual Guide to a Healthy Weight

2 tsp. firmly packed brown sugar

1 tsp. ground allspice

1 tsp. ground cinnamon

½ tsp. ground ginger

½ tsp. onion powder

½ tsp. garlic powder

¼ tsp. cayenne pepper

⅛ tsp. ground cloves

¾ tsp. salt

½ tsp. freshly ground black pepper

1 pork tenderloin, about 1 lb., trimmed of visible fat

2 tsp. white vinegar

1½ tsp. dark honey

1 tsp. tomato paste

1. In a small bowl, combine the brown sugar, allspice, cinnamon, ginger, onion powder, garlic powder, cayenne, cloves, ½ tsp. of the salt, and the black pepper. Rub the spice mixture over the pork and let stand for 15 minutes.

2. In another bowl, combine the vinegar, honey, tomato paste, and remaining ¼ tsp. salt. Whisk to blend. Set aside.

3. Prepare a hot fire in a charcoal grill or preheat a gas grill or broiler to medium-high or 400 F. Away from the heat source, lightly coat the grill rack or broiler pan with cooking spray. Position the cooking rack 4 to 6 inches from the heat source.

4. Place the pork on the grill rack or broiler pan. Grill or broil at medium-high heat, turning several times, until browned on all sides, 3 to 4 minutes total. Move to a cooler part of the grill or reduce the heat and continue cooking for 14 to 16 minutes. Baste with the glaze and continue cooking until the pork is slightly pink inside and an instant-read thermometer inserted into the thickest part reads 160 F, 3 to 4 minutes longer. Transfer to a cutting board and let rest for 5 minutes before slicing.

5. To serve, slice the pork tenderloin crosswise into 16 pieces and arrange on a warmed serving platter, or divide the slices among individual plates.

This recipe is one of 150 recipes collected in *The New Mayo Clinic Cookbook*, published by Mayo Clinic Health Information and Oxmoor House and available in bookstores in the United States and Canada.

Minted Mediterranean fruit mix
SERVES: 6 • PREPARATION: 20 minutes

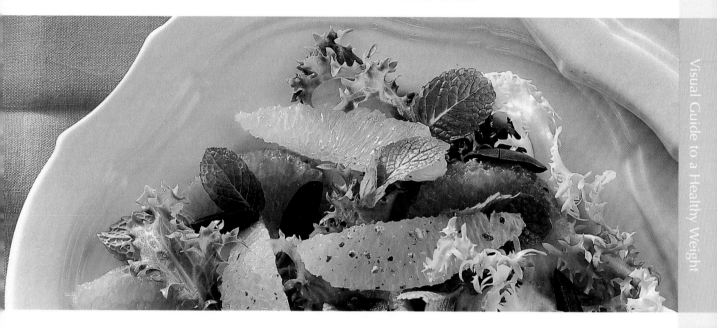

2 large Ruby Red grapefruits
3 large navel oranges
2 c. fresh mint leaves
¼ c. kalamata olives, pitted and sliced
1 tbsp. walnut oil
¼ tsp. ground pepper
6 curly endive leaves

1. Working over a sieve set in a large bowl, peel and segment the grapefruits and oranges. Remove and discard any seeds.

2. Pour off all but 2 tbsp. juice, add the grapefruit and orange segments, mint, olives, oil and pepper. Toss gently to combine.

3. To serve, arrange the endive leaves on individual plates and top with the fruit mixture.

This recipe is reprinted from *The Mayo Clinic | Williams-Sonoma Cookbook*, with permission of Weldon Owen, Inc.

Chocolate pudding pie

SERVES: 8 • PREPARATION: 30 minutes • COOKING: 30 minutes • CHILLING: 2 hours

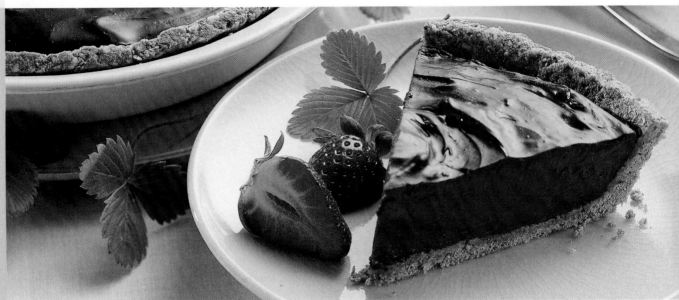

Crust

8 whole graham crackers

⅔ c. 100 percent unprocessed wheat bran

2 tbsp. sugar

¼ tsp. ground cinnamon

2 egg whites

Filling

⅓ c. cornstarch

⅓ c. sugar

⅓ c. unsweetened cocoa powder

3½ c. fat-free milk

2 tsp. vanilla extract

16 strawberries, hulled

1. Preheat the oven to 350 F. Coat a 9-inch pie pan with nonstick cooking spray.

2. To make the crust, in a food processor, process the graham crackers and wheat bran to fine crumbs. Add the sugar, cinnamon and egg whites and process until all the crumbs are dampened. Put the mixture in the prepared pan and firmly pat and press it over the bottom and sides of the pan, taking care not to make the edges too thick.

3. Bake until crust is lightly browned, feels firm and gives to moderate pressure, about 15 minutes. If overbaked, it will be brittle when cold. Cool completely, about 1 hour.

4. To make the filling, into a heavy saucepan, sift together the cornstarch, sugar and cocoa powder. Gradually whisk in the milk. Place over medium heat and cook, whisking constantly, until the mixture thickens and boils, about 7 minutes. Reduce heat to medium-low and boil gently, whisking constantly, 2 minutes longer. Remove from heat and press a piece of plastic wrap directly onto the surface of the mixture to prevent a skin from forming. Cool 30 minutes.

5. Remove the plastic from the filling and stir in the vanilla. Pour the filling into the crust and refrigerate until set, at least 2 hours.

6. Cut into wedges to serve and garnish with strawberries.

This recipe is reprinted from *The Mayo Clinic | Williams-Sonoma Cookbook*, with permission of Weldon Owen, Inc.

weeklong program, including potatoes, fruit juices and some vegetables.

The only problem is that cabbage soup proponents report feeling lightheaded and weak because the diet is too low in protein, vitamins and complex carbohydrates. You may lose weight, but you'll probably be too queasy to enjoy it.

Others

Many other fad diets exist. If you were to try all of them, you'd be busy dieting and doing nothing else. Followers of the raw foods diet, for example, consume only uncooked food. The caveman diet allows you to eat only what Stone Age people ate. And the plan in *The Body Code*, by Jay Cooper and Kathryn Lance, divides dieters into warriors, nurturers, communicators and visionaries.

Gwen Shamblin's *The Weigh Down Diet* advises using spirituality to avoid overeating. Harvey and Marilyn Diamond's *Fit for Life* recommends eating foods in specific combinations at certain times of the day. And Suzanne Somers' books touting "Somersizing" involve specific combinations of foods and the elimination of sugars and alcohol. You get the idea.

MEAL PROVIDERS

Some people have a difficult time knowing exactly what they're supposed to eat in order to lose weight. Busy schedules can leave little time for meal preparation or even keep you from trying new recipes. In such cases, relying on ready-made meals eaten at home may deserve consideration. Remember, however, that some of these services can be expensive. Examples include the following:

Jenny Craig

The Jenny Craig weight-loss business started in 1983 by providing its clients with frozen meals. It has since branched into cookbooks and programs that encourage clients to make food choices from readily available foods, as well as an at-home program for people who don't live close to a Jenny Craig center. Jenny Craig also encourages long-term weight loss through exercise, stress reduction and individual support.

Food is shipped to your home overnight. You can receive personal consultations over the telephone if you need support. Using frozen meals is convenient, and the meals contain the right proportion of fats, carbohydrates, proteins and other necessary nutrients you need.

NutriSystem

NutriSystem also delivers frozen meals to your door for a set price based on a 28-day program. You select what you want for each meal, as well as desserts and snacks. NutriSystem's foods emphasize low-glycemic-index carbohydrates, optimal protein and low fat content. Other NutriSystem products such as salad dressings, gelatins, crackers, rolls, beverages and skim milk alternatives are available as meal supplements.

MEAL REPLACEMENTS

Meal replacements provide fewer than 400 calories a meal and are nutritionally complete. Slim-Fast is an example.

Slim-Fast

Slim-Fast is mainly known for its meal replacement drinks, but the company also offers a selection of meals and snack bars. On the Slim-Fast plan, you replace two meals a day, such as breakfast and lunch, with a Slim-Fast shake, meal bar or other Slim-Fast food. The plan calls for you to eat one sensible meal, between 600 and 700 calories, of your own choosing, and it recommends that you eat healthy snacks between meals. Slim-Fast also encourages you to drink plenty of water and to exercise at least 30 minutes a day. Studies have shown people on the Slim-Fast plan can lose at least as much weight as they would on a calorie-controlled diet.

GROUP APPROACHES

Even when you decide the best way to lose weight comes from eating low-calorie foods in moderate amounts and adding more physical activity, you don't have to go it alone. Commercial group programs can support your efforts, giving you eating plans, exercise recommendations and support from others on the same path.

These dietary approaches inspire camaraderie, and they're different from fad diets in what they recommend. You usually won't find weird food combinations or the tiresome consumption of any one food item, for example. You won't be able to eat all the meat and cheese you want, but you won't grow sick at the sight of cabbage soup either.

Here's a sampling of group approaches that may help you make the kind of lifestyle changes that will ultimately reward you with a healthy weight you can maintain.

Weight Watchers

Since its founding in 1963, Weight Watchers has assisted millions of people in their quest to lose unwanted pounds. Today more than 1 million members gather each week at group meetings around the world.

Weight Watchers believes in a healthy, comprehensive weight management program that includes plans for food, activity and behavior modification. Once you join, you attend a weekly meeting for a private weigh-in, group information or activity session, and supportive conversation with fellow participants.

The program involves a three-step approach encompassing the foods you eat, your activity levels and the use of specific strategies that promote long-term healthy weight. The initial focus is on a 10 percent reduction in your weight. Once you reach that goal, you receive instruction and encouragement for continued weight loss. Eventually you reach your healthy weight, and the focus of the program moves to maintenance.

TOPS Club

TOPS (Taking Off Pounds Sensibly) Club was launched in 1948 and now has members in over 10,000 chapters in the United States and other countries. Mainly a support group, TOPS doesn't tell you what foods to eat or how much to consume, nor does it watch over your exercise levels. It's a nonprofit, noncommercial group that's run solely by volunteers.

Weekly meetings begin with a confidential weigh-in and include a program from a TOPS leader or member, or perhaps a physician, dietitian or psychologist. Participants can share their successes and challenges in sessions afterward.

Before getting started, TOPS urges you to see your doctor for food and exercise plans, as well as an appropriate goal weight. The group does recommend an exchange dietary plan and publishes a healthy lifestyle guide that includes a full description of how to use the plan. Annual membership includes a monthly magazine delivered to your home.

Overeaters Anonymous

Are you a compulsive overeater? According to Overeaters Anonymous (OA), you're in the best position to decide whether your eating is out of control. If food has become unmanageable for you, Overeaters Anonymous can help. This is a program designed for people who regard themselves as recovering compulsive overeaters. The approach is identical to that of Alcoholics Anonymous, with 12 steps and 12 traditions. Its goals are to

help members avoid compulsive overeating and to carry its message to others who may need it.

OA takes no position on issues unrelated to overeating. It's not affiliated with private or public groups, ideologies or doctrines. The group is self-supporting, relying on contributions from members — there are no fees or dues. Donations are not solicited from nonmembers.

NOW'S THE TIME

If you have an eating disorder (see pages 22-23) or if you feel you're depressed, treatment from a licensed mental health professional may be beneficial. Ask your doctor for a referral. Some of these professionals specialize in treating people with weight or eating problems.

No matter what route you take on your journey toward achieving a healthy weight, it's important just to get started. Determine the eating plan that will work for you over the long haul, decide on activities that you enjoy doing and identify a support system that will help you when the going gets tough.

CHAPTER 13

Medications
for weight loss

Current medications for weight loss may sound like a dieter's dream. Some make you feel full before you've eaten much. One blocks your body's ability to absorb some of the fat you eat. But medications for weight loss aren't for everyone who's overweight. In fact, some hospitals reserve them for people with weight-related health problems, such as high blood pressure, high cholesterol or diabetes.

It's best to lose weight through a healthy diet and regular exercise. Some people, though, have physical limitations that keep them from exercising. Others need extra help reducing their calorie intake. If you're among those who struggle to lose weight and the excess weight

has produced medical problems — which can be improved by losing weight — medications may be able to help you.

Typically, the most popular prescription medications — combined with fewer calories and more activity — can help you lose anywhere from 5 percent to 10 percent of your total body weight within a year. However, by the second year, some of the weight tends to come back. In addition, the effectiveness and safety of the most popular prescription drugs haven't been tested beyond two years. So long term, it's the changes in diet and activity that ultimately decrease weight and improve health. Drugs should be looked at as a tool to help make changes in diet, not as the answer to the problem.

WHO'S A CANDIDATE?

Doctors stress that medications for weight loss are most appropriate for obese or overweight people who have health complications related to weight. They're not for casual use. Along with the drugs, a weight-control program that emphasizes behavior treatment, healthy nutrition and physical activity is also recommended.

The main goal in using weight-loss medication is to improve your health, not your appearance. If you're one of the several million overweight Americans with medical complications, modest weight loss can improve your health, including lowering your blood pressure, cholesterol and blood sugar level. There's no compelling evidence to suggest that the use of these drugs by otherwise healthy overweight people will prevent weight-related complications.

If you start a weight-loss medication, you may need to take it indefinitely, or as long as it's effective and the side effects are tolerable. Studies show that when drug treatment is stopped, much or all of the excess weight generally returns. The dilemma is that long-term effects of the most commonly used prescription drugs are unknown.

In general, doctors will consider you a candidate for medication treatment in the following two situations:

- Other methods of weight loss haven't worked for you, your body mass index (BMI) is greater than 27 and you have medical complications of obesity.

- Other methods of weight loss haven't worked for you and your BMI is 30 or higher, regardless of other complications.

Be aware that weight-loss drugs might not work for you. Studies suggest that if you don't lose at least 4 pounds within the first month on a particular drug, it may be ineffective. In that case, your doctor may adjust the dosage, take you off the drug or perhaps try another.

POPULAR PRESCRIPTION DRUGS

Two prescription drugs are approved by the Food and Drug Administration (FDA) for long-term weight loss. These drugs work in different ways and have different side effects. But in general, both appear moderately effective.

The 'I feel full' drug

Sibutramine (Meridia) doesn't seem to decrease your appetite, but it changes your brain chemistry, affecting the chemicals serotonin and norepinephrine, and makes you feel full more quickly.

You generally take Meridia once a day with a full glass of water, with or without food. The recommended dose is 10 milligrams (mg), although your doctor may adjust the dosage if it's too much for you to tolerate, or doesn't work. Common side effects of Meridia include headache, dry mouth, constipation and insomnia.

In several one-year studies, people who followed a reduced-calorie diet and took Meridia generally lost 5 percent to 8 percent of their body weight over a six-month period, about two to three times that observed in those on a reduced-calorie diet and placebo. A large two-year study suggests that Meridia may also help you maintain your weight loss. The best results with Meridia were achieved when the drug was combined with diet and lifestyle education and support.

Meridia isn't without risks. It can cause a small increase in blood pressure that, for some people, may warrant discontinuing the drug. Meridia isn't recommended for people with uncontrolled high blood pressure, heart disease, irregular heartbeat or a history of stroke. If you do take the drug, you should carefully monitor your blood pressure. Avoid Meridia if you're pregnant or breast-feeding, because it's still uncertain whether the drug can harm your child. And you probably shouldn't take Meridia if you take medications such as some antidepressants, that affect serotonin in the brain.

The fat blocker

Rather than work through your central nervous system, orlistat (Xenical) acts only in your digestive tract, and then passes out of your body, unabsorbed. Xenical blocks natural enzymes needed to digest fat in the foods you eat. So just as indigestible fiber passes completely through your digestive system, so does about 30 percent of the fat you eat when you take Xenical. The recommended dose is 120 mg up to three times a day, with meals that contain fat.

Average weight loss is modest — and similar to what you could expect with Meridia. In clinical trials, most people on reduced-calorie diets who took Xenical for a year lost between 5 percent and 10 percent of their initial weight. Studies lasting up to two years, though, show that around a third of the weight lost in the first year is generally regained in the second year. Still, the overall weight loss is often enough to improve your health.

Because your body doesn't absorb the drug, you can avoid potentially serious side effects, especially with a low-fat diet. The side effects may include:

- Oily rectal seepage or spotting
- Passing gas with discharge
- Sudden bowel movements
- Fatty or oily stools

These problems affect about one in five people taking Xenical, but they're generally mild and short-lived. Studies show that by the second year, or even sooner, the symptoms have disappeared.

Because Xenical blocks absorption of some nutrients, your doctor may also recommend that you take a multivitamin. This should be taken two hours before or after taking Xenical.

Medications for short-term use

Several prescription medications are available for the short-term treatment of obesity. Examples include benzphetamine (Didrex), diethylpropion (Tenuate, generics), phendimetrazine (Bontril, generics) and phentermine (Adipex-P, Ionamin, generics). These drugs suppress appetite, but their effects usually decrease quickly. So they're typically used only for a short time while you're learning new ways to eat and exercise.

Side effects may include dry mouth, a false sense of well-being, dizziness and lightheadedness. In addition, use within 14 days of taking a monoamine oxidase (MAO) inhibitor may result in sudden, extreme high blood pressure.

POPULAR NONPRESCRIPTION DRUGS

Over-the-counter (OTC) diet products are a huge success — for the companies that manufacture them. Sales have climbed steadily, creating an over $17 billion-a-year industry. Unfortunately, you can't count on these drugs to lighten anything but your wallet. Worse, some OTC diet drugs can do far more harm than good.

Most of these products promise to help you shed pounds by raising your metabolism or suppressing your appetite. Some may help you lose a small amount of weight temporarily, but the side effects can be dangerous.

The problem with dietary supplements is not only that they may or may not work, but also that they may not be safe. Dietary supplements don't have to meet FDA standards before being put on the market. Thus, the manufacturers are responsible for the products' safety and effectiveness, and most of these products don't go through extensive testing. For the consumer, it's hard to be sure of what you're getting, or even if the list of ingredients matches what's in the bottle.

Here's a look at some of the more popular OTC diet medications and what they can and can't do for you.

5-hydroxy-L-tryptophan (5-HTP)

The plant seed extract 5-hydroxy-L-tryptophan (5-HTP) — sold under brand names such as Natrol, Nature's Way and Nutraceutical Sciences Institute (NSI) — may have a slight effect on body weight but its safety is in question. The extract is a breakdown product of tryptophan, a once popular supplement that was linked to a serious blood and muscle disorder called eosinophilia-myalgia syndrome. Research suggests that the same contaminant linked to the serious problems with tryptophan may also be found in some 5-HTP products. Until more is known, consumers are warned to avoid using 5-HTP.

Caffeine

Because caffeine can suppress appetite, some coffee drinkers assume that they'll eat fewer calories. But the appetite-suppressant effect of caffeine doesn't last long enough to lead to significant weight loss.

Caffeine is also a diuretic, which acts to help your body lose water by increasing the amount of urine. This water loss may decrease body weight, but the weight you lose isn't body fat. In addition, many caffeinated beverages, such as soft drinks, contain sugar, which adds calories and contributes to weight gain.

Chitosan

Chitosan is a dietary supplement made from chitin, a starch found in the skeletons of shellfish. Because chitosan (KI-to-sun) isn't digested, it passes through your intestinal tract unabsorbed. The chemical nature of chitosan suggests that it might bind with fatty foods you eat, removing some of this fat from your body. For this reason, it has been compared to the prescription drug orlistat. But several studies on humans have not shown this to be true. Without reducing calories, chitosan doesn't seem to cause weight loss.

Ephedra

In the late 1990s, some of the most popular OTC weight-loss products contained a natural substance called ephedra, also called ma-huang. Ephedra can also be made synthetically. This synthetic version is usually referred to as ephedrine. It's regulated as a drug and has long been used in asthma medicine.

Although ephedra can slightly suppress your appetite, you'd have to continue taking the product indefinitely to maintain any weight loss.

Studies have found that products containing ephedra are linked to high blood pressure, heart rate irregularities, insomnia, nervousness, tremors, seizures, heart attacks, strokes and death. Because of these concerns, the FDA published a final ruling in early 2004 prohibiting the sale of dietary supplements containing ephedra.

Be cautious of any products similar to ephedra. For example, CortiSlim contains the ingredient synephrine, which is similar to ephedrine. The FDA has warned manufacturers of CortiSlim about unsubstantiated claims regarding weight loss.

Herbal laxatives and diuretics

Herbal laxatives and diuretics include herbs such as aloe, rhubarb, cascara (buckthorn), senna, parsley, juniper, licorice and dandelion. Some of these herbs are incorporated into dieters' teas. These products are often taken with the belief that increased urination or bowel movements will prevent absorption of calories. But their effects take place in your colon and kidneys, after calories have been absorbed by the small intestine. Any weight that you're losing is fluid, not fat.

Chronic use of laxatives can cause diarrhea, nausea and vomiting, which can lead to dehydration. Excessive loss of fluid can lower your blood potassium levels, eventually causing heart and muscle problems. In addition, if you use laxatives too often, your bowels start depending on them in order to function properly.

Hydroxycitric acid

A common ingredient in herbal weight-loss products is hydroxycitric acid (HCA), or garcinia. HCA supplements come in various forms, such as tablets, powder, snack bars and chewing gum. Evidence regarding its efficacy is conflicting. Some studies found that HCA enhances weight loss, other studies observed no effect at all. One of the largest and most rigorous studies found that people taking HCA and eating a low-calorie diet lost no more weight than did people on the same diet and taking a placebo. The long-term safety of taking HCA is still unknown.

Phenylpropanolamine

Phenylpropanolamine (PPA) is a stimulant that was used in cough and cold medicines and nonprescription appetite suppressants. Because it has been linked to an increased risk of bleeding in the brain (hemorrhagic stroke), the FDA has asked drug manufacturers to stop selling products containing PPA. The FDA has also advised consumers to stop using such products. You can often determine whether a product contains PPA by reading the list of ingredients on the label. If you're unsure, ask your pharmacist.

Pyruvate

Pyruvate is a popular weight-loss dietary supplement that may have a slight effect on weight, according to various studies. But large amounts of the supplement — at least 10 grams a day — are required to have an effect, and the actual weight loss is small. Pyruvate, in the form of pyruvic acid, is found in various foods, such as red apples, cheese and red wine. Pyruvate seems safe, but claims of it boosting metabolism, decreasing appetite and weight loss need further study.

St. John's wort

St. John's wort is an herbal medicine said to have an effect on levels of the brain chemical serotonin. Some people believe it may be capable of suppressing your appetite, but no well-designed studies have been able to verify this. In addition, St. John's wort may lessen the effectiveness of some prescription medications, so talk to your doctor before taking the herb if you currently take other drugs.

Green tea

There are potential mechanisms by which green tea may help weight loss. Animal studies have shown an effect, and one human study showed increased energy expenditure. But there have been no clinical trials in humans to suggest that it can actually bring about weight loss.

A word to the wise

Whether you have 5 or 100 pounds to lose, you ultimately have to eat right and exercise to control your weight. OTC diet drugs can't help you with anything beyond short-term, temporary weight loss — if that. Don't believe everything that you read or hear. Often these diet products don't produce the kind of results you expect and may do more harm than good.

You can find out more about dietary supplements at Web sites such as:

- Center for Food Safety and Applied Nutrition
  www.cfsan.fda.gov/~dms/supplmnt.html
- Office of Dietary Supplements
  http://dietary-supplements.info.nih.gov
- MedlinePlus
  http://medlineplus.gov

CHAPTER 14

Surgery for weight loss

Surgery is no easy fix for your weight problem, but sometimes it can accomplish what exercise and diet alone can't. Surgery for weight loss is generally reserved for people who are severely overweight and who have health problems as a result.

The most common weight-loss surgery does three things. First, it blocks off part of your stomach, limiting how much you can comfortably eat. Second, depending on the type of surgery and how it's done, food moves through the digestive system faster, resulting in fewer calories being absorbed. Third, it discourages you from eating high-calorie sweets because of a side effect of the surgery, which is known as dumping syndrome. For example, on an empty stomach, a soft drink can move through your digestive system too quickly, causing nausea, abdominal cramps, diarrhea and other signs and symptoms of dumping syndrome.

Surgery alone won't solve your weight problem. But if you're truly committed to losing weight and the surgery is accompanied by the combination of a healthy diet, exercise and a positive outlook, you have an excellent chance of losing much of your excess weight and keeping it off. The average weight loss after one of the most effective types of surgery — the Roux-en-Y gastric bypass — ranges from 65 percent to 75 percent of excess weight. This means you may weigh approximately 35 percent of your initial weight.

IS SURGERY RIGHT FOR YOU?

Before you can answer this question, you'll want to make sure you've made every effort to exercise and change any eating behaviors that have contributed to weight gain. Surgery is not a replacement for these. In fact, the success of your surgery will depend at least partly on your commitment to following the guidelines given to you about diet and exercise.

For these reasons, candidates for weight-loss surgery meet with several health care professionals. Typically, preparation will include the following: A physician nutritionist will evaluate your need for surgery, explain how the surgery will change the way your body receives and handles nutrients and discuss with you the importance of carefully following nutritional guidelines you'll receive. He or she will also arrange a long-term monitoring program you'll need to follow after surgery.

A dietitian will help you make healthy food selections before and after surgery, and a psychologist will discuss social and psychological problems you may face, as well as help you make lifestyle changes that encourage exercise and healthy eating. A surgeon will evaluate you as a surgical candidate. If he or she thinks that you're a good candidate, the surgery will be scheduled. Insurance preapproval is usually necessary.

Even after your surgery, you'll continue to meet with health care professionals at least every three months for the first year, and then at least annually, to monitor the changes in your life.

Generally, you may be a candidate for surgery if both of the following conditions apply: you have a body mass index above 40, and you have a weight-related health problem.

Body mass index above 40

A body mass index (BMI) above 40 indicates severe obesity. BMI is a ratio of a person's weight and height. A man of average height (5 feet, 9 inches) generally reaches a BMI of 40 when he weighs 270 pounds. For a woman of average height (5 feet, 4 inches), this point is reached at about 230 pounds. To calculate your BMI, see page 18.

Weight-related health problems

Doctors at Mayo Clinic generally won't perform the surgery simply because you have a BMI above 40. You'll typically have a weight-related health problem that will likely improve once you lose weight. Excessive weight can produce many medical problems, including high blood pressure, heart disease, diabetes, degenerative joint disease, obstructive sleep apnea and other conditions.

In some cases, Mayo Clinic doctors will perform surgery if your BMI is as low as 35 if your related health problem warrants it. Some medical centers will perform surgery if you have no weight-related health problem — as long as your BMI is above 40 — because potential health problems might be avoided with surgery.

YOUR DIGESTIVE SYSTEM

Once you understand how your digestive system works, it's easier to see how surgery can help reduce weight. After you chew and swallow your food, muscles in your esophagus propel it into your stomach. Food is held in the stomach about an hour, during which time digestive juices and the churning action of stomach muscles create a mostly liquid mixture.

The stomach contents are then gradually released through a small opening (the pyloric valve) into your small intestine, which is about 18 feet long. Here is where most food nutrients and water are absorbed into your bloodstream.

After food residue passes through your small intestine, it enters your large intestine — your colon — which eliminates undigested and unabsorbed particles and other waste products from your body.

OPTIONS TO CONSIDER

Weight-loss operations fall into one or both of two categories: restrictive surgery and malabsorptive surgery.

Restrictive surgery dramatically inhibits the amount of food your stomach can hold. This type of operation uses a band or staples to create a small pouch at the top of your stomach, where food enters from your esophagus. With some surgeries, the pouch can hold only about an ounce or two of food initially. After the operation, you can eat only small portions of food at a time without feeling nausea or discomfort.

Malabsorptive surgery restricts the amount of calories your body absorbs. It does this by bypassing parts of your small intestine, where nutrients are generally absorbed. Instead, the nutrients, and the calories they contain, are redirected to the colon and eliminated from your body.

The following are descriptions of specific operations.

Gastric bypass

Gastric bypass, also called Roux-en-Y gastric bypass, is the weight-loss surgery most often used in the United States. It combines both types of surgery — restrictive and malabsorptive — by using a small pouch and adding a bypass around parts of your stomach and small intestine.

The surgeon staples your stomach all the way across the top, creating a tiny pouch of the uppermost part of your stomach. The pouch holds about half an ounce. Then the surgeon cuts the small intestine in half and attaches a part of it directly onto the upper pouch. This redirects the food, bypassing most of your stomach and the first section of your small intestine. Food flows directly into the middle section of your small intestine, limiting your ability to absorb calories.

Even though food never enters the lower part of your stomach, the stomach stays healthy and continues to supply digestive juices to your small intestine.

Most surgeons prefer this procedure because it's safe and has fewer complications than do some other surgeries. In addition, research shows that weight loss is encouraging and usually maintained. Most people maintain a loss of at least half their excess weight, even 10 years after surgery. In other words, for the right person, the benefits of the surgery substantially outweigh its risks.

Some of the complications that may occur right after any surgery include bleeding, infection at the incision site and blood clots in your legs (venous thrombosis). Such a blood clot may travel up to your lungs and block an artery, restricting blood flow and causing tissue damage. If the blood clot completely blocks the lung artery, it can be fatal. The chances of this happening, though, are extremely low and occur in about one or two out of 1,000. Moving your legs or walking after surgery can help prevent blood clots from forming. There's also a small chance of a leak at one of the staple lines in the stomach. Antibiotics are typically prescribed to prevent any infection.

Potential long-term complications specific to gastric bypass surgery include dumping syndrome, a hernia at the incision site and a bleeding sore (ulcer) that might develop where your small intestine is attached to the upper part of your stomach. An ulcer occurs in only 1 percent to 2 percent of recipients and can often be healed with medicine, although corrective surgery might be needed. Finally, vomiting can occur if you eat more than the stomach pouch can handle.

A rare but possible complication is a

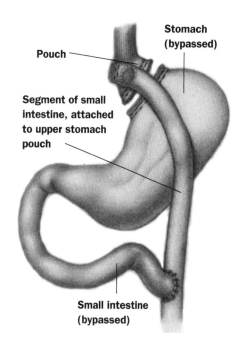

Gastric bypass creates a small pouch at the top of your stomach and a bypass around most of your stomach and part of your small intestine.

narrowing of the opening between your stomach and small intestine. This may require corrective surgery or, more commonly, an outpatient procedure that stretches the opening with a dilating tube.

Other common but less serious side effects include deficiencies of iron, vitamin B-12 and calcium. These occur because of decreased intake and restricted absorption of nutrients within the digestive system. People undergoing gastric bypass should take calcium supplements and multivitamins containing vitamin B-12 for the rest of their lives. Supplemental vitamin B-12 is often prescribed and comes in injection form or as a nasal or oral spray. If you're premenopausal, you may be especially vulnerable to iron deficiency. Taking pills that contain iron can reverse this deficiency.

Some surgeons perform this operation by using a laparoscope — a small, tubular instrument with a camera attached at the tip — through short incisions in the abdomen. The tiny camera allows the surgeon to see inside your abdomen.

Compared with open gastric bypass done through an incision, the laparoscopic technique usually shortens your hospital stay and leads to a faster recovery. In addition, people who undergo laparoscopic surgery seem to have fewer wound-related problems. However, overall complications are similar to the open procedure. Laparoscopic gastric bypass isn't for everyone. Your doctor can advise whether this approach is right for you.

Vertical banded gastroplasty

Vertical banded gastroplasty, or VBG, is a purely restrictive surgery designed to partition the stomach into two parts. There is no bypass. The surgeon, using staples, divides your stomach into upper and lower sections. The upper pouch is small and empties into the lower pouch, which is the rest of your stomach. The small size of the upper pouch is intended to limit the amount of food you eat.

This procedure is called a vertical banded gastroplasty because the staple line separating the pouches is placed vertically (up and down) on the stomach. At the dime-size opening where the upper pouch empties into the rest of your stomach, the surgeon wraps the tissue with a piece of nonexpandable plastic. This plas-

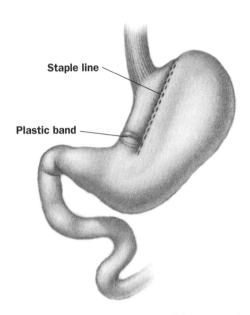

Staple line

Plastic band

A vertical banded gastroplasty divides your stomach into upper and lower sections. The upper pouch holds only 1 ounce of food. An opening into the lower pouch is reinforced by a plastic band.

tic banding helps prevent the opening from stretching. If the opening stretches enough, the two pouches essentially become one again, defeating the restrictive purpose of the surgery.

The average weight loss is less than with gastric bypass, especially long term. One reason for less than expected weight loss is what's termed maladaptive eating behavior. With VBG, the small size of the upper stomach pouch and the narrowness of the opening into the rest of the stomach can limit the amount of "meat and potatoes" you're able to eat. However, ice cream, milkshakes and other high-calorie liquids or soft sweets can slide through the opening with little resistance. Intake of such high-calorie foods prevents adequate weight loss. With VBG, as with other weight-loss operations, surgery

Small bowel bypass

The first operation for obesity was the small bowel bypass, also called a jejunoileal bypass. This type of malabsorptive surgery takes your food on a bypass from your stomach to your colon, skipping almost all of your small intestine. As a result, most of the food you eat never comes in contact with the absorptive area of your intestine, so most nutrients are lost.

People lose a large amount of weight with this surgery, but many also experience severe complications: liver failure, arthritis, kidney stones and severe diarrhea. For this reason, this operation is no longer performed. Many doctors recommend that people who underwent this operation have it reversed if they have active complications. Even if you don't have any complications, lifetime follow-up is crucial to maintaining your health if the surgery isn't reversed.

alone isn't enough. Healthy eating patterns must be maintained for the procedure to be successful.

Because VBG can produce unsatisfactory results, especially compared with gastric bypass, it's used less frequently.

Gastric banding

Gastric banding, also a purely restrictive technique, is popular in Europe, Australia and Latin America. One form of banding — the Lap-Band — was approved in the United States in 2001. With this procedure, the surgeon uses a band instead of staples to partition the stomach into two parts. The band is wrapped around the upper part of your stomach and pulled tight, like a belt, creating a tiny channel between the two pouches. The band is hollow and filled with a saline solution, allowing it to be adjusted by increasing or decreasing the amount of saline solution via an injection port placed just under the skin. The band can stay in place indefinitely. The surgery is almost always done laparoscopically.

Evidence of long-term effectiveness is still lacking for this procedure, but several studies with follow-up of longer than five years have shown promising results. For example, one study found a 57 percent average excess weight loss six years after the surgery. So far most studies have been done outside of the United States.

Side effects include nausea, vomiting, heartburn, abdominal pain, and problems related to the migration, erosion and slippage of the band. The need for another operation — often an outpatient procedure — ranges from 2 percent to 41 percent. Improved surgical technique and experience seem to decrease such complications. One of the advantages of this procedure is the ability to adjust the device as needed. At the same time, this requires follow-up and frequent adjustments.

Gastric pacing

A new, experimental procedure called gastric pacing involves implanting a pacemaker-like device in the abdomen, with electrical leads attached to stomach wall muscle. The device stimulates the stomach with electrical impulses. Although researchers aren't sure why, the impulses make you feel full, resulting in lower food intake and weight loss. Unlike bypass procedures, gastric pacing doesn't alter the normal anatomy of the digestive tract. The implantable gastric stimulation device is still under investigation, but in initial tests the approach appears safe.

Biliopancreatic diversion

Biliopancreatic diversion is mostly a malabsorptive procedure, although it does include some restriction of the stomach pouch. In this procedure, a portion of your stomach is removed. The remaining pouch is connected directly to your small intestine, but completely bypasses your duodenum and jejunum where most nutrient absorption takes place. Biliopancreatic diversion results in greater sustained weight loss than other weight-loss surgeries do, but it also causes increased nutrient deficiencies. Side effects include frequent bowel movements and diarrhea.

A modified version of this technique is called the biliopancreatic diversion with duodenal switch, which keeps a portion of your duodenum within your working digestive tract. This allows you to eat more normal amounts of food and preserves your pyloric sphincter, which regulates the rate at which your stomach is emptied, thus preventing dumping syndrome. It's also thought to cause less nutritional deficiency than does the original biliopancreatic diversion.

Biliopancreatic diversion is more radical than are other weight-loss surgeries. In the United States, it's generally reserved

for people whose weight is life-threatening — more than 450 pounds in men and more than 400 pounds in women.

SIDE EFFECTS OF SURGERY

No matter what surgery you have, in the first months you may experience one or more of the following changes as your body reacts to acute weight loss:

- Feeling tired, as if you have the flu
- Feeling cold
- Dry skin
- Hair loss (temporary)
- Changes in mood

These side effects go away in time.

A hernia or abdominal wall bulge may also develop at the site of your incision. This happens in about 15 percent of people who have weight-loss surgery. The hernia will usually require future surgical repair, depending on the symptoms and the extent of the bulge. The use of laparoscopic techniques substantially decreases the rate of hernia complications.

Another side effect is that the faster you lose weight, the more muscle and lean tissue you lose along with fat. That's why it's important to exercise while losing weight. The exercise helps you maintain your muscles while you lose fat tissue.

MAKING THE ADJUSTMENTS

Many people underestimate the adjustments they'll have to make after surgery.

Cost-benefit analysis of weight-loss surgery

Benefits

- Potential to lose at least half of your excess weight
- Improved blood sugar levels, blood pressure, cardiovascular function, cholesterol levels and sleeping patterns
- Improved mobility and quality of life
- In women, improved sex hormone balance, fertility and menstrual regularity, and decreased stress incontinence

Costs

- Radically changed eating behavior, primarily in terms of the amount of food you're able to eat
- Physical and psychological adjustments to improve your chances of success
- Possibility of side effects such as nausea, diarrhea and dumping syndrome
- Need to eat a balanced diet and take vitamin and mineral supplements in order to avoid nutritional deficiencies
- Women need to avoid becoming pregnant in the first year after surgery
- Possibility that you may need a second surgery to correct complications
- A very small chance of fatality

You'll have a stomach about the size of a small egg. Immediately after surgery, you won't be allowed to eat or drink for two or three days so that your stomach has time to heal. After that, you'll follow a specific dietary progression for about 12 weeks. This begins with liquids only, then proceeds to puréed and soft foods, and finally regular foods. Eventually, you'll be able to eat larger quantities and more varieties of foods. A key component is eating slowly and chewing thoroughly before swallowing. This helps prevent some of the side effects of having a small stomach, such as vomiting and nausea.

Dinner parties and eating out can be especially difficult. Everyone else is eating a regular meal, when all you're able to eat is a few bites. The change in your body image also may require adjustments. Your new appearance can affect your relationships, producing tension, anxiety and depression. This is one of the reasons you'll be asked to see a psychologist before and sometimes after your surgery.

IT TAKES MORE THAN SURGERY

Surgery for weight reduction is not a miracle procedure. Although you can expect to lose weight, especially if you have a gastric bypass, the changes needed in your eating and exercise habits are essential to keeping weight off. But the feeling of accomplishment as you lose weight, as well as the awareness of improved health, are significant benefits.

Action Guide
to Weight-Loss Barriers

Long-term success with a weight program sometimes follows a bumpy, uneven path. Many obstacles arise that can keep you from achieving a more healthy weight.

Learning to identify potential roadblocks and to confront personal temptations is an important part of your journey to better health. To make it past the rough spots along the way, it's important to have strategies ready to guide your response as problems arise and to help you stay on course.

In this easy-to-use action guide, we identify common weight-loss barriers and provide specific strategies for overcoming them. If you find a strategy that helps you, consider including it with the personal action plan that you create for building a healthy lifestyle.

We have grouped the barriers into three categories: nutrition, physical activity and behaviors. To lose weight — and maintain a healthy weight — it's important that you address all three of these key weight-loss components.

Obstacle:

I don't have time to make healthy meals.

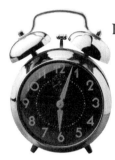 Lack of time is a common problem in our society. For many people, having too little time to cook is a common obstacle to healthy eating. Now is the time to prioritize your health needs. Even when meal preparations are rushed, you can find ways to eat healthier. Healthy meals don't require a lot of cooking time, but they do require that you plan ahead.

Strategies:

Here are tips to help you eat well on a busy schedule.

- Plan a week's worth of meals at a time. Make a detailed grocery list to eliminate last-minute trips to the grocery store.
- Devote time on the weekend to preparing meals for the coming week. Consider making several meals and freezing them in meal-size batches.
- Remember that healthy meals don't have to be complicated. Serve a fresh salad with fat-free dressing, a whole-grain roll and a piece of fruit.

- Keep staple ingredients on hand to make basic, healthy meals. For example, you can quickly mix together rice, beans and spices for a Tex-Mex casserole.
- Have family members help out in the kitchen. Split up the tasks to save time.
- On days when you don't have time to make a healthy meal, stop at a deli or grocery store and purchase a healthy sandwich, soup or prepared entree that's low calorie and low fat.

ACTION GUIDE

NUTRITION

Obstacle:

I don't like to cook.

Not interested in becoming a gourmet chef? No problem. Many people are reluctant to change their diets because they worry that a more healthy eating plan means spending too many hours in the kitchen or struggling with complicated recipes. Healthy eating doesn't require advanced cooking skills, and many healthy meals can be made with minimal time and effort.

Strategies:

If you don't enjoy cooking, here are some suggestions to help you eat well without a lot of culinary effort.

- Purchase a cookbook that offers quick and easy healthy meals, or check one out at your local library.
- Base your meals on fresh fruits and vegetables, none of which take much preparation or cooking time.
- Try out a variety of cooking techniques. You might not like baking, but microwaving or grilling may be your thing.

- Be creative. Use shortcuts such as prepackaged salad greens or raw vegetables, or precooked and ready-to-eat lean meats.
- Eat out or order in. It's OK to eat at a restaurant, order in dinner or buy something ready-to-eat on your way home as long as you choose items that are healthy and you eat moderate portions.

Obstacle:

I don't like vegetables and fruits.

Some people find vegetables and fruits to be bland and boring. A common opinion is that vegetables and fruits don't have much taste, or that they all taste the same. Not true. Vegetables and fruits can be tasty — you just have to know which ones to eat, or how to prepare them. Much of what you eat is conditioned — that is, over time, you've learned to like it. In the same respect, you can learn to like new foods, such as vegetables and fruits.

Strategies:
To learn to like vegetables and fruits, you can experiment.
Here are some suggestions.

- Keep in mind that you don't need to like all vegetables and fruits, just some.

- Instead of the familiar apples and oranges, buy fresh fruits that you haven't tried before, perhaps kiwi, mango, Bing cherries and apricots.

- Try different ways of preparation. For example, grill pineapple or make fruit smoothies.

- If you don't care for raw vegetables, lightly cook them and see if you prefer them with a softer texture. Sprinkle them with herbs for flavor.

- To get more vegetables and fruits into your diet, incorporate them with other foods or recipes: Add vegetables to one of your favorite soups, replace some of the hamburger in casseroles with vegetables, add peppers and onions to your pizza, include fresh fruit with your morning cereal, stir fruit in with yogurt or cottage cheese.

ACTION GUIDE

NUTRITION

Obstacle:

When eating out, I like to eat my favorite foods, not something healthy.

Not a problem, unless you eat out a lot. It's OK to treat yourself to your favorite food on occasion. However, if you dine out frequently, it's important that you make healthy meals a part of your restaurant experience.

Strategies:

Here are tips you might consider so that you can enjoy your favorites and still limit calories.

- Eat only half of your favorite food and save the other half for the next day. That way, you consume only half the calories and you get to enjoy the food more than just once.
- Limit other things you eat before or during your meal, such as appetizers, bread, side dishes or high-calorie beverages.

- Look for ways to make your favorite foods more healthy. For example, if your favorite dish comes with a rich sauce, you might ask for the sauce on the side. That way you can control how much of it you eat.
- If you know that you'll be eating out and eating extra calories, increase your exercise for that day.

Obstacle:

Healthy foods, such as fresh produce and fish, are expensive. I can't afford them.

Although fresh produce and fish can be more expensive, your overall grocery bill may actually be less because you're eating less of other foods, such as chips, cookies and ice cream. These processed foods can also be costly. Plus, you may find that you're eating more meals at home and fewer in restaurants — this, too, can save you money.

Strategies:

Here are suggestions to prevent your healthy eating plan from adding up at the grocery store.

- A recent report indicated that, with planning, the recommended daily servings of fruits and vegetables can be obtained at a very limited price. Check out your grocery store options and watch for specials.

- Buy grains such as oatmeal and brown rice in bulk. Food co-ops are often good for offering foods in bulk.

- Visit farmers markets for summertime deals. You can usually pick up the freshest produce at the lowest prices.

- Consider growing some of your own produce. It's not as hard as you might think. If you don't have room for a garden, you can grow items such as tomatoes and peppers in outdoor pots.

- Eat simple meals at times. A whole-wheat peanut butter sandwich or a bowl of soup and a few pieces of fruit don't cost much.

Obstacle:

My family doesn't like to try new things, and it's too much work to make two different meals.

Family support is important, but don't let your family stop you from trying new foods or exploring different ways of preparing favorite foods. If your family sees you eating differently, your good habits may eventually rub off on them, too. People underestimate their ability to change tastes. For example, when people first try skim or low-fat milk, they often say that it tastes like water. But after they stick with it for a while, most of these same people say that whole milk tastes like cream.

Strategies:

Here are some changes that may help both you
and your family get on the right track.

- Take it slow. Don't try to overhaul your family's diet overnight. Make a few small changes each week. In time, these small changes will add up, and soon you'll all be following a healthier eating plan.
- Keep more fruits and vegetables in the house, and keep fruit in a location where it's visible. When looking for a snack, make it easy to grab a banana, pear or some grapes.

- Try preparing a favorite dish using a different cooking method. For example, instead of frying pork chops or chicken breasts, bake or grill them.
- Involve your family. Ask family members what they'd like to try that's different and healthy. If they can choose, they might be more willing to experiment.

Obstacle:

I can't resist certain foods that I shouldn't eat, such as chocolate and junk food.

To achieve any goal, you have to be flexible. As you prepare your healthy eating plan, ask yourself how you can fit occasional sweets or junk food into the plan without destroying your overall weight goal. Instead of avoiding these foods, give yourself permission to eat them on occasion and in moderation. If you try to resist and completely avoid your favorite foods, you'll feel deprived that you can't have them, which can lead to a loss of willpower and binge eating.

Strategies:

Here are suggestions to help you learn how to incorporate your favorite unhealthy foods into your healthy eating plan.

- Plan ahead for events occurring during the week when you might be around sweets or junk food. In appropriate situations — such as going out to dinner with friends — enjoy some of your favorite foods in moderate portions.

- Know that once you've sampled a favorite food, you may crave more. So it's important to determine in advance how much you'll eat and stick with your plan.

- Eat healthy foods first so that when it comes time to enjoy your favorites, you won't be so hungry.

- Don't keep chocolate or junk food at home. If you get an urge to eat such foods, but you have to go and buy them first, the urge might pass. If you do buy chocolate or junk food, buy only a small amount, such as a single serving.

Obstacle:

I travel a lot, and I often have to eat at airports, hotels or business events.

It can be a bit more difficult to eat healthy when traveling, but it's certainly not impossible. You can eat well when you're away from home. Part of the solution may be your mind-set. Avoid rationalizations such as, "I'm traveling, so I'll have to eat whatever is available."

Strategies:

Eating well on the road often requires a little planning.

- If you travel by car, pack a cooler with healthy foods, such as sandwiches, yogurt, fruit and raw vegetables.
- If you travel by plane, pack snacks such as nuts and fruit in your carry-on bag.
- Ask hotel employees about restaurants that have healthy foods on their menus, or that offer grilled or broiled foods in addition to fried foods. You might also ask if there's a grocery store nearby where you can purchase fruit and easy-to-fix items.

- At business events, use portion control. Allow yourself small servings of some higher calorie foods so that you don't feel deprived, but eat larger servings of lower calorie foods.
- Focus your mind on how eating healthy will give you the energy you need during your trip.

Obstacle:

I'm not hungry in the morning, and I often skip breakfast.

Breakfast is an important meal. Research suggests that people who eat breakfast get more nutrients and manage their weight better than do people who don't eat breakfast. Even if you're not hungry, try to eat a little something in the morning. Just as your body got used to not eating breakfast, it can get used to eating it again. A good breakfast also helps keep you from becoming ravenous later in the day, when you shouldn't eat as much.

Strategies:
To eat a good breakfast, even if you're not hungry, try these tips.

- Start gradually. The first week, plan to have breakfast twice. The next week, aim for breakfast three days a week. Your eventual goal is to eat breakfast every day.
- If time is an issue, put out your breakfast the evening before. Place a box of cereal, a bowl and a spoon on the table. Or have a breakfast shake that comes in a can or that you mix yourself.

- Keep on hand food that you can take with you and eat in the car, on the train or bus, or at work. Convenient foods for this are apples, bananas, whole-grain bagels and low-fat yogurt in single-serving containers.
- If you don't like traditional breakfast foods, fix a sandwich.

ACTION GUIDE

NUTRITION

Obstacle:

Healthy eating involves too much busy work — measuring food, keeping records and figuring out calories.

Nobody said it would be easy! Losing weight does take time and effort. But the time and effort you spend gradually lessens as you become familiar with serving sizes and can gauge in your head the amount of calories you consume each day. Initially, though, it's important to get in the habit of keeping records because many people find that they eat far more calories each day than they thought they did. If you get frustrated by all of the details, try to focus on the big picture — what it is you're trying to accomplish.

Strategies:

Here are suggestions for limiting the time you spend each day keeping records.

- Keep your food record where you have easy access to it. Write your entries after each meal instead of doing them at the end of the day and then trying to remember everything you ate that day.
- Keep a serving-sizes chart on hand that you can refer to for substitutions in recipes and for portion control.

- Don't worry about accurately recording serving sizes for vegetables and fruits. You can eat, within reason, unlimited amounts of these foods. The main reason for keeping records is to make sure that you get enough servings of vegetables and fruits each day.

Obstacle:

I'm not good at menu planning. I never have the right ingredients around the house to make a healthy meal.

It helps if you plan ahead, but you can still wing it and eat well. Remember that healthy eating doesn't have to be complicated or involve hard-to-find ingredients. When you go to the grocery store, stock up on some of the basics. If you have on hand foods and ingredients such as those suggested below, you'll be able to prepare a good meal.

Strategies:

Here are examples of good foods and ingredients to have on hand.

- Plenty of fruits and vegetables, including canned tomato products and vegetable soups and broth.
- Lentils and beans such as black beans, kidney beans and garbanzos.
- Low-fat or fat-free milk, low-fat or fat-free cottage cheese, and reduced-fat cheeses.
- Whole-grain bread, bagels and pita bread, low-fat tortillas, oatmeal, brown and white rice, whole-grain pasta, and whole-grain cereals that aren't pre-sweetened.

- Skinless chicken and turkey, unbreaded fish, extra-lean ground beef, and round or sirloin beef cuts.
- Condiments, seasonings and spreads such as low-fat or fat-free salad dressings, herbs, spices, flavored vinegars and salsa.
- Nonstick cooking spray, olive oil and trans-fat-free margarine.
- A list of kitchen staples for the Healthy Weight Program is on page 187. The weekly shopping lists add fresh produce, meat, dairy and bakery products.

Obstacle:

I was slowly losing weight, but now I'm not anymore, and I haven't changed my diet.

You may have reached what is often referred to as a plateau. You may have lost all of the weight that you will lose based on the amount of calories you're eating each day and the amount of time you're exercising. Sticking to your current eating and exercise plan will help you maintain this weight, but it may not cause you to lose more. At this point, you need to ask yourself if you're satisfied with your current weight — that is, if you can live with it and be happy — or if you want to lose more weight. If you want to lose additional pounds, you'll need to adjust your weight program.

Strategies:
To get beyond a plateau, try these suggestions.

- Reduce your daily calorie intake by 200 calories — provided this doesn't put you below 1,200 calories. Fewer than 1,200 calories may not provide you with enough food, causing you to feel hungry all of the time. Hunger increases the risk of constant nibbling and binge eating.

- Gradually increase the amount of time you exercise by an additional 15 to 30 minutes. You might also increase the intensity of your exercise, if you feel that's possible. Additional exercise will cause you to burn more calories.

- Aside from exercise, increase your physical activity throughout the day. For example, use your car less or plan to do more yardwork and gardening projects.

- If you find these changes difficult or unsuccessful, re-examine your weight-loss goal. Maybe the weight you're striving for is unrealistic for you. Consider the positives of what you've accomplished so far. Chances are you've reduced your risk of diabetes and heart disease and, maybe, you've reduced your blood pressure medication dosage. These are all significant accomplishments.

- Don't throw in the towel. Just because you may have reached a point where further weight loss is more difficult, don't revert back to your old eating and exercise habits. That may cause you to regain the weight that you've lost.

Obstacle:

I don't have time to exercise.

Much as with your diet, time is a common obstacle, but with creativity and planning, you can make time for physical activity. Perhaps you have more time than you realize. For example, the average American watches four hours of television each day. Add to that the time you may spend surfing the Web or watching your child participate in an activity, and there's bound to be some time for exercise. In most cases, time really isn't the issue, rather it's a matter of determining priorities. To become more physically active, it may be that you need to give up another habit.

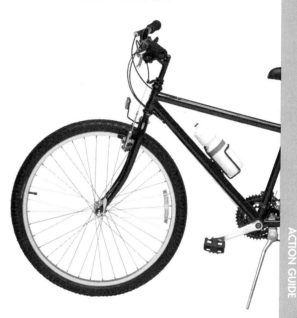

Strategies:

If you can't find 30 minutes to an hour during your day to exercise, look for 10-minute windows. Exercising for 10 minutes three times a day is beneficial, too. Here are strategies you might try.

- Walk for 10 minutes over your lunch hour, or get up a few minutes earlier in the morning and go for a short walk.
- Take the stairs instead of the elevator, at least for a few floors.
- Take regular activity breaks. Get up from your desk to stretch and walk around.
- Use the community pool to swim laps or do water workouts.
- Schedule time with a friend to do physical activities together on a regular basis.

- Develop a routine that you can do at home. While watching your favorite television program or reading, walk on a treadmill, or bike on a stationary bicycle.
- Instead of always looking for the shortcut from one destination to another, look for opportunities to walk and get more physical activity in your day.
- While your child is at soccer practice or taking piano lessons, go for a walk or jog.

Obstacle:

I'm too tired to exercise.

Maybe that's because you're not exercising enough. Many people find they're less tired once they're involved with a regular exercise program. That's because regular physical activity gives you more energy and because fatigue is more often mental than it is physical. If you're fatigued due to stress, exercise is a great stress reliever.

Strategies:
To incorporate more physical activity into your day, try these tips.

- Begin with just five to 10 minutes of activity. Keep in mind that a little activity is better than none. And once you start, chances are you'll keep going for the full 10 minutes — if not longer.
- Exercise in the morning. This will give you more energy throughout the day.

- When you get home from work, don't sit down to watch television or read the newspaper. Instead, put on your walking shoes as soon as you arrive home and go for a walk.
- Keep motivational messages where you need them to remind you of your goal.

Obstacle:

I don't like to exercise.

People who don't like to exercise generally view physical activity as painful or boring. It doesn't have to be either. From among the many forms of physical activity, you're bound to find something enjoyable. You need to experiment. Find something that piques your interest and try it out.

Strategies:

Here are things you can do to help make exercise more enjoyable.

- Try not to focus on exercise only. Think of enjoyable things to do in which you're physically active, such as working in your flower garden or helping a friend with a building project. How you frame physical activity in your mind can make a big difference.

- Exercise with a friend or a group. That way, you can socialize while you exercise, which may make the time go faster and the task seem less boring or painful.

- Mix things up. Don't feel tied to one activity, such as walking. On occasion, try biking or swimming instead. For more ideas on different activities, see page 258.

- Listen to music while you exercise. Upbeat music can rev you up and make your workout seem easier. It can also make the time pass more quickly.

- Take advantage of introductory classes or exercise videos to learn basic skills and techniques.

- Focus on the benefits of activity instead of the activity itself. Think of your workout time as personal time for you. Reflect on your goals and remind yourself how good it'll feel to achieve them.

Obstacle:

I'm too old to exercise.
I might hurt myself.

You're never too old or out of shape to be physically active, and it's never too late to start. Moderate physical activity can help you achieve or maintain a healthy weight. Moderate physical activity can also help delay age-associated illnesses and conditions such as heart disease, high blood pressure, diabetes and bone loss.

Strategies:

If you haven't been physically active, it's important to see your doctor before you begin exercising, especially if you have some health concerns. Once your doctor gives you the OK, here are suggestions for getting started.

- Start slowly and give your body a chance to get used to increased activity, and then gradually increase your activity level.
- Walking is a good starter exercise. Or try a stationary bike with no resistance. Water exercise is another good option.
- Stretch. Staying flexible is key to improving or maintaining range of motion in your joints and muscles. It's best to do stretching exercises after a brief warmup period of light activity.

- Do things you enjoy. Activities such as dancing and gardening also can provide effective workouts.
- Consider light-resistance exercises, such as use of elastic bands. Studies have shown that even people in their 80s can double their strength.
- Muscle soreness after exercise is common, especially if it's a new activity. Pain during exercise may send a different signal. For more on exercise red flags, see page 62.

Obstacle:

I start out fired up, but I have trouble staying motivated.

The most common mistake people make is starting an activity program at too high an intensity and progressing too quickly. If your body isn't accustomed to exercise, your muscles and joints may become sore and stiff, which can be frustrating. Boredom is another major reason why people quit exercising, often because they repeat the same activity day after day.

Strategies:

Even if you've tried in the past to make exercise a regular part of your day and it hasn't worked, you can try again. The following tips can help you stay motivated for the long haul.

- Do activities you enjoy. Instead of the more traditional forms of exercise, maybe you'd prefer enrolling in a dance class or participating in water aerobics.
- Choose activities that fit your lifestyle. If you prefer solitude, consider activities such as walking or jogging. If group activities appeal to you, you might join an aerobics class or a golf league.
- Focus on small steps. Set realistic, attainable goals that you can achieve and feel good about. For example, a short-term goal might be to take the stairs at work instead of the elevator three days a week or to walk to the neighborhood store or post office instead of drive.

- Think long term. In addition to short-term goals, set your sights on a goal such as a 5-kilometer run. Map out your weekly goals to help you be successful.
- Reward yourself. When you meet your goals, give yourself a small reward. Feeling good about your accomplishments — even if they seem small — can help keep you motivated. Once you've achieved your goal, set a new, more challenging one.
- Seek social support. Exercising with a friend or a family member can help keep you motivated. You might also join an exercise group.

Obstacle:

I don't like to exercise when it's cold, rainy or hot.

Choose activities that you can do regardless of the weather, and be flexible with your exercise routine. On days when the weather isn't conducive to your normal outdoor activity, have plans ready for an alternate activity. You might also want to vary your exercise routine according to the seasons.

Strategies:

Here are some suggestions you might consider.

- Have options for moving your routine indoors. If you bicycle, cycle inside on a stationary bicycle. If you like to walk, walk indoors at a nearby mall or school.
- Be willing to try something different. Instead of jogging, do indoor aerobics or strength exercises.
- Swimming in the summer keeps you cool and provides a great aerobic workout.

- In colder climates, take advantage of wintertime activities such as ice-skating, snowshoeing or cross-country skiing.
- Check out the local health club as an option for exercise. Some don't require that you have a membership but rather allow you to pay per visit.

Obstacle:

I worry that other people will think I look funny when I exercise.

Try to put aside such thoughts. Most active people will give you credit for exercising and not make fun of you. Ask yourself which is more important: avoiding possible embarrassment or losing weight. Once you get started, you may find exercise isn't as embarrassing as you thought it would be.

Strategies:

If you're concerned about exercising in front of others, consider these suggestions.

- Most of your embarrassment will disappear as exercise becomes more routine and you become more confident.
- Exercise early in the morning or late in the evening, when fewer people are around.
- Buy an exercise video or an exercise machine, such as a stationary bicycle or a treadmill, so that you can work out in the privacy of your own home.

- Sign up for an exercise class that includes other people trying to lose weight.
- Ask an exercise professional to demonstrate proper technique and provide information on appropriate exercises so that you can feel confident in your abilities.

Obstacle:

I travel a lot, so exercise is inconvenient.

Travel, whether for business or pleasure, doesn't have to interrupt your exercise routine. It's easier than you may think to incorporate physical activity into your trips away from home. And doing so can increase your energy level and help you better handle the stress of travel.

Strategies:

Healthy habits travel easily. Here are strategies for staying fit on the road.

- Call your hotel and ask about fitness facilities on-site or nearby. Knowing what's available will help you pack the right workout clothes.
- Remember that walking can be done almost anywhere. Walk around the airport terminal while you're waiting to board your flight. If you're driving, take an occasional break and get out and walk around a rest area.

- Do exercises in your hotel room. Pack an exercise band or jump-rope or do exercises that don't require equipment, such as sit-ups or squats.
- If you're able to, rent a bicycle and do sightseeing. Or, just get out and explore the neighborhood.

Obstacle:

I can't exercise because of painful arthritis in my knees.

For many people with pain problems, exercise can be beneficial. Physical activity can help you manage the symptoms of many chronic conditions. In the case of arthritis, proper exercise can help you better maintain joint mobility.

Strategies:

The key is to know which exercises are helpful to your condition and which are harmful. If you have arthritis:

- Try water exercises. The buoyancy of water takes the weight off your joints. You can swim laps on your own or you might try a water aerobics class.
- Use a stationary or recumbent bicycle. This takes pressure off your knees.
- Consider joining a basic yoga or tai chi class to increase strength and flexibility in your joints.

- See a physical therapist who can offer recommendations on the best type of exercises for you and teach you how to do them properly to avoid injury and further pain.

ACTION GUIDE

PHYSICAL ACTIVITY

Obstacle:

Exercise makes me hungry.

Studies show that people may eat a little more when they start to exercise regularly. However, they're usually burning more calories with the exercise than they're taking in with the increased eating. Most people who exercise find that about an hour or so after they're done exercising, they're hungry. There's certainly nothing wrong with eating afterward, but you don't want to negate all of the benefits of physical activity by mindlessly eating high-calorie snacks.

Strategies:
Here are some suggestions for maintaining the benefits of exercise, while still satisfying your hunger.

- Before you exercise, eat foods that stick with you longer, such as whole-grain bread, cereal, pasta and brown rice.
- Prepare a small healthy snack for after your workout, such as fruit, yogurt or whole-grain crackers.

- Drink plenty of water before, during and after your workout.

Obstacle:

I have trouble controlling how much I eat.

For many people, one of the main goals of achieving and maintaining a healthy weight is learning how to eat less. Part of the problem is that they don't have a realistic idea of what constitutes a serving. In an era of jumbo meals, supersizing and free refills, overgenerous portions of food and beverages have become the norm. In addition, eating habits that you learned from a young age — that it's OK to have seconds, that you should clean your plate, that dessert always follows a meal — can be difficult to break. But difficult doesn't mean impossible.

Strategies:

You can train your body to feel full with less, just as it became accustomed to needing more. Try these suggestions.

- Serve meals already dished onto plates instead of placing serving bowls on the table. This allows you to think twice before having a second portion.
- Try using a smaller plate or bowl to make less food seem like more.
- Eat slowly and savor each bite. When you eat too fast, your brain doesn't get the signal that you're full until too late and you've already overeaten.
- Eat foods that are healthy and low in calories first. You can eat a lot of these foods without taking in a lot of calories.
- When eating, focus on your meal and your company. Watching television, reading or working while you eat can distract you. Before you know it, you've eaten much more than you wanted to.

- Stop eating as soon as you begin to feel full. Don't feel as if you need to clean your plate.
- Designate one area of the house to eat meals, such as the kitchen table, and sit down to eat your meals.
- If you're still hungry after you've finished what's on your plate, nibble on something low in calories, such as fresh vegetables, fruit or crackers.
- When ordering at a restaurant, request a take-home container. When you receive your meal, put part of it in the container. Or ask that one-half of your meal be put into a container before the meal is served. Portion sizes in restaurants can be two to three times the amount you need.

Obstacle:

I've tried to lose weight before, but it didn't work. So, I don't have a lot of confidence that it'll work this time.

For many people, losing weight is one of life's most difficult challenges. Don't be discouraged if you've tried to lose weight in the past and you weren't able to — or you lost weight but you gained it all back. Many people experiment with several different weight-loss plans before they find an approach that works.

Strategies:
Following these tips may help you succeed this time around.

- Think of losing weight as a positive experience, not a negative one. Approaching weight loss with a positive attitude will help you succeed.
- Set realistic expectations for yourself. Focus on behavioral changes and don't overly focus on your weight.
- Make small, not drastic, changes to your lifestyle. Adjustments that are too intense or vigorous can make you uncomfortable and cause you to give up.

- Accept the fact that you'll have setbacks. Believe in yourself. Instead of giving up entirely, simply start fresh the next day.
- Use problem-solving techniques. Write down the obstacles that you experienced in previous attempts to lose weight, and come up with strategies for dealing with those obstacles.

Obstacle:

I eat when I'm stressed, depressed or bored.

Sometimes the strongest longings for food happen right when you're at your weakest point emotionally. Many people turn to food for comfort — be it consciously or unconsciously — when they're dealing with a difficult problem or looking for something to keep themselves occupied.

Strategies:

To help keep food out of your mood, try these suggestions.

- Try to distract yourself from eating by calling a friend, running an errand or going for a walk. When your mind is occupied with something else, the cravings quickly go away.
- Don't keep comfort foods in the house. If you tend to eat high-fat, high-calorie foods when you're upset or depressed, don't keep them around.

- Identify your mood. Often the urge to eat can be attributed to a specific mood and not to physical hunger.
- When you feel down, make an attempt to replace negative thoughts with positive ones. For example, write down all of the positive qualities about yourself and what you want to achieve with weight loss.

Obstacle:

I have a hard time not eating something when I'm watching television or when I'm at the movies or a sporting event.

There's nothing inherently wrong with doing this, but when you're distracted by a TV show, movie or event, you tend to eat thoughtlessly — which typically translates into eating more than you intend. If you can't break this habit, at least make sure you're munching on something low in calories and try to limit how much you eat.

Strategies:
Here are suggestions you might consider.

- If you're at a movie theater or sporting event, order a small bag of popcorn with no butter and work on it slowly.
- Eat something healthy before you leave home so that you're not real hungry when you arrive.
- Drink water or a calorie-free beverage instead of having a snack.

- Try to reduce the amount of time that you spend watching television each day. Studies show that TV watching contributes to increased weight.
- Find something else to do with your hands when you're watching television. Fold clothes or work on a hobby.

Obstacle:

When I go to parties, I can't resist all of the hors d'oeuvres.

In most social situations where food is around, the key is to treat yourself to a few of your favorite hors d'oeuvres, in moderation. If you try to resist the food, your craving will only get stronger and harder to control. By following a few simple strategies, you can enjoy yourself without overeating.

Strategies:

Next time you step up to the hors d'oeuvre table, try these strategies.

- Make only one trip and be selective. Decide ahead of time how much you'll eat and choose only foods that you really want.
- Treat yourself to one or two samples of high-calorie or fatty foods. Fill up on vegetables and fruits, if you can.
- Take only small portions. A taste may be all that you need to satisfy your craving.

- Nibble. If you eat slowly, you'll likely eat less — but don't nibble all night long.
- Don't stand next to or sit near the hors d'oeuvre table. As the old saying goes, "Out of sight, out of mind."
- Eat something healthy before you arrive. If you arrive hungry, you'll be more inclined to overeat.

ACTION GUIDE

BEHAVIORS

Obstacle:

While I'm cooking, I have a hard time not sampling what I'm making.

Many people who enjoy cooking find that they consume a lot of calories each day by sampling what they're preparing — especially if they're making something that's high in fat or high in calories. Most people are surprised by how quickly a few bites here and there add up. The best way to reduce these unwanted extra calories is to stay out of the kitchen except for mealtime, but that's not always possible.

Strategies:

When you're preparing meals or preparing food for other people or events, try these suggestions to keep yourself from sampling the goods.

- Chew gum or suck on a mint or a calorie-free piece of candy while you're baking or cooking.
- Have fruits or vegetables on hand that you can munch on while you're cooking.
- If you're preparing a food in which you need to taste-test the batter to make sure you have the ingredients right, have someone else do the taste-testing for you.

- Avoid the temptation. If you need to bring an item such as cookies or a dessert to a social function, consider buying the food at a bakery or grocery store.

Obstacle:

I'm a late-night snacker.

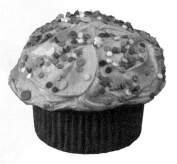

You want to avoid eating late at night because loading up on calories right before bed only intensifies overeating challenges. It's better to eat during the day or early in the evening so that your body has plenty of time to digest the food before you go to bed.

Strategies:

Here are suggestions if you often find yourself
battling the late-night munchies.

- Make sure you eat three good meals during the day, including a good breakfast. This will help prevent you from snacking late at night, simply because you won't be so hungry.

- Don't have snack foods around the house to tempt you. If you get the late-night munchies, eat fruits, vegetables or other healthy snacks.

- Find something else to keep you busy in the hours before bedtime. Your snacking may be more of a habit than actual hunger.

Obstacle:

When I sabotage my eating plan, it's hard for me to get back on track.

Lapses happen. Many times a minor slip — a bad day when you just couldn't keep to your eating plan or get exercise — leads to more slips. That doesn't mean, though, that you're a failure and all is lost. Instead of beating yourself up over your lapse, accept that you're going to have bumps along the way and put it behind you. Everyone makes mistakes. Think back to the steps you took when you first began your weight program and put them to use again to help you get back on track.

Strategies:

Here are suggestions to prevent a lapse from turning into a full-blown collapse.

- Tell yourself that mistakes happen and remind yourself that every day is a new opportunity to start again.
- Guilt from the initial lapse often leads to more lapses. Being prepared for mistakes and having a plan to deal with them is important to your success.

- Keep your response simple. Focus on things that you know you can do and stick with them. Gradually add more healthy changes until you're back on track.
- Open up an old food record and follow it. Those meals can be used like a menu to help you get back to your eating routine.

Obstacle:

Some of my friends aren't supportive. They seem uncomfortable when I exercise or try to eat healthy.

This isn't uncommon. Sometimes friends, and even spouses, can undermine your efforts. Some people are intimidated by the efforts of others to lose weight or improve their health. Others simply may not know how to be supportive. But it's up to you to stick to your program. It may be as simple as saying no thanks to an offer of pie and ice cream, or it can be more complicated. If they're good friends, open communication may work. Tell them how you feel and ask for their support.

Strategies:

If you're not getting support from your friends, try these suggestions.

- Let your friends know how important their support is to you.
- Be specific as to how your friends can help you, such as by going on a walk with you or just listening to you.
- Don't let unsupportive friends distract you from your goals. Join a group, such as an aerobics class or golf league, in which you're around others who have the same goals as you do and who are willing to provide support.

Obstacle:

I get frustrated when I lose just a pound or two after I've tried really hard all week.

Many people long for a secret potion or magic pill that will take off excess weight instantly. Unfortunately, such a remedy doesn't exist. Losing 1 or 2 pounds a week is a more realistic weight-loss goal. That pace can be frustrating if your expectations are too high. But slow and steady is the healthiest way to go, and the weight is much more likely to stay off.

Strategies:
Follow these tips to keep yourself on track.

- Don't focus all of your attention on the bathroom scale. Instead, concentrate on eating better, exercising more and improving your health.
- Don't consider yourself to be "on a diet." Instead, try to adopt a more positive outlook with the goal of a healthier lifestyle.
- Make a list of all the benefits of losing weight, such as having more energy, improving your health and feeling better about yourself. Refer to this list if your motivation wanes.

- Don't use life's ups and downs as an excuse to quit. If stressful events occur, cut yourself some slack if you need to, but stay with the program.
- Remind yourself that 1 to 2 pounds a week equates to 50 to 100 pounds a year!

Obstacle:

I don't like my body image.

How you feel about your body can be central to how you feel about yourself. Many people despair between the way they look and the way they feel they should look, and then hurt themselves emotionally as a result. Having a positive view of your body — no matter how imperfect it may be — is important. To feel good about the accomplishments you're making in losing weight and improving your health, you have to feel good about your body.

Strategies:

Here are suggestions to help you view your body in a more positive light.

- Think of your body as a gift. It allows you to live, move and accomplish many things. If you focus on the good things about your body, it becomes less of an adversary.

- Don't equate body image with self-esteem. The assumption that how you look is who you are can be very damaging. Your appearance is only one aspect of your life. You can be a success at many things in life, regardless of your appearance — or how you think you appear. Focus on those things that you're good at.

- Don't avoid looking at your body. Many people who don't like their bodies avoid mirrors and windows so that they won't have to look at themselves. Instead of avoiding your body, try to find a way to think of your body as a friend.

- Write a list of positive things about yourself and add to it often. In addition, post self-affirming messages ("I'm beautiful!") on your bathroom mirror, in your car or at your desk at work.

- Spend time with people who are positive and supportive.

- Remember that appearance is independent of health. Some people are slender but they have increased health risks. Conversely, others may not have a picture-perfect appearance, but their attitudes and spirits may be wonderful. Beauty comes from within. When you feel good about yourself, it will shine through.

The Mayo Clinic
Healthy Weight Program

WELCOME TO THE PROGRAM

The Mayo Clinic Healthy Weight Program is a practical guide to weight control. The program requires your full commitment and a willingness to make important lifestyle changes. But it's also a program that you can enjoy. The food you eat is intended to be appealing and tasty. The physical activities recommended should be enjoyable and challenging. And the lifestyle changes you're encouraged to make should leave you feeling more energetic and in control.

The focus of the Healthy Weight Program is on your health, not on the number of pounds you wish to lose. But by following the program, you will lose weight — slowly and safely. The program is structured to help you lose about 1 or 2 pounds a week over a 12-week period. If you wish to lose more weight, you simply can continue the program beyond the initial 12 weeks outlined here. The program also provides information on how to maintain the weight loss once you've reached your weight goal.

This weight-loss program isn't a quick fix that you follow for a short period of time and then return back to your old habits. Its focus is on making permanent behavior changes. Throughout 12 weeks, you'll be asked to assess your eating and exercise habits and to develop strategies for changing unhealthy behaviors. You'll be encouraged to set achievable goals each week. It's an eating and exercise program intended to last you a lifetime.

Getting ready to start

To start the Mayo Clinic Healthy Weight Program, you'll need to work through the steps described in this introduction. Think of these steps as comparable to preflight checks that airline pilots undertake before take-offs to ensure all systems are ready. Your "preflight check" requires you to:

1.) Assess your readiness to start a weight-loss program
2.) Establish your weight goal
3.) Identify your daily calorie goal
4.) Determine your daily food servings
5.) Assess your fitness level

Seems like a lot of work just to get started? Actually, each step only takes a few minutes of your time.

There are other preflight tasks to take care of. These involve making sure that you have all of the resources you'll need for the program, such as stocking your kitchen to make meal preparation more efficient, and having appropriate shoes and clothing for exercise. These you can do as soon as you're able.

What's left for you to get started? Only to pick a start date. Once you start the Healthy Weight Program, you'll work through weekly units that explain vital topics such as serving sizes and exercise programs in more detail. But you don't have to wait until you get to those units to start eating better and exercising more. Begin making improvements now and along the way you'll learn more specific strategies to help you succeed.

ARE YOU READY TO LOSE WEIGHT?

You need to decide whether now is the right time to start a weight program. It's OK if it's not. Starting before you're ready can set you up for failure. But don't put off your start date any longer than necessary. The following questions may help you make this decision.

1. How motivated are you to lose weight?
   a. Extremely motivated
   b. Quite motivated
   c. Somewhat motivated
   d. Slightly motivated or not at all

2. Considering the amount of stress affecting your life right now, to what extent can you focus on weight loss and on making lifestyle changes?
   a. Can focus easily
   b. Can focus well
   c. Uncertain
   d. Can focus somewhat or not at all

3. Weight loss is recommended at a rate of 1 to 2 pounds a week. How realistic do you think your expectations are about how much weight you would like to lose and how quickly you want to lose it?
   a. Very realistic
   b. Moderately realistic
   c. Somewhat realistic
   d. Somewhat or very unrealistic

4. Aside from holiday feasts, have you ever eaten a large amount of food rap-idly and felt afterward that this eating was out of control?
   a. No
   b. Yes

5. If you answered *yes* to question 4, how often have you eaten like this during the last year?
   a. About once a month or less
   b. A few times a month
   c. About once a week
   d. About three times a week or more

6. Do you eat for emotional reasons, for example, when you feel anxious, depressed, angry or lonely? Do you celebrate good feelings by overeating?
   a. Never or rarely
   b. Occasionally
   c. Frequently
   d. Always

7. How confident are you that you can make and sustain changes in your eating habits?
   a. Completely confident
   b. Highly confident
   c. Somewhat confident
   d. Slightly confident or not at all

8. How confident are you that you can exercise regularly?
   a. Completely confident
   b. Highly confident
   c. Somewhat confident
   d. Slightly confident or not at all

Evaluating your readiness to lose weight

- If your responses to most of the questions on the previous page are **a** and **b**, it appears you're ready to start.
- If your responses to most of these questions are **b** and **c**, consider if you're ready to start a weight-loss program or if you should wait for a better time.

- If your responses to most of these questions is **d**, you may want to hold off on your start date. Reassess your readiness again in a short while.
- If your answer to question 5 was **b**, **c** or **d**, you may want to discuss this with your doctor.

ESTABLISH YOUR WEIGHT-LOSS GOAL

How much weight would you like to lose? Perhaps you want to lose 10 to 20 pounds. Or maybe your goal is more ambitious — you'd like to lose 50 or even 100 pounds.

Now ask yourself, is your goal realistic? If you think your goal may be unrealistic, decide on a number that you feel confident that you can achieve. Maybe instead of 100 pounds, your goal might become 30 or 40 pounds.

For many overweight people, a reasonable goal is to lose about 10 percent of their starting body weight. That amount is generally achievable. And many people experience noticeable improvements in their health when they lose 10 percent of their body weight.

To calculate what 10 percent is, take your current body weight and divide your weight by 10. How does the number you get compare with the number of pounds you'd like to lose?

Remember that weight control is an ongoing process. Once you reach your weight goal, you can set another goal until you achieve the weight you want to be at. What you don't want are expectations that are too high and that set you up for disappointment.

Once you've determined your weight-loss goal, write it down in the space provided here.

WEIGHT-LOSS GOAL:
··

IDENTIFY YOUR DAILY CALORIE GOAL

To meet your energy needs and reach your weight-loss goal, how many calories should you eat each day? If you eat 500 calories less each day than the number of

calories you burn, you should lose about 1 pound a week. Five hundred fewer calories a day for seven days is 3,500 fewer total calories, which equals 1 pound of body fat. But if you don't know how many calories you consume each day, this may be difficult to determine.

Here's a simpler approach. If you weigh less than 250 pounds and you want to lose weight, a daily goal of 1,200 calories generally works best for women, and 1,400 calories works best for men. These levels can be adjusted, based on your individual health risks and on how quickly you want to lose weight. If you feel exceptionally hungry, or you lose

weight too quickly, you may consider jumping to the next higher calorie level indicated on the table below.

Fewer than 1,200 daily calories for women and 1,400 daily calories for men generally isn't recommended for weight loss. Although it's tempting to starve yourself to lose weight quickly, you may not be getting enough of the nutrients you need for good health. If you weigh more than 250 pounds, you'll need slightly higher calorie goals (see the table).

Your daily calorie level for healthy weight loss

	Weight in pounds	Starting calorie level			
		1,200	1,400	1,600	1,800
Women	250 or fewer	X			
	251 to 300		X		
	301 or more			X	
Men	250 or fewer		X		
	251 to 300			X	
	301 or more				X

DETERMINE YOUR DAILY FOOD SERVINGS

Now that you know your daily calorie goal, the next step is to determine how much you should eat each day.

To lose weight — while still getting the nutrients your body needs — you want consume a specific number of servings from each of the food groups. This ensures that you're eating healthy.

The chart at the top of the following page indicates how many servings you should eat from each of the food groups. To learn more about what foods are included within each of the groups, review pages A7-A11 of the Visual Guide. Using these lists, you can make sure that you meet your daily food servings until

Daily serving recommendations for calorie levels

Food group	Daily calorie goals				
	1,200	1,400	1,600	1,800	2,000
Vegetables	4 or more	4 or more	5 or more	5 or more	5 or more
Fruits	3 or more	4 or more	5 or more	5 or more	5 or more
Carbohydrates	4	5	6	7	8
Protein/Dairy	3	4	5	6	7
Fats	3	3	3	4	5

HOW FIT ARE YOU?

In general, the Healthy Weight Program encourages you to do 30 to 60 minutes of moderately intense physical activity daily to maintain your health and your weight.

However, you don't want to undertake activity that's too strenuous or tiring, especially if it's been awhile since you've been physically active. Your responses to the five questions below can help determine your current level of fitness.

Evaluating your fitness level

- If most of the boxes you checked were *rarely* or *sometimes,* consult your doctor for recommended activities.
- If most of the boxes you checked were *sometimes* and *usually,* you want to gradually increase your activity level.
- If most of the boxes you checked were *usually* and *always,* focus on maintaining your current fitness level.

	Rarely	Sometimes	Usually	Always
I am physically active for at least 30 minutes each day.				
I can easily carry on a conversation while doing light physical exertion.				
I go for short walks on a regular basis.				
I can do housework on my own without difficulty.				
I have little trouble reaching for objects above or picking up objects on the floor.				

INTRODUCTION

GETTING PREPARED TO START

Two factors that frequently work against a healthy diet are lack of time and lack of ingredients. These factors often work in tandem. How often has this scenario occurred: You return home bone-tired at the end of a long day. You're scrambling to get a meal ready and you haven't gone grocery shopping in days. After scanning what's available in the refrigerator and cupboard, you find little to choose from that's fresh and healthy. So you appease your hunger with handfuls of snack food from an open bag.

The best way to avoid this scenario is to have a kitchen that's arranged to suit your needs and is well-stocked with healthy ingredients. This doesn't mean loading up on fancy appliances and expensive foods. Keep it simple. A clean, organized workspace and a few high-quality utensils will usually suffice. It's also important to have available certain foods — so-called staples — that are regularly used in food preparation. Having what you need on hand gives you greater flexibility and allows you to prepare quick, healthy meals in little time. Read Chapter 7 for more details on creating an efficient kitchen.

Listed on the following page are foods that you should always have in your kitchen. You'll find that most are used in the 12 week's worth of menus in the Mayo Clinic Healthy Weight Program. These staples will likely be part of other dishes that you prepare.

Before starting the program, do an inventory of your cupboards and refrigerator and check to see if you have these foods available. How much you need will depend on how many people you're cooking for. Anytime you go to the grocery store, replenish these ingredients if you feel that you're running low.

A key part of losing weight — and keeping it off — is daily physical activity. Therefore, it's also important to be prepared for daily exercise. You'll be getting started on regular walks in the first week of the program and you'll increase your activity from there. Not having the right attire can lead to blisters, sore muscles, dehydration and fatigue. When you exercise, make sure that you:

- Have good shoes that provide protection and stability. Page A4 of the Visual Guide shows you what features to look for in a walking shoe.
- Dress in comfortable clothing appropriate for the weather. It doesn't have to be expensive or fancy. Use a windbreaker for cool, windy days and layers of clothing in cold weather. To ensure others can see you, especially if you exercise outside early in the morning or late in the evening, wear bright colors trimmed in reflective fabric or tape.
- Protect yourself from the sun with sunscreen, sunglasses and a wide-brimmed hat.
- Carry a water bottle to replenish fluids lost during exercise.

KITCHEN STAPLES

Keep your kitchen stocked with the following ingredients. When you notice that you're running short of a particular item, please add it to your weekly shopping list.

Baking powder and baking soda
Beans (kidney and black)
Bouillon cubes (chicken and vegetable)
Breakfast cereal, whole-grain
Cooking spray, vegetable
Corn, frozen
Cornmeal
Cornstarch
Crackers (whole-grain, wheat, saltine)
Croutons, seasoned
Flour, all-purpose
Honey
Jam or jelly, any flavor
Ketchup
Lemon juice
Margarine, trans-fat free
Mayonnaise, reduced-calorie
Molasses, light
Mustard (regular, Dijon, honey)
Nuts (almonds and peanuts)
Oatmeal
Oil (canola, extra-virgin olive, sesame, peanut)
Pasta, whole-grain (linguine, spaghetti, shells)
Peanut butter
Peas, frozen
Raisins
Rice (brown and wild)

Salad dressings, reduced-calorie
Seeds (sesame and sunflower)
Soy sauce, low-sodium
Stock or broth (chicken and vegetable)
Sugar (brown and white)
Syrup
Tomato paste and tomato sauce
Tomatoes, canned (diced and whole)
Tortilla chips, baked
Tortillas, fat-free (corn or flour)
Tuna, canned, water-packed
Vinegar (balsamic, cider, white and red wine, herb-flavored)
Wine, for cooking (white and red)

Herbs, seasonings and spices (dry)
Basil
Bay leaf
Celery seed
Chili powder
Cinnamon, ground
Cloves, ground
Cumin
Dill weed
Garlic powder
Ginger, ground
Mustard, dry
Onion powder
Oregano
Parsley
Pepper (black, cayenne, garlic and lemon)
Rosemary
Salt
Thyme

Not all margarine is the same

The menus that follow recommend use of margarine. It's important to note that some margarines are healthier than others. A number of margarines contain trans-fatty acids, which can lower your high-density lipoprotein (HDL or "good") cholesterol. Look for margarines labeled as "trans-fat free" or that are made from canola oil. Stick margarines are generally higher in trans-fatty acids than tub varieties. Margarines high in trans fats are generally no better for you than butter, and may actually be worse.

HOW TO PROCEED WITH THE WEEKLY UNITS

After having worked through this introduction, you now have the basic elements for starting the Mayo Clinic Healthy Weight Program:

- You feel that you're motivated and ready.
- You've decided on the number of pounds you'd like to lose.
- You've determined your daily calorie goal.
- You've determined your daily serving totals from the food groups of the Mayo Clinic Healthy Weight Pyramid.
- You understand that you need some physical activity each day, and you're ready to get active. (If you're worried that you're out-of-shape — especially if you have health concerns — it would be a good idea to talk with your doctor before beginning the program.)

You can now move on to Week 1 of the program. Each week focuses on one of 12 topics that can help you successfully control your weight, whether this involves losing pounds or maintaining the weight you're at right now. Weekly topics include serving sizes, record keeping, healthy eating, physical activity, changing behaviors and coping with setbacks.

Each week, you'll be asked to set short-term goals related to the topic. You'll often be referred to specific pages within the book that can help you better understand the topic. Assessments and strategies are included in each week to help you implement this knowledge.

Each unit contains menus for all seven days of the week, along with recipes. You don't need to follow the menus exactly. It's OK to follow them only partially and substitute your own meals whenever you like. Regardless, it's important that you meet your requirements for the daily food servings. For example, with a daily goal of 1,200 calories, always aim for at least four vegetable servings and three fruit servings, as well as four carbohydrate servings, three protein and dairy servings and three fats servings. Use the servings lists in the Visual Guide (see pages A7-A11) to develop your own healthy menus.

Throughout the 12 weeks — especially during the first few weeks — you'll be asked to keep records. Studies show that people who keep records of what they eat and how much they exercise generally have better success with weight control.

In Week 1, you'll start a weight record. A blank form can be found on the following page. Photocopy this form. You'll be expected to make an entry on the record at least once a week.

In Week 3, you'll start a food record and an activity record. These blank forms can be found on pages 190 and 191. Like the weight record, the easiest way to use these forms may be to make photocopies of them. You'll need to make daily entries on each of these forms for a couple of weeks to establish your routine. Later, you may find you only need to make occasional entries

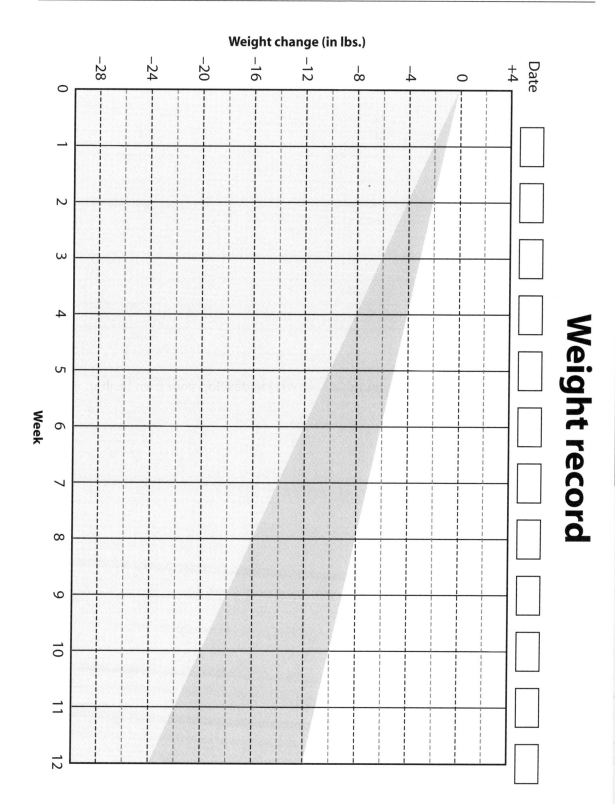

Weight record

INTRODUCTION

Daily food record

	Food	Amount	Servings	Food groups
Breakfast				
Snack				
Lunch				
Snack				
Dinner				
Snack				

Sweets
(75 calories daily
or 500 calories per week)

Serving goals for my _____-calorie diet

Fats:_____servings

Protein/Dairy:_____servings

Carbohydrates:_____servings

Fruits:_____servings
Vegetables:_____servings

Mayo Clinic Healthy Weight Pyramid

Activity record

Date____/____/____ to ____/____/____

	Goal	Week total
Minutes	_____	_____
Steps	_____	_____

Day 1

Activity	Minutes	Steps	Calories
Total			

Day 2

Activity	Minutes	Steps	Calories
Total			

Day 3

Activity	Minutes	Steps	Calories
Total			

Day 4

Activity	Minutes	Steps	Calories
Total			

Day 5

Activity	Minutes	Steps	Calories
Total			

Day 6

Activity	Minutes	Steps	Calories
Total			

Day 7

Activity	Minutes	Steps	Calories
Total			

INTRODUCTION

Week 1

Getting started

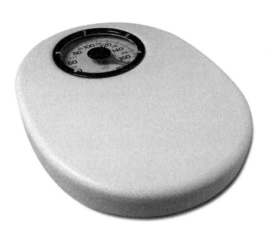

The introduction provided you with all of the information you'll need to start the Mayo Clinic Healthy Weight Program. You now know your weight goal, your daily calorie goal and how many daily servings you should eat from each of the food groups. This week, you can put the program into action.

Throughout the next 12 weeks, remember that slow and steady wins the race. Weight loss is best when it's gradual. Your aim, with this program, is to lose no more than 1 to 2 pounds a week. That's realistic, achievable and less stressful on you physically and emotionally. A loss of just 5 percent to 10 percent of your body weight — no matter what your weight — brings important benefits to your health and to your quality of life.

Too many people think that the number of pounds they lose is the only way to judge their progress in a weight program. But success is not only measured by a bathroom scale. Consider the fact that, even with minor weight loss, you're healthier, you have more energy, and you feel better about yourself. These are all important indications that you're getting your weight under control.

Weighing in is often a highly emotional experience. If you find that you've gained weight, you may feel devastated and convinced that you should quit the program. If your weight stays the same, you may become frustrated, disillusioned or bored. If you lose more weight than expected, elation may lead to slackened commitment. Try to view the scale as a helpful tool in your weight program, and not as a harsh judge of your efforts.

How regularly should you weigh yourself? That depends. Checking the scale too

Weight record

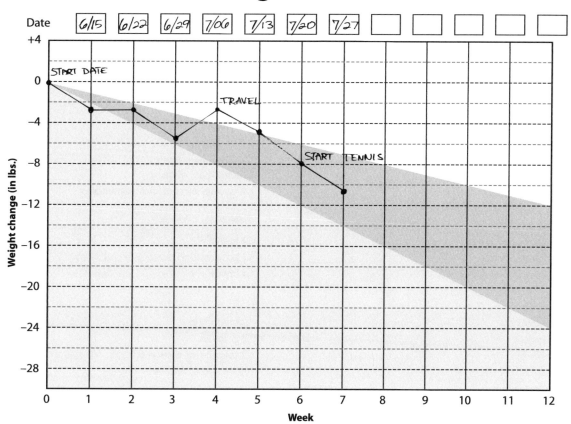

often can cause people to obsess about daily weight fluctuations. Not checking enough may indicate a lack of commitment. A good rule of thumb is to weigh yourself once a week. But if you feel that you should weigh in more often — several times a week or even daily — go for it. Remember to keep track of the general trend in your weight, not just the week-to-week changes.

What's most important is that you're consistent from week to week. Choose a day and a time for a weigh-in and stick to that schedule. And remember to record the pounds lost or gained in your weight record. If it's helpful, you can include comments with your recording, as shown above.

You'll weigh yourself twice in Week 1: on your start date and later at the end of the week. Your weight on the start date is the only number you'll need to remember — write it down somewhere. It's marked as "0" on your Weight Record (use a photocopy of the form on page 189).

Use each weekly weigh-in as a time to review your progress. If you didn't meet your goals, don't be too hard on yourself. Try to identify situations that may have worked against your progress and see what you can do to avoid or prevent a recurrence of these situations.

Week 1 shopping list

This shopping list includes many of the fresh ingredients and general grocery items you'll need on hand for the Week 1 menus. It does not include the kitchen staples listed on page 187 — make sure you have them in stock. If you replace any of the recipes with a selection of your own, you'll need to adjust the shopping list.

Fresh vegetables   QTY

❑ asparagus spears   _____
❑ bell peppers, any color   _____
❑ broccoli   _____
❑ carrots, regular and baby   _____
❑ celery   _____
❑ green beans   _____
❑ lettuce or mixed greens   _____
❑ mushrooms, portobello   _____
❑ onions, green   _____
❑ onions, yellow   _____
❑ onions, pearl   _____

                                           QTY

❑ peas   _____
❑ shallots, large   _____
❑ spinach leaves, baby   _____
❑ tomatoes   _____
❑ tomatoes, cherry   _____
❑ tomatoes, plum   _____
❑ favorite or seasonal vegetables _____

Fresh herbs

❑ fennel   _____
❑ parsley   _____
❑ thyme   _____

Fresh fruits

❑ apples   _____
❑ bananas   _____
❑ berries   _____

❑ cantaloupe   _____
❑ oranges   _____
❑ favorite or seasonal fruits _____

Carbohydrates

❑ bread, whole-grain   _____
❑ muffin, small, any flavor   _____
❑ pita bread, whole-grain   _____

❑ potatoes, baking   _____
❑ potatoes, red-skinned or white _____
❑ roll, whole-grain   _____

Protein & dairy

❑ beef stew meat, lean, boneless   _____
❑ chicken breast, boneless, skinless _____
❑ halibut or other fish fillet   _____
❑ pork tenderloin   _____
❑ shrimp or other fish   _____
❑ turkey, smoked, sliced   _____

❑ cheese, cheddar, low-fat   _____
❑ cheese, mozzarella, low-fat   _____
❑ cheese, Parmesan   _____
❑ egg   _____
❑ milk, skim   _____
❑ vanilla yogurt, fat-free, reduced-calorie _____

Fats

❑ avocado   _____

❑ vegetable dip, reduced-calorie _____

General groceries

❑ applesauce   _____
❑ cranberry sauce   _____
❑ mandarin orange sections   _____
❑ orange juice   _____
❑ pineapple, crushed   _____

❑ pizza crust, 12-inch   _____
❑ spaghetti sauce, meatless   _____
❑ tuna, water-packed, canned   _____
❑ water chestnuts   _____

WEEK 1

DAY 1 MENU

Breakfast

½ c. cooked oatmeal *Carbohydrates* ●
2 tbsp. raisins *Fruit* ●
1 c. skim milk *P/D* ●
Calorie-free beverage

Lunch

Southwestern salad *Fruit* ●, *Vegetables* ●●,
   P/D ●, *Fat* ●●
Top 2 c. shredded lettuce with 2½ oz. shredded
cooked chicken, 1 c. chopped green peppers and
onions, ½ c. crushed pineapple, ⅙ avocado, and
2 tbsp. low-calorie Western-style salad dressing.
½ whole-grain pita bread *Carbohydrates* ●
Calorie-free beverage

Dinner

Spaghetti with marinara sauce *Carbohydrates* ●●,
   Protein ●, *Vegetables* ●●
Top 1 c. cooked whole-grain spaghetti with ½ c.
meatless spaghetti sauce from a jar and 4 tbsp.
Parmesan cheese.
* ¼ small cantaloupe *Fruit* ●
Calorie-free beverage

Snack

7 whole almonds *Fat* ●

* The serving size stated is the minimum amount.
  Eat as much as you wish.

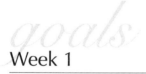

Week 1

You can adapt this week's goals or substitute different goals that are more to your liking. When you
meet a goal, check the corresponding box.

❑ **Weigh yourself.** Start your weight record using a
photocopy of the form on page 189. Your weight
at your start date will be indicated by "0" on the
record. Weigh yourself at the end of this week
and mark the difference in pounds lost or gained
on the record. Generally, it's only necessary to
weigh yourself once a week, but you can do it
more often if you feel that works better for you.

❑ **Get active.** Choose one or two strategies to help
increase the amount of physical activity in your
day and put them into practice. Try to get at least
15 minutes of new activity daily, or you can set
your own goal, if you prefer. What's important
is that you're moving more.

❑ **Start walking.** Schedule time to go for a 15-minute
walk on several days this week. Consider devising
more than one walking route. For example, use
an indoor shopping mall for times when the
weather is bad. The track at a nearby school or
college may also provide a convenient alternative.

❑ **Eat more vegetables and fruits.** Look for ways to
increase the amount of vegetables and fruits you
eat each day. Aim for at least one more serving
of vegetables and one more serving of fruits daily,
or set your own goal. Remember that you can eat
unlimited servings of vegetables and fresh fruits.

❑ **Use this week's Healthy Weight menu.** Follow the
suggested menus for this week. These menus are
devised for a 1,200-calorie diet. At this calorie
level, you'll eat a minimum of four servings each
of vegetables and carbohydrates, and three servings each of fruits, protein and dairy, and fats. If
your daily calorie goal is higher, you'll need to
adjust the menus accordingly. See page 185.

Daily recommended servings

Vegetables (no limit)	●●●●
Fruits (no limit)	●●●
Carbohydrates	●●●●
Protein & Dairy (P/D)	●●●
Fats	●●●

DAY 2 MENU

Breakfast

Pancake *Fruit* ●, *Carbohydrates* ●, *Fat* ●
*Top a 4-inch-diameter pancake with ¾ c. berries,
1 tsp. margarine and 1½ tbsp. syrup.*
1 c. skim milk *P/D* ●
Calorie-free beverage

Lunch

1 serving dilled pasta salad with spring
vegetables *Vegetables* ●, *Carbohydrates* ●●,
Fat ●
* 1 small apple *Fruit* ●
Calorie-free beverage

Dinner

Rosemary chicken *P/D* ●●, *Fat* ●
*Brush 5-oz. boneless, skinless chicken breast with 1 tsp.
each olive oil, lemon juice and rosemary. Grill or bake.*
⅓ c. brown rice mixed with ½ c. chopped
green onion *Carbohydrates* ●, *Vegetables* ●
* 1½ c. green beans *Vegetables* ●●
* 1 medium orange *Fruit* ●
Calorie-free beverage

Snack

* 1 serving favorite fruit

* The serving size stated is the minimum amount.
Eat as much as you wish.

recipe serves 8

Dilled pasta salad with spring vegetables

3 c. shell pasta (medium-sized)
8 asparagus spears, cut into ½-inch pieces
1 c. halved cherry tomatoes
1 c. sliced green peppers
½ c. chopped green onions

For the dressing:
¼ c. olive oil
2 tbsp. lemon juice
2 tbsp. rice or white wine vinegar
2 tsp. dill weed
Cracked black pepper, to taste

- Cook pasta according to package directions.
  Drain into a colander and rinse with cold water.
  Put into a large serving bowl.
- In a small saucepan, cover asparagus with water.
  Bring to a boil and cook only until tender-crisp,
  3 to 5 minutes. Drain and rinse under cold water.
  Add asparagus, tomatoes, green peppers and
  onions to pasta.
- In a small bowl, whisk together the ingredients for
  the dressing. Pour dressing over the pasta and veg-
  etables. Toss to coat. Cover, refrigerate and serve.

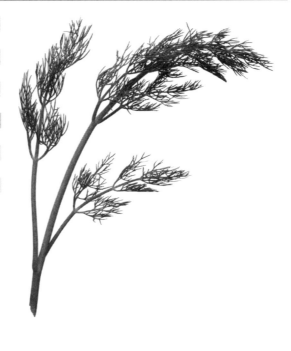

DAY 3 MENU

Breakfast

1 poached egg *P/D* ●
1 slice whole-grain toast *Carbohydrates* ●
1 tsp. margarine *Fat* ●
½ c. orange juice *Fruit* ●
Calorie-free beverage

Lunch

Tuna salad pita *Carbohydrates* ●, *P/D* ●, *Fat* ●
Fill ½ whole-grain pita bread with mixture of 3 oz. water-packed tuna, chopped celery and onion, and 1 tbsp. reduced-calorie mayonnaise.
* 1 medium bell pepper, sliced *Vegetables* ●
* 1 small apple *Fruit* ●
Calorie-free beverage

Dinner

¼ **classic tomato-basil pizza** *Carbohydrates* ●●, *P/D* ●, *Vegetables* ●
Top a prepared 12-inch pizza crust with 1 c. diced plum tomatoes, fresh basil, 1⅓ c. shredded low-fat mozzarella cheese. Bake at 400 F about 10 minutes.
* 2 c. lettuce *Vegetables* ●
2 tbsp. low-calorie salad dressing *Fat* ●
* ¼ small cantaloupe *Fruit* ●
Calorie-free beverage

Snack

* 1 serving favorite vegetable *Vegetables* ●

* The serving size stated is the minimum amount. Eat as much as you wish.

Dietitian's tips

- When in a pinch, frozen pancakes or waffles may be substituted for homemade. Check the label for calorie content and serving size.
- Frozen berries (strawberries, raspberries, blueberries) can be used in place of fresh berries. However, don't expect the same appearance and texture.
- A number of recipes this week call for vegetables, such as peas and green beans. Fresh vegetables generally provide the best texture and taste, but if you don't have access to fresh vegetables, it's OK to use frozen vegetables. Canned vegetables also may be substituted, but watch for added salt or sugar.
- To help save yourself time, you may want to cook an extra chicken breast or two for upcoming meals. Cooked chicken may be safely used for up to two days if kept covered and refrigerated. Also, if time is an issue, precooked, packaged chicken breasts can be used in a variety of salads and sandwiches.
- If you don't have fresh herbs on hand, you can use dried herbs instead. However, because dried herbs have a more intense flavor, you want to use less of them. Add only one-third to one-half the amount called for.
- Throughout the 12 weeks of menus, you will see the term *calorie-free beverage*. This includes beverages such as water, sparkling water, coffee, hot tea, calorie-free iced tea and diet soda. For more on the amount of calories in various beverages, see page 297.
- Keep in mind that frozen vegetables (broccoli, cauliflower, green beans) can be quickly thawed under running water and added to salads — or dipped into your favorite reduced-calorie dressing or vegetable dip.

DAY 4 MENU

Breakfast

Fruit yogurt parfait *Fruit* ●, *P/D* ●
*Combine 1 c. reduced-calorie, fat-free vanilla yogurt
with 1 serving of fruit.*
1 small muffin, any flavor *Carbohydrates* ●
1 tsp. margarine *Fat* ●
Calorie-free beverage

Lunch

Spinach fruit salad *Fruit* ●, *Vegetables* ● ●
*Top 2 c. baby spinach with ¹/₂ c. green pepper
strips and water chestnuts and ¹/₂ c. mandarin
orange sections.*
2 tbsp. low-calorie French dressing *Fat* ●
6 whole-grain crackers *Carbohydrates* ●
1 c. skim milk *P/D* ●
Calorie-free beverage

Dinner

3 oz. shrimp or fish, broiled or grilled *P/D* ●
²/₃ c. cooked brown rice *Carbohydrates* ● ●
* 1 c. steamed broccoli *Vegetables* ●
* 2 c. lettuce *Vegetables* ●
2 tbsp. reduced-calorie salad dressing *Fat* ●
* 1 c. mixed berries *Fruit* ●
Calorie-free beverage

Snack

* 1 serving favorite fruit *Fruit* ●

* The serving size stated is the minimum amount.
Eat as much as you wish.

strategies

10 ways to add physical activity to your day

*A great way to control your weight is to increase your
level of physical activity. Look for ways to walk and
move around a few minutes more each day. It doesn't
have to be a lot more — even a bit of added activity
helps. If a fitness center isn't your scene or just the
thought of jogging makes your blood run cold, then
try some of the following lifestyle activities instead:*

- Take the stairs instead of the elevator or escalator, for at least a few floors.
- Walk or bike to nearby destinations instead of always driving.
- At the mall, park your car farthest from where you intend to shop.
- Get off the bus a few blocks early or park three blocks from work.
- Exercise while watching television, especially during commercials.
- Hide your remote control and get up to change TV channels or adjust the volume.
- Busy yourself with housework, such as vacuuming, washing the floors, polishing the furniture or washing the windows.
- Take the dog for a walk.

- Work in the garden or yard, such as weeding or pruning the bushes.
- Wash or wax the car in your driveway rather than take it to the automatic carwash.

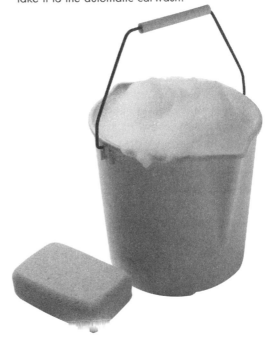

DAY 5 MENU

Breakfast
2 slices whole-grain toast *Carbohydrates* ● ●
1 tbsp. peanut butter *Fat* ● ●
½ c. orange juice *Fruit* ●
Calorie-free beverage

Lunch
2 oz. low-fat cheddar cheese *P/D* ●
10 whole-grain crackers *Carbohydrates* ● ●
* ½ c. raw baby carrots *Vegetables* ●
2 tbsp. reduced-calorie ranch dressing *Fat* ●
* 1 small apple *Fruit* ●
Calorie-free beverage

Dinner
4 oz. pork tenderloin, roasted or grilled
   P/D ● ●
* 1½ c. cooked green beans *Vegetables* ● ●
* ½ c. applesauce with cinnamon *Fruit* ●
Calorie-free beverage

Snack
* 1 serving favorite vegetable *Vegetables* ●

* The serving size stated is the minimum amount.
Eat as much as you wish.

strategies

10 ways to eat more vegetables and fruits

Many people think that weight control means food restrictions: "You can't eat that" and "Don't eat too much of this." That's not the case with fresh vegetables and fruits, where the precept is, "Eat all you want." Fresh vegetables and fruits are the foundation of a healthy diet and successful weight loss. However, for some people, making sure they have a few servings of vegetables and fruits in their diets every day is a struggle. Here are tips that might help change that:

■ Add a banana, strawberries or another favorite fruit to your cereal or yogurt at breakfast.
■ Include a small salad with one of your main meals of the day.
■ When eating a full meal, work on your vegetable portions right away, rather than reserving them for the end after you've finished other items.
■ Stir-fry vegetables with a small portion of poultry, seafood or meat.
■ Use fresh fruit and fruit sauces as toppings on desserts and pancakes.
■ When you're in a hurry, have ready-to-eat frozen vegetables handy as a quick addition to a meal. Use fresh vegetables and fruits that require little

preparation, such as baby carrots, cherry tomatoes, broccoli, cauliflower, grapes and apples.
■ Liven up your sandwiches with vegetables such as tomato, lettuce, onion, peppers and cucumber.
■ When you have a craving for chips, have a small handful with lots of fresh salsa.
■ For dessert, have baked apples or grilled pineapple.
■ Experimenting with new tastes keeps you challenged. Try vegetables and fruits that you're unfamiliar with, perhaps mango, papaya, tomatillo, jicama and star fruit, which can be obtained at most grocery stores or specialty food stores.

Limit dried fruit and fruit juice
One of the basic premises of the Healthy Weight Program is unlimited servings of fresh vegetables and fruits. You can basically eat as much as you want. This, however, doesn't apply to dried fruit, such as raisins and dates, or to fruit juice, such as orange or apple juice. That's because these items are higher in calories and unlimited servings could cause a significant increase in daily calories.

DAY 6 MENU

Breakfast

Fruit yogurt parfait *Fruit* ●, *P/D* ●
Combine 1 c. reduced-calorie, fat-free vanilla yogurt with 1 serving fruit.
1 small muffin, any flavor *Carbohydrates* ●
1 tsp. margarine *Fat* ●
Calorie-free beverage

Lunch

Chicken wrap *Fruit* ●, *Carbohydrates* ●, *P/D* ●
Combine 2 1/2 oz. shredded cooked chicken, 2 tbsp. raisins, 3 tbsp. cranberry sauce and shredded lettuce. Wrap in 6-inch corn tortilla.
1 sliced tomato *Vegetables* ●, *Fat* ●
Drizzle tomato with 1 tsp. extra-virgin olive oil and balsamic vinegar to taste.
Calorie-free beverage

Dinner

1 serving beef stew *Vegetables* ● ● ●,
Carbohydrates ●, *P/D* ●
1 small whole-grain roll *Carbohydrates* ●
1 tsp. margarine *Fat* ●
Calorie-free beverage

Snack

* 1 serving favorite fruit *Fruit* ●

* The serving size stated is the minimum amount. Eat as much as you wish.

recipe serves 6

Beef stew with fennel and shallots

3 tbsp. all-purpose flour
1 lb. boneless lean beef stew meat, trimmed of visible fat and cut into 1 1/2-inch cubes
2 tbsp. olive oil or canola oil
1/2 fennel bulb, trimmed and thinly sliced vertically
3 large shallots, chopped
1 1/2 tsp. salt
3/4 tsp. pepper
2 fresh thyme sprigs
1 bay leaf
3 c. vegetable stock or broth
1/2 c. red wine (optional)
4 large carrots, peeled and cut into 1-inch chunks
4 large red-skinned or white potatoes, peeled and cut into 1-inch chunks
18 pearl onions, about 10 oz. total weight, halved crosswise
3 portobello mushrooms, brushed clean and cut into 1-inch chunks
1/3 c. finely chopped fresh flat-leaf (Italian) parsley

■ Place the flour on a plate. Dredge the beef cubes in the flour. In a large, heavy saucepan, heat the oil over medium heat. Add the beef and cook, turning as needed, until browned on all sides, about 5 minutes. Remove the beef from the pan and set aside.

■ Add the fennel and shallots to the pan and sauté over medium heat until softened and lightly golden, 7 to 8 minutes. Add 1/2 tsp. of the salt, 1/4 tsp. of the pepper, the thyme sprigs, and the bay leaf and sauté for 1 minute. Return the beef to the pan and add the vegetable stock and the wine, if using. Bring to a boil, then reduce the heat to low, cover, and simmer gently until the meat is tender, 40 to 45 minutes.

■ Add the carrots, potatoes, onions and mushrooms. (The liquid won't cover the vegetables completely, but more liquid will accumulate as the mushrooms soften.) Simmer gently until the vegetables are tender, about 30 minutes longer. Discard the thyme sprigs and bay leaf. Stir in the parsley and the remaining 1 tsp. salt and 1/2 tsp. pepper.

■ Ladle into individual bowls and serve.

This recipe is one of 150 recipes collected in "The New Mayo Clinic Cookbook," published by Mayo Clinic Health Information and Oxmoor House and available in bookstores.

DAY 7 MENU

Breakfast
$^1/_2$ c. whole-grain cereal *Carbohydrates* ●
* 1 small banana *Fruit* ●
1 c. skim milk *P/D* ●
Calorie-free beverage

Lunch
Turkey sandwich *Carbohydrates* ● ●, *P/D* ●
Top two slices whole-grain bread with 3 oz. smoked turkey, Dijon mustard, lettuce and tomato slices.
* 2 c. mixed greens *Vegetables* ●
2 tbsp. reduced-calorie salad dressing *Fat* ●
* 1 small apple *Fruit* ●
Calorie-free beverage

Dinner
3 oz. grilled halibut or other fish *P/D* ●
Sprinkle with lemon and season with garlic pepper.
* $^1/_2$ c. peas *Vegetables* ● ●
$^1/_2$ medium baked potato *Carbohydrates* ●
1 tsp. margarine *Fat* ●
* 1 c. berries *Fruit* ●
Calorie-free beverage

Snack
* 1 serving favorite vegetable *Vegetables* ●
3 tbsp. reduced-calorie vegetable dip *Fat* ●

* The serving size stated is the minimum amount.
Eat as much as you wish.

strategies

Find a walking route

Walking is one of the most convenient ways to fit physical activity into your day. Take a brief stroll over your lunch hour and use your legs rather than your car for short errands. It's also good to take longer walks, perhaps several times a week.

Many people like to have a planned route in mind when they go for a walk. That way, they can gauge approximately how far they've traveled and how much energy they expend. They also feel assured that the paths are safe and that they won't get lost. Take time to plan a walking route in your neighborhood or in a location that you like to visit, such as a park. You may prefer a loop path or an out-and-back path. If you're not in shape, start with a 15-minute route but try to work your way up to 30 minutes.

Here are a few guidelines to keep in mind as you plan your walking route:

■ **Look for a route that's close by and accessible.**
Being able to step out your door to start your walk is convenient and motivating. If that's not possible, try to avoid long drives in order to exercise. Use stores, downtown areas or public spaces as different destinations.

■ **Make personal safety your top priority.** Carrying a cell phone, whistle or walking stick can protect and reassure you. Try to walk in the daytime or in well-lighted areas after dark. Make note of locations along or near your route that may be useful, such as public restrooms, emergency phones and stores that sell water. Finding a walking partner is an excellent precaution.

■ **Choose a route that's varied.** Make your route interesting, but don't involve too many stops, turns and busy intersections. You'll benefit most, and lose more calories, from a sustained, steady stride. Note where there are uneven sidewalks, inclines or loose gravel. Dirt paths can become slick and muddy after a rain. Have proper attire and shoes ready for any situation. Explore alternative portions of your path, if they look inviting. Hills can add intensity to your walk but include them at the beginning, while you're still fresh, rather than at the end of the walk — and use the top of a hill to enjoy a beautiful view.

Week 2

Serving sizes

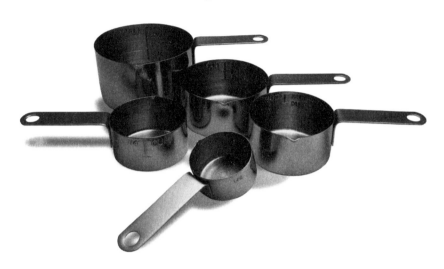

You may think servings are simply generous amounts of food put on your plate for a meal. So long as the food is tasty and satisfies your hunger, considerations about the quantity of food you eat are easily overlooked. Yet, inattention to how much you consume can lead to overeating and weight gain.

In fact, a *serving* is an exact amount, defined by common measurements such as cups, ounces, tablespoons or pieces, for example, a medium apple or a large egg. That's different from a *portion*, which is defined as the amount of food put on your plate — and usually greater than a single serving.

Serving sizes in the Mayo Clinic Healthy Weight Program are based on calories. All foods within each group are relatively equal in calories per serving. The total number of servings you have

each day from each food group will determine the total calories you consume.

The number of calories you need may vary from day to day, depending on how many calories you expend. But if you eat the recommended number of servings from each food group — with the proper serving sizes in mind — you can be sure to get all of the nutrients your body needs and avoid overeating and weight gain.

You don't need the mind of a mathematician to estimate serving sizes, and there's no need to carry measuring cups and spoons with you at all times to make sure that your calculations are exact. It is important, though, that you understand the important role serving sizes play in successful weight control. Take time to do the assessment on the next page and, if you haven't already, read Chapter 5.

Do you know serving sizes?

Answer the questions below to assess your current knowledge of serving sizes. If you feel like you're lost and don't have a clue, just give your best guess and don't be discouraged. The more you try, the easier it becomes. Keep in mind, a "cup" in these questions refers to an exact measurement.

1. How many dairy servings are in 1 cup of low-fat milk?

   Answer: One cup of low-fat milk is a single serving of dairy.

2. How many carbohydrate servings are in 2 cups of cooked pasta?

   Answer: Four servings, because $1/2$ cup of cooked pasta is a single serving.

3. How many protein servings are in a 9-ounce grilled steak?

   Answer: Six servings, because $1^1/2$ ounces of beef is a single serving.

4. Which choice provides one serving of fruit: a medium orange or $1/2$ cup of orange juice?

Answer: A medium orange and $1/2$ cup of orange juice each provide one fruit serving. Note that the size equivalents of different fruits vary. For example, a small apple and a large peach are one fruit serving.

5. Approximately how many vegetable servings would you get from a simple dinner salad consisting of 2 cups of lettuce, a medium tomato, $1/2$ cup of cucumber and a sprinkling of shredded carrot?

   Answer: Approximately three servings of vegetables because each of the following amounts equals one serving: 2 cups of lettuce, one medium tomato, and a combination of $1/2$ cup cucumber and $1/2$ cup carrot.

   If you don't have a lot of experience with serving sizes, don't expect to get all of the responses correct. If your estimates were close on at least one or two of the questions, you did a great job. It's very common for people to underestimate the number of servings they're actually eating.

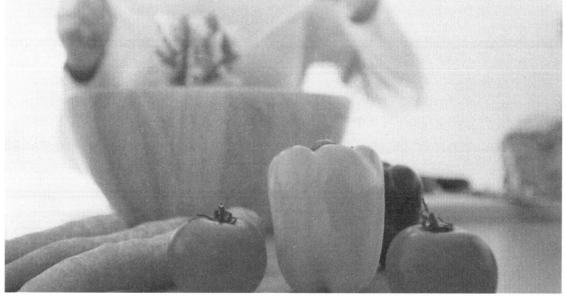

Week 2 shopping list

This shopping list includes many of the fresh ingredients and general grocery items you'll need on hand for the Week 2 menus. It does not include the kitchen staples listed on page 187 — make sure you have them in stock. If you replace any of the recipes with a selection of your own, you'll need to adjust the shopping list.

Fresh vegetables	QTY		QTY
❑ asparagus spears	_____	❑ onions, red and yellow	_____
❑ bean sprouts	_____	❑ spinach leaves, baby	_____
❑ bell peppers, green, red and yellow	_____	❑ tomatoes	_____
❑ broccoli	_____	❑ tomatoes, cherry	_____
❑ cabbage	_____	❑ favorite or seasonal vegetables	_____
❑ carrots	_____		
❑ celery	_____	*Fresh herbs*	
❑ cucumbers	_____	❑ basil	_____
❑ eggplant	_____	❑ garlic	_____
❑ lettuce or mixed greens	_____	❑ ginger	_____
❑ onions, green	_____	❑ mint	_____

Fresh fruits	QTY		QTY
❑ apples	_____	❑ grapes	_____
❑ bananas	_____	❑ limes	_____
❑ berries	_____	❑ oranges	_____
❑ grapefruit	_____	❑ favorite or seasonal fruit	_____

Carbohydrates	QTY		QTY
❑ bagels, whole-grain	_____	❑ bun, whole-grain	_____
❑ bread, sourdough	_____	❑ English muffins, whole-grain	_____
❑ bread, whole-grain	_____	❑ sweet potatoes	_____

Protein & dairy	QTY		QTY
❑ beef, lean	_____	❑ tuna or other fish fillet	_____
❑ chicken breast, boneless, skinless	_____	❑ turkey, smoked, sliced	_____
❑ chicken breast, sliced	_____	❑ cheese, Gouda, low-fat	_____
❑ ham, lean, sliced	_____	❑ cheese, mozzarella, part-skim	_____
❑ orange roughy or other fish fillet	_____	❑ milk, skim	_____
❑ pork roast, lean	_____		

Fats	QTY
❑ vegetable dip, reduced-calorie	_____

General groceries	QTY		QTY
❑ black beans, canned	_____	❑ pretzel sticks	_____
❑ diced tomatoes, canned	_____	❑ Ramen noodles	_____
❑ kidney beans, canned	_____	❑ tofu	_____
❑ mandarin oranges	_____	❑ tuna, water-packed	_____
❑ marinara sauce	_____	❑ vegetable juice	_____
❑ pineapple chunks, unsweetened	_____		

WEEK 2

DAY 1 MENU

Breakfast
* * 1 small banana *Fruit* ●
  ½ whole-grain English muffin *Carbohydrates* ●
  1 tsp. margarine *Fat* ●
  1 c. skim milk *P/D* ●
  Calorie-free beverage

Lunch
* Bagel sandwich *Carbohydrates* ●●, *P/D* ●
  Spread 1 whole-grain bagel with mustard. Top with
  2 oz. lean ham, lettuce, tomato and onion slices.
* * 2 c. raw mixed vegetables *Vegetables* ●●
  Calorie-free beverage

Dinner
  ¼ recipe Chinese noodles and vegetables
  Carbohydrates ●, *Vegetables* ●●, *Fat* ●●

Prepare 1 package ramen noodles as directed. Rinse
and set aside. Sauté 1 tbsp. grated ginger and 1 tbsp.
chopped garlic in 1 tbsp. sesame oil and 1 tbsp.
peanut oil. Add ½ c. broccoli florets and sauté 3 minutes. Add ½ c. of each: bean sprouts, fresh spinach
and cherry tomato halves. Add noodles and toss.
Sprinkle with chopped green onions and soy sauce.
* * ½ c. pineapple chunks *Fruit* ●
  1 c. skim milk *P/D* ●
  Calorie-free beverage

Snack
* * 1 serving favorite fruit *Fruit* ●

* * The serving size stated is the minimum amount.
  Eat as much as you wish.

goals

Week 2

You can adapt this week's goals or substitute different goals that are more to your liking. When you
meet a goal, check the corresponding box.

❑ **Become familiar with serving sizes.** Study the lists
of serving sizes for the different food groups on
pages A7-A11 of the Visual Guide. Take a few
minutes before each meal to gauge the number of
servings on your plate before you begin to eat. At
first, it might be helpful to measure them to see
how close your estimates are. Before you can
effectively control your food portions, you'll need
to know serving sizes.

❑ **Reduce your portion sizes.** Try some of the strategies listed on page 208. Choose one or two that
will help you control the amount of food you eat
daily. Your purpose is to satisfy your hunger and
meet your dietary needs but not to overeat.

❑ **Assemble visual cues.** Collect everyday objects that
can serve as visual cues for serving sizes. Keep
these cues handy in your kitchen area for reference. An example would be a tennis ball, the size
of which is equivalent to one serving of fruit. Other
visual cues are shown on A6 of the Visual Guide.

❑ **Increase your walking pace slightly.** Increased
intensity can increase the aerobic benefits of
walking. Do this only if it causes no discomfort or
pain. Avoiding injuries and enjoying your exercise are key factors in keeping you motivated.
❑ **Update your Weight Record.** Weigh in at your regular time and record the number of pounds lost or
gained this week on the Weight Record.
❑ **Use Week 2's Healthy Weight menu.** These menus
are devised for a 1,200-calorie diet. If your daily
goal varies from this calorie level, you'll need to
adjust the menus accordingly. See page 185.

Daily recommended servings

Vegetables (no limit)	●●●●
Fruits (no limit)	●●●
Carbohydrates	●●●●
Protein & Dairy (P/D)	●●●
Fats	●●●

DAY 2 MENU

Breakfast

½ c. whole-grain cereal *Carbohydrates* ●
1 c. skim milk *P/D* ●
* 1 small banana *Fruit* ●
Calorie-free beverage

Lunch

1 serving pineapple chicken salad with balsamic
  vinaigrette *Fruit* ●, *Vegetables* ●●, *P/D* ●,
  Fat ●●
6 wheat crackers *Carbohydrates* ●
½ c. vegetable juice *Vegetables* ●
Calorie-free beverage

Dinner

3 oz. grilled tuna or other fish *P/D* ●
Brush with lemon juice and top with fresh minced basil.
½ baked sweet potato *Carbohydrates* ●
1 tsp. margarine *Fat* ●
* Cucumber and tomato salad *Vegetables* ●●
*Combine 1 c. thinly sliced cucumber and 8 cherry
tomatoes, halved. Sprinkle with balsamic, rice wine or
herb-flavored vinegar to taste.*
* 1 c. grapes *Fruit* ●
Calorie-free beverage

Snack

30 pretzel sticks *Carbohydrates* ●

* The serving size stated is the minimum amount.
  Eat as much as you wish.

recipe serves 4

Pineapple chicken salad with balsamic vinaigrette

4 c. fresh baby spinach leaves
1 can (8 oz.) unsweetened pineapple chunks
2 cooked boneless, skinless chicken breasts, cubed
2 c. broccoli florets
½ c. thinly sliced red onion

For the dressing:
¼ c. olive oil
2 tbsp. balsamic vinegar
2 tsp. sugar
¼ tsp. cinnamon

- Wash baby spinach leaves and pat dry. Drain the
  pineapple (reserve 2 tbsp. juice). Combine the
  cooked chicken, broccoli, spinach and onions in a
  large serving bowl.
- Prepare dressing. In a small bowl whisk together the
  oil, vinegar, reserved pineapple juice, sugar and
  cinnamon. Pour over the salad. Serve immediately.

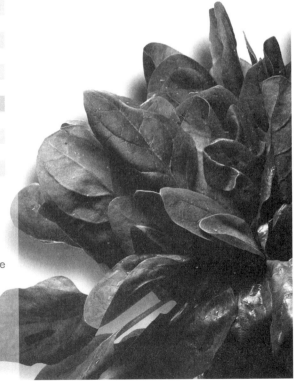

WEEK 2

DAY 3 MENU

Breakfast
1 slice whole-grain toast *Carbohydrates* ●
1 tsp. margarine *Fat* ●
* 1 medium orange *Fruit* ●
Calorie-free beverage

Lunch
Open-faced turkey sandwich *Carbohydrates* ●,
   P/D ●, *Fat* ●
Spread 1 tbsp. reduced-calorie mayonnaise on a slice
of sourdough bread. Top with 3 oz. smoked turkey,
2 oz. low-fat Gouda cheese, 1 slice tomato and
chopped basil.
* 1 c. carrot and celery sticks *Vegetables* ●
Calorie-free beverage

Dinner
¼ recipe vegetarian chili *Carbohydrates* ●●,
   P/D ●●, *Vegetables* ●●●
Sauté ½ c. onion in olive oil. Add 12 oz. tofu pieces, 2
14-oz. cans diced tomatoes, 2 14-oz. cans kidney
beans and 1 14-oz. can black beans (drained), 3 tbsp.
chili powder, 1 tbsp. oregano. Simmer 30 minutes.
* 1 c. grapes *Fruit* ●
Calorie-free beverage

Snack
1 sliced apple with 1½ tsp. peanut butter
   Fruit ●, *Fat* ●

* The serving size stated is the minimum amount.
Eat as much as you wish.

Dietitian's tips

*Fish is an important part of a healthy diet and it's
generally recommended that you eat fish twice a
week. Here are simple ways to vary your menu:*

Seasonings you can use with fish
- Bay (seafood) seasoning
- Cajun (blackening) spice
- Dill
- Italian seasoning
- Garlic-herb blend
- Lemon pepper
- Lemon-dill seasoning
- Paprika and onion
- Teriyaki or soy sauce
- Smoke (Plank fillets onto untreated cedar, apple-
  wood or maple planks, or use similar wood chips,
  and grill. Seaweed or kelp also may be used.)

Marinades you can use with fish
*Mix the ingredients from one of the bullet points in
the following list. Place the mixture along with the fish
fillets in a covered dish or plastic bag and marinate
for about 30 minutes in the refrigerator (turning the
fillets once):*

- 1 tsp. olive oil, 2 green onions including green
  tops (chopped), ¼ c. rice wine vinegar
- ¼ c. each: soy sauce, rice wine vinegar, 1 tbsp.
  ginger (chopped)
- 1 tsp. olive oil, juice from 1 lemon, ½ tsp. dried
  basil, 2 cloves garlic (chopped)
- ½ c. orange juice, 1 tbsp. Dijon mustard,
  ¼ tsp. cracked black pepper
- ¼ c. each: orange juice, teriyaki or soy sauce,
  ½ tbsp. garlic (chopped)

Flavorful companions for fish
*In a covered baking dish, bake fish at 325 F,
topped with one of the following:*
- 4 green onions (chopped), lemon slices and
  ½ c. chicken broth
- 1 bay leaf (broken into several pieces), 3 sprigs
  fresh parsley (chopped), ½ c. chicken broth
- 1 tomato (sliced), ¼ tsp. oregano, ¼ tsp. basil,
  crushed black pepper, ½ c. chicken broth
- 1 stalk celery, ¼ c. lemon juice, 1 tsp. dill,
  ½ c. chicken broth

DAY 4 MENU

Breakfast

1 slice whole-grain toast *Carbohydrates* ●
1½ tsp. peanut butter *Fat* ●
* 1 small banana *Fruit* ●
1 c. skim milk *P/D* ●
Calorie-free beverage

Lunch

Tuna salad bagel *Carbohydrates* ●, *P/D* ●, *Fat* ●
Spread on 1 bagel a mixture of 3 oz. water-packed
tuna, chopped celery and onion, and 1 tbsp. reduced-
calorie mayonnaise.
* 1 c. sliced bell pepper *Vegetables* ●
* 1 small apple *Fruit* ●
Calorie-free beverage

Dinner

Beef fajita *Vegetables* ● ●, *P/D* ●, *Fat* ●
Sauté 1½ oz. lean beef strips in 1 tsp. extra-virgin
olive oil. Add ½ c. sliced onion and 1 c. sliced green,
red and yellow bell peppers. Season with chili powder
and lime juice as desired.
2 tortillas *Carbohydrates* ● ●
* ½ c. mandarin orange sections *Fruit* ●
Calorie-free beverage

Snack

* 1 serving favorite vegetable *Vegetables* ●

* The serving size stated is the minimum amount.
Eat as much as you wish.

strategies
Limit how much you eat

*Being familiar with serving sizes helps you meet —
and not exceed — your daily calorie needs. Other
strategies to help control the amount of food you
eat are described below:*

- **Eat slowly.** Quick eating creates a time lag
  between when you stop eating and when your
  brain registers that you're full. That makes it easy
  to overeat before you feel the consequences.

- **See what you eat.** Eating directly from a container
  gives you no sense of portion size. Seeing food
  on a plate or in a bowl keeps you aware of how
  much you're eating.

- **Try to eat three meals at regular times.** Skipping a
  meal during the day can cause extreme hunger,
  which can lead to indiscriminate snacking.

- **Focus on your food.** Avoid distractions. Meals
  eaten with the television on or while you're
  reading can lead to mindless eating.

- **Serve smaller portions.** At the beginning of a
  meal, take slightly less than what you think you'll
  eat. You can always have seconds, if necessary.

- **Don't feel obligated to clean your plate.** Stop eating as soon as your stomach feels full. Those extra

bites of food that you're trying not to waste add
unneeded calories.

- **Keep snacking under control.** Eating high-calorie,
  high-fat snacks often affects your enjoyment of
  regular meals.

- **Share a meal.** As generous as most restaurant portions are, you and a dining companion may be
  able to divide a single entree from the menu and
  satisfy both your appetites.

- **Ask for a carryout bag.** Make it a habit at restaurants to ask that a portion of your meal be boxed
  up to take home.

DAY 5 MENU

Breakfast

1 c. whole-grain cereal *Carbohydrates* ● ●
1 c. skim milk *P/D* ●
* 1 medium orange *Fruit* ●
Calorie-free beverage

Lunch

Open-faced grilled cheese sandwich
     Carbohydrates ●, *P/D* ●
*Top ½ whole-grain bagel with a tomato slice and 1 ½
oz. mozzarella cheese. Broil until cheese melts.*
1½ c. shredded cabbage and ½ c. shredded
     carrots *Vegetables* ● ●
Toss with cider vinegar, celery seed and ½ tsp. sugar.
* 1 medium apple *Fruit* ●
Calorie-free beverage

Dinner

2 oz. lean pork *P/D* ●
½ medium baked sweet potato *Carbohydrates* ●
1 tsp. margarine *Fat* ●
6 steamed asparagus spears, topped with
     4 tsp. sliced almonds *Vegetables* ●, *Fat* ●
* ½ c. pineapple cubes *Fruit* ●
Calorie-free beverage

Snack

* 1 serving favorite vegetable *Vegetables* ●
3 tbsp. low-calorie vegetable dip *Fat* ●

* The serving size stated is the minimum amount.
Eat as much as you wish.

strategies

Make sense of servings

Estimating your servings at meals is a great way to
control the calories you consume. Unfortunately, the
eye can be deceiving. Most people habitually, and
unintentionally, underestimate the number of servings
they eat. This means they consume more calories
than they think they're getting, and they can't understand why they're gaining weight. Here's an exercise to help you get a better sense of servings.

Pour dry cereal into a bowl until you have what
you think is about ½ cup. Don't use a measuring
device, just depend on your own estimation. Now
pour the cereal out of the bowl and into a measuring cup. How close did you come to ½ cup? If you
overestimated, don't feel discouraged. Most people
imagine ½ cup being a greater amount than it actually is. Try this exercise a few more times to see if
you can get a closer estimate. One serving of dry
cereal is the equivalent of ½ cup.

You can try this same exercise the next time you're
cooking pasta or rice. After you've drained the
cooked pasta or rice, try putting approximately ½
cup into a bowl, then put it into a measuring cup.
One serving of cooked pasta or rice is the equivalent of ½ cup.

Try this exercise with favorite foods that you frequently eat. The more you practice, the more control
you'll have over portion sizes when you're getting
ready for meals.

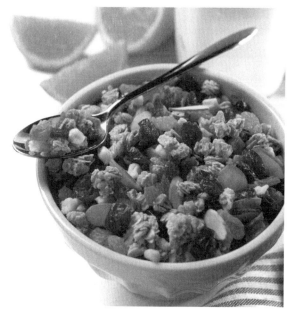

DAY 6 MENU

Breakfast

½ English muffin *Carbohydrate* ●
1 tsp. margarine *Fat* ●
* 1 large grapefruit *Fruit* ● ●
Calorie-free beverage

Lunch

Simple pizza *Vegetables* ● ●, *Carbohydrates* ● ●,
   P/D ● ●

Top two English muffin halves each with ¼ c. marinara sauce, ½ c. sliced onion and green pepper, and ⅓ c. shredded part-skim mozzarella cheese. Broil until cheese melts.
Calorie-free beverage

Dinner

1 serving chicken stir-fry with eggplant and basil
   P/D ●, *Fat* ●, *Vegetables* ● ● ●
⅓ c. cooked brown rice *Carbohydrates* ●
* ½ c. pineapple cubes *Fruit* ●
Calorie-free beverage

Snack

7 smoked almonds *Fat* ●

* The serving size stated is the minimum amount. Eat as much as you wish.

recipe serves 4

Chicken stir-fry with eggplant and basil

¼ c. coarsely chopped fresh basil
2 tbsp. chopped fresh mint
¾ c. chicken stock or broth
3 green (spring) onions, including tender green tops, 2 coarsely chopped and 1 thinly sliced
2 cloves garlic
1 tbsp. peeled and chopped fresh ginger
2 tbsp. extra-virgin olive oil
1 small eggplant, with peel, diced (about 4 c.)
1 yellow onion, coarsely chopped
1 red bell pepper, seeded and cut into julienne
1 yellow bell pepper, seeded and cut into julienne
1 lb. boneless, skinless chicken breasts, cut into strips ½-inch wide and 2 inches long
2 tbsp. low-sodium soy sauce

■ In a blender or food processor, combine the basil, mint, ¼ c. of the stock, the chopped green onions, garlic and ginger. Pulse until the mixture is minced but not puréed. Set aside.

■ In a large, nonstick frying pan, heat 1 tbsp. of the olive oil over medium-high heat. Add the eggplant, yellow onion and bell peppers and sauté until the vegetables are tender, about 8 minutes.

Transfer the sautéed vegetables to a bowl and cover to keep warm.

■ Add the remaining 1 tbsp. olive oil to the pan and heat over medium-high heat. Add the basil mixture and sauté for about 1 minute, stirring constantly. Add the chicken strips and soy sauce and sauté until the chicken is almost opaque throughout, about 2 minutes. Add the remaining ½ c. stock and bring to a boil. Return the vegetable mixture to the pan and stir until heated through, about 3 minutes. Transfer to a serving dish and garnish with the sliced green onion. Serve immediately.

This recipe is one of 150 recipes collected in "The New Mayo Clinic Cookbook," published by Mayo Clinic Health Information and Oxmoor House and available in bookstores in the United States and Canada.

DAY 7 MENU

Breakfast

½ c. whole-grain cereal *Carbohydrates* ●
1 c. skim milk *P/D* ●
* ½ large grapefruit *Fruit* ●
Calorie-free beverage

Lunch

Chicken sandwich *Carbohydrates* ● ●, *P/D* ●
Spread 1 whole-grain bun with honey mustard. Add 2½ oz. grilled, boneless, skinless chicken breast, lettuce and tomato slices.
* 2 c. mixed spring greens *Vegetables* ●
1 tbsp. sunflower seeds *Fat* ●
2 tbsp. low-calorie ranch dressing *Fat* ●
* 1 small banana *Fruit* ●
Calorie-free beverage

Dinner

3 oz. orange roughy or other fish *P/D* ●
½ c. linguine topped with ¼ c. marinara sauce
    Carbohydrates ●, *Vegetables* ●
* 1 c. steamed broccoli *Vegetables* ●
* 1 c. berries *Fruit* ●
Calorie-free beverage

Snack

* 1 serving favorite vegetable *Vegetables* ●
3 tbsp. reduced-calorie vegetable dip *Fat* ●

* The serving size stated is the minimum amount.
Eat as much as you wish.

review

Week 2

You're just completing the second week of your Healthy Weight Program. How is it going so far? As you take steps to change your eating behaviors and to get more active, take time every once in a while to assess how your efforts are paying off:

■ **Evaluate your progress.** Review the goals you set for yourself at the start of this week. Were you able to successfully use one or two strategies that helped you control portion sizes? With practice and the use of visual cues, are you better able to estimate serving sizes? Think about what worked and what didn't work for you in the Healthy Weight menu. Try to find ways to better adapt the menus to your personal preferences and tastes.

■ **Understanding energy density.** Serving size relates directly to energy density, a foundation of the Healthy Weight Program. Energy density is the number of calories contained in a given amount of food. Most vegetables and fruits have a low energy density, which means that you can eat a large volume and receive relatively few calories. That's why the number of daily servings of

vegetables and fruits is unlimited in the program. Fats and sweets have a high energy density, which is why servings from both groups are so restricted. For more on energy density, see pages 41-42.

■ **Looking forward.** Next week's unit gets you started on a daily food record. The knowledge of serving sizes that you gained this week will allow you to keep a more accurate and useful record. Collecting information about your food intake over a period of time guides your weight program, helps you control portions and ensures you're getting a balanced, healthy diet.

Week 3

Record keeping

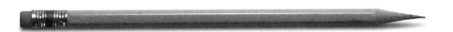

Most food pyramids encourage you to eat a varied diet based on a certain number of servings from each of the different food groups. It's one thing to know the number of servings in a single meal. It's another thing to keep track of food servings for an entire day. And how do you know if you're getting enough variety in your diet over a period of several weeks or months?

One approach is to write down the servings you eat at each meal in a record book. Over time, this record lets you compare daily serving totals and determine if you're getting the nutrients you need from all the food groups. The third week of the Mayo Clinic Healthy Weight Program gets you started on record keeping, which can be a valuable tool for weight control. During the week, read pages 68-73 to learn other strategies that

you may use along with a food record to help control your weight.

Record keeping is also a valuable tool for tracking your activity level. Instead of numbers of servings, you may be recording minutes of activity. Keeping track helps you spread those minutes between a variety of activities and exercises that form your daily routine.

Record keeping may help you identify problem patterns in your eating behavior or recurring situations or moods that lead to poor food choices, overeating or putting off exercise. Sometimes, these patterns or situations become apparent only after comparing several weeks' worth of entries.

The routine of keeping records can also motivate you to stay with your eating and exercise programs. Seeing your progress over several months can build confidence and inspire you to set higher goals.

Getting started

Keeping records requires good organization to reduce your time and effort. Your entries can be as simple or complex as you wish. What's important is that the record book is easy to use and gathers useful information.

An example of a food record entry is illustrated below. On this record, you indicate everything you ate throughout the day, including the types of food, the amounts and the servings. At the end of each day, compare the servings in each food group with your nutritional goals.

A blank copy of this food record can be found on page 190. Make photocopies of the page to use each day.

When keeping a food record, it's important that you record everything you eat or drink during the entire day, including snacks and even a "bite" of something.

To help keep accurate records, carry a small notepad with you wherever you go and enter the information immediately. Don't wait for a "convenient" time — you'll forget the details.

Keep a daily record for at least the first two weeks of the Healthy Weight Program. That should be adequate time to establish your eating routine and allow you to notice patterns that may contribute to poor food choices. After these initial weeks, you decide if you think a food record is helpful.

WEEK 3

Daily food record

	Food	Amount	Servings	Food groups
Breakfast	Oatmeal	1/2 cup	1	Carbohydrates
	Skim milk	1 cup	1	Protein/Dairy
	Banana	1 large	1 1/2	Fruits
Snack	Orange	1 medium	1	Fruits
Lunch	Greek salad			
	Tomato, cucumber	1 1/2 cups	1	Vegetables
	Green pepper	1/2 cup	1	Vegetables
	Olive oil	2 tsp	1	Fats
	Bread (whole-grain)	1 slice	1	Carbohydrates
Snack	Walnuts	4 halves	1	Fats
Dinner	Salmon	3 ounces	1	Protein/Dairy
	Salad (lettuce with olive oil)	2 cups	1	Vegetables, Fats
	Pasta (whole-grain)	1/2 cup	1	Carbohydrates
	Tomato sauce	1/2 cup	1	Vegetables
	Broccoli	1 cup	1	Protein/Dairy
	Bread (whole-grain)	1 slice	1	Carbohydrates
Snack	Grapes	1 cup	2	Fruits

Week 3 shopping list

This shopping list includes many of the fresh ingredients and general grocery items you'll need on hand for the Week 3 menus. It does not include the kitchen staples listed on page 187 — make sure you have them in stock. If you replace any of the recipes with a selection of your own, you'll need to adjust the shopping list.

Fresh vegetables	QTY		QTY
❑ bell peppers, red and green	_____	❑ peas	_____
❑ broccoli	_____	❑ summer squash	_____
❑ carrots, regular and baby	_____	❑ tomatoes, regular and cherry	_____
❑ celery	_____	❑ zucchini	_____
❑ cucumbers	_____	❑ favorite or seasonal vegetables	_____
❑ green beans	_____	*Fresh herbs*	
❑ lettuce (romaine) or mixed greens	_____		
❑ mushrooms	_____	❑ basil	_____
❑ onions, pearl	_____	❑ dill	_____
❑ onions, red	_____	❑ garlic	_____
❑ onions, yellow	_____	❑ parsley, flat-leaf (Italian)	_____

Fresh fruits			
❑ apples	_____	❑ grapes	_____
❑ bananas	_____	❑ lemons	_____
❑ berries	_____	❑ pears	_____
❑ cantaloupe	_____	❑ favorite or seasonal fruit	_____
❑ grapefruit	_____		

Carbohydrates			
❑ bread, whole-grain and sourdough	_____	❑ hamburger buns, whole-grain	_____
❑ breadstick, baked	_____	❑ pita bread, whole-grain	_____
❑ bulgar wheat	_____	❑ potatoes, baby, red-skinned	_____
❑ English muffins, whole-grain	_____		

Protein & dairy			
❑ chicken breast, boneless, skinless	_____	❑ cheese, Gouda, low-fat	_____
❑ cod or other fish fillet	_____	❑ egg	_____
❑ flank steak	_____	❑ egg substitute	_____
❑ ground beef, extra-lean	_____	❑ milk, skim	_____
❑ salmon or other fish fillet	_____	❑ soy milk, plain	_____
❑ turkey, smoked, sliced	_____	❑ yogurt, frozen, fat-free	_____
❑ turkey breast, boneless, skinless	_____	❑ yogurt, reduced-calorie, fat-free	_____
❑ cheese, Gouda, low-fat	_____		

Fats			
❑ cream cheese, fat-free	_____	❑ vegetable dip, reduced-calorie	_____
❑ olives	_____	❑ whipped topping, nondairy	_____
❑ sour cream, low-fat	_____		

General groceries			
❑ artichoke hearts, frozen	_____	❑ salsa	_____
❑ garbanzos, canned	_____	❑ smokey BBQ sauce	_____
❑ lentil soup, canned	_____	❑ tomatoes, diced, canned	_____
❑ orange juice	_____	❑ tuna, water-packed, canned	_____

WEEK 3

DAY 1 MENU

Breakfast

½ whole-grain English muffin *Carbohydrates* ●
1 tbsp. honey
* ½ large grapefruit *Fruit* ●
Calorie-free beverage

Lunch

Tuna salad sandwich *Carbohydrates* ●●,
P/D ●, *Fat* ●
Top 2 slices whole-grain bread with mixture of 3 oz. water-packed tuna, chopped celery and onion to taste, and 1 tbsp. reduced-calorie mayonnaise.
2 c. bell peppers and cucumbers, sliced
Vegetables ●●
* 1 c. grapes *Fruit* ●
Calorie-free beverage

Dinner

2½ oz. grilled chicken breast, boneless
and skinless *P/D* ●, *Fat* ●
Top with 4 tsp. sliced almonds.
* 1 c. steamed broccoli *Vegetables* ●
1 6- to 8-inch breadstick *Carbohydrates* ●
½ c. fat-free frozen yogurt topped with 1 c.
berries *P/D* ●, *Fruit* ●
Calorie-free beverage

Snack

* 1 serving favorite vegetable *Vegetables* ●
2 tbsp. reduced-calorie vegetable dip *Fat* ●

* *The serving size stated is the minimum amount. Eat as much as you wish.*

goals

Week 3

You can adapt this week's goals or substitute different goals that are more to your liking. When you meet a goal, check the corresponding box.

❏ **Keep records.** Start tracking your diet and activity level. Consider using photocopies of the blank forms provided in this book, or something equivalent. You may want to collect your records in a binder, or use whatever type of record book is most convenient for you. Keep daily records for about two weeks to establish your routine. Then you may choose to record only two or three days a week to monitor your progress.

❏ **Increase your daily steps.** With the use of a pedometer, find out approximately how many steps you take each day for three consecutive days. Add the daily totals and divide by three to determine the average number of steps you take each day. Set a goal to increase your average number of steps, by either 2,000 or 3,000 steps a day. Your ultimate goal would be to reach 10,000 total steps each day.

❏ **Update your Weight Record.** Weigh in and record the number of pounds gained or lost on your

Weight Record. If you feel as though you're struggling to lose weight, take time to re-examine your barriers to weight loss.

❏ **Use Week 3's Healthy Weight menu.** The menus provided here are devised for a 1,200-calorie diet. At this calorie level, you'll eat a minimum of four servings each of vegetables and carbohydrates, and three servings each of fruits, protein and dairy, and fats. If your daily calorie goal is higher, you'll need to adjust the menus accordingly. See page 185.

Daily recommended servings

Vegetables (no limit)	●●●●
Fruits (no limit)	●●●
Carbohydrates	●●●●
Protein & Dairy (P/D)	●●●
Fats	●●●

DAY 2 MENU

Breakfast

2 slices whole-grain toast *Carbohydrates* ● ●
1½ tsp. peanut butter *Fat* ●
½ c. orange juice *Fruit* ●
Calorie-free beverage

Lunch

California burger *Vegetables* ●, *Carbohydrates* ● ●,
P/D ● ●, *Fat* ●
*Top 3 oz. cooked extra-lean ground beef patty with
½ grilled onion, lettuce and tomato slices. Serve on
a small whole-grain bun spread with 1 tbsp. reduced-
calorie mayonnaise.*
* 1 small apple *Fruit* ●
Calorie-free beverage

Dinner

3 oz. cod or other fish topped with salsa
P/D ●, *Vegetables* ●
* ¾ c. green beans *Vegetables* ●
* 1 c. cubed cantaloupe *Fruit* ●
Calorie-free beverage

Snack

* 4 celery sticks spread with 1½ tsp. peanut
butter *Vegetables* ●, *Fat* ●

* The serving size stated is the minimum amount.
Eat as much as you wish.

Dietitian's tips

■ The menu for Day 3 includes lentil soup. Lentils
are a type of legume. Legumes can be a healthy
substitute for meat in many recipes. For more on
legumes, see page 92. Here are suggestions to
help you select, store and serve legumes:

Select legumes with a deep, almost glossy
color. Dry-looking or faded legumes may have
been stored for a long time and not taste as fresh.

Look for legumes of a uniform size and condition. Similar-sized legumes cook more evenly.
Check that the legumes are free of mold and
aren't broken or cracked.

Place dried legumes away from heat, light and
moisture after purchase. They keep well for up to
one year in an airtight container.

Keep canned legumes such as beans in a cool,
dry place. They safely store for two to five years.

Sort and rinse legumes carefully before use.
Bags of legumes may include a few small stones,
fibers or misshapen or discolored items. Remove
these before cooking.

Soak most dried legumes before cooking. Beans
and other large, dried legumes require soaking in
room-temperature water overnight, a step that

rehydrates them for more even cooking. Split
peas and lentils require no soaking.

Use canned legumes for convenience. Rinse them
to remove any sodium added during processing.

■ Soup is a favorite meal. When you don't have
enough time to make your own, it's OK to use
canned or dried soups. To help keep calories in
check, add water or skim milk instead of whole
milk to soup concentrate. And select soups that
are loaded with vegetables.

■ The main ingredient in hummus is garbanzos, also
known as chickpeas. Commercially prepared varieties are nutritionally similar to homemade. They
often come seasoned in a variety of ways — scal-
lion, garlic, red pepper, dill.

■ According to the American Heart Association,
people may consume three to four egg yolks a
week and stay within cholesterol recommendations. This allows occasional "sunny-side up"
breakfasts. In recipes, in place of one whole egg
you can substitute two egg whites or the specified
amount of cholesterol-free egg substitute.

DAY 3 MENU

Breakfast

* ½ large grapefruit *Fruit* ●
  1 c. reduced-calorie, fat-free yogurt *P/D* ●
  Calorie-free beverage

Lunch

  1 c. canned lentil soup *P/D* ●
  10 baked tortilla chips *Carbohydrates* ●
* ¼ c. salsa *Vegetables* ●
* 1 c. grapes *Fruit* ●
  Calorie-free beverage

Dinner

  1 serving spring pasta salad *Vegetables* ● ● ●,
  Carbohydrates ● ●, *Fat* ●

  1 slice whole-grain bread *Carbohydrates* ●
  1 tsp. margarine *Fat* ●
  1 c. skim milk *P/D* ●
  Calorie-free beverage

Snack

* 1 serving favorite fruit *Fruit* ●
  ½ c. nondairy whipped topping *Fat* ●

* The serving size stated is the minimum amount.
  Eat as much as you wish.

recipe serves 6

Spring pasta salad

6 c. cooked pasta
1 tbsp. olive oil
¼ c. chicken broth
1 clove garlic, chopped
2 medium onions, chopped
1 28-oz. can tomatoes in juice
1 lb. mushrooms, sliced
1 red bell pepper, sliced
1 green bell pepper, sliced
2 medium zucchinis, shredded
½ tsp. basil
½ tsp. oregano
Several leaves of romaine lettuce

*The pasta can be any shape — elbows, spirals,
bow ties — or any color.*

■ Fill a large kettle with water and heat until boiling.
  Add the pasta and cook until al dente. Don't over-
  cook. Remove from heat and drain the pasta.
  Place pasta in a large bowl. Add the olive oil and
  toss. Set aside.
■ In a large skillet, add the chicken broth and heat.
  Add the garlic, onions and tomatoes. Cook until

the onions are transparent. Add the remaining
vegetables and cook for about 5 minutes or until
they're tender-crisp. Stir in the basil and oregano.
Pour over the pasta, mix and refrigerate. Serve on
a leaf of romaine lettuce.

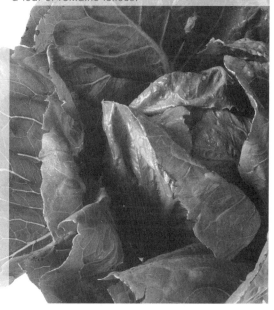

DAY 4 MENU

Breakfast

1 whole-grain English muffin *Carbohydrates* ● ●
1 tbsp. peanut butter *Fat* ● ●
1/2 c. orange juice *Fruit* ●
Calorie-free beverage

Lunch

Open-faced turkey sandwich *Carbohydrates* ●,
  P/D ● ●, *Fat* ●
*Spread 1 tbsp. reduced-calorie mayonnaise on a slice
of sourdough bread. Top with 3 oz. smoked turkey,
2 oz. low-fat Gouda cheese, 1 slice tomato and
chopped basil.*
* 2 c. carrots and celery sticks *Vegetables* ● ●
Calorie-free beverage

Dinner

1/4 recipe marinated flank steak *P/D* ●
*Place 6 oz. flank steak in plastic bag with 1/2 c. smoky
barbecue sauce. Refrigerate several hours. Grill steak
or sear on stove. Slice and top with barbecue sauce.*
3 baby red-skinned potatoes *Carbohydrates* ●
* 1 1/2 c. summer squash *Vegetables* ● ●
* 1 c. berries *Fruit* ●
Calorie-free beverage

Snack

* 1 serving favorite fruit *Fruit* ●

* The serving size stated is the minimum amount.
  Eat as much as you wish.

strategies

Your activity record

An activity record can be as simple or complex as a food record, depending on the kind of information you find useful. An example of an activity record is shown below. The example requires you to list different activities of the day, including household chores, hobbies, recreation and exercise, and the minutes involved in each. If you're using a pedometer, you can also record the number of steps you took. Total the minute column and step column at the end of the day. Compare these to the daily or weekly activity goals you've established for yourself.

If you're able to determine the number of calories burned per minute of activity, you can include that figure with your record. This information is not always available. A listing of calories burned during certain activities is shown on page A5 of the Visual Guide.

A blank copy of this activity record can be found on page 191. Photocopy the page and each week you can enter information on a different page in a similar manner to what's shown here.

Daily activity record

Activity	Minutes	Steps	Calories
House chores	15	1,200	
Gardening	30	500	
Walking	30	2,500	200
Miscellaneous		2,350	
Total	75	6,550	

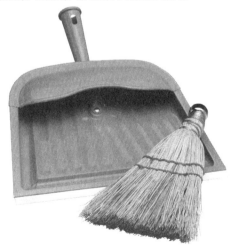

DAY 5 MENU

Breakfast

Omelet *Vegetables* ●, *P/D* ●
Mix ¹/₂ c. egg substitute with ¹/₂ c. diced onions, tomatoes, green peppers and mushrooms, and cook until set.
1 slice whole-grain toast *Carbohydrates* ●
1 tsp. margarine *Fat* ●
* 1 small banana *Fruit* ●
Calorie-free beverage

Lunch

1 whole-grain pita bread with hummus
    Carbohydrates ● ●, *P/D* ●, *Fat* ●
Combine ¹/₃ c. mashed garbanzos with 1 tsp. olive oil. Add garlic, cumin, lemon and parsley to taste.
* Cucumber and tomato salad *Vegetables* ● ●

Combine 1 c. thinly sliced cucumber and 8 cherry tomatoes, halved. Add balsamic, rice wine or herb-flavored vinegar to taste.
* 1 small pear *Fruit* ●
Calorie-free beverage

Dinner

3 oz. salmon or other fish *P/D* ●
Season with lemon juice and dill.
¹/₂ c. cooked pasta with 1 tsp. olive oil and
    black pepper *Carbohydrates* ●, *Fat* ●
* 1 c. steamed broccoli *Vegetables* ●
Calorie-free beverage

Snack

* 1 serving favorite fruit *Fruit* ●

* The serving size stated is the minimum amount. Eat as much as you wish.

strategies

Record-keeping tips

Your food record

■ Include an estimated amount of each item you eat. For each piece of fresh vegetable or fruit, note its approximate size (small, medium or large). For pasta, rice, cooked vegetables, soups, beverages, sauces and gravies, indicate the number of measuring cups or spoons. For baked goods, use approximate dimensions. For meat, poultry and fish, use approximate weight or size.

■ For mixed entrees such as casseroles, try to list the separate ingredients — or those greater than a teaspoon — and estimate the approximate amount of each. Refer to ingredient lists in recipes or on package labels, if available.

■ Pay attention to accompaniments such as spreads, gravies and condiments, such as ketchup, that may come with a food item. Accompaniments may have the most calories of anything you eat.

■ You may include the approximate time of day with each of your entries.

■ If known, include the method of preparation, such as fried, baked or broiled.

■ Include all beverages, including water, milk, juice and alcohol.

Your activity record

■ Indicate the total amount of time for each activity. Enter only those activities that last five minutes or longer.

■ Be aware of how intense an activity feels to you at the time you're doing it. Don't try to mentally re-create the experience later. Indicate the intensity of your activity on the record, such as slow, medium or fast.

■ Along with a small notebook, you may find it helpful to carry a watch or pedometer.

■ If you're walking or jogging, it helps to estimate the approximate distance you covered.

■ You may wish to include other information that you feel is important to your program, such as weather conditions, type of terrain or muscle and joint aches.

■ At the end of each day, compute the total amount of time you spent being physically active.

DAY 6 MENU

Breakfast

1 whole-grain English muffin *Carbohydrates* ● ●
3 tbsp. fat-free cream cheese *Fat* ●
* 1 medium apple *Fruit* ●
Calorie-free beverage

Lunch

Chicken Caesar salad *Vegetables* ●, *P/D* ●, *Fat* ●

Combine 2 c. romaine lettuce with 2½ oz. grilled boneless, skinless chicken breast strips, 2 tbsp. low-calorie Caesar dressing and 1 tbsp. seasoned croutons.

6 whole-grain crackers *Carbohydrates* ●
Calorie-free beverage

Dinner

1 serving turkey pot pie with baby vegetables *Vegetables* ● ●, *P/D* ● ●, *Carbohydrates* ●, *Fat* ●
* 1 c. mixed fruit *Fruit* ● ●
Calorie-free beverage

Snack

* 1 serving favorite vegetable *Vegetables* ●

* The serving size stated is the minimum amount. Eat as much as you wish.

recipe *serves 8*

Turkey pot pie with baby vegetables

10 baby carrots
1 c. pearl onions
⅓ lb. fresh white mushrooms
1¼ c. frozen artichoke hearts, thawed
¼ c. plus 2 tbsp. olive oil
1 tsp. dry mustard
¾ c. all-purpose (plain) flour
2½ c. chicken stock or broth
1 clove garlic, minced
2 lb. skinless, boneless turkey breast, diced
1 c. peas
1 tomato, seeded and diced
1 tbsp. each fresh chopped dill and basil
¼ c. low-fat sour cream
1½ tsp. salt
½ tsp. fresh ground pepper
½ c. cornmeal
1½ tsp. baking powder
¾ c. plain soy milk
1 tbsp. dark honey

■ Halve and slice carrots crosswise. Boil onions in water about 2 minutes, drain, and plunge in cold water. Cut root ends off onions, slip off the skins, and cut a shallow X in the root end of each. Clean and slice mushrooms. Quarter artichokes lengthwise. Set the vegetables aside.

■ In a large pan or Dutch oven, heat ¼ c. olive oil over low heat. Add mustard and ¼ c. of flour. Cook, whisking continuously for 1 to 2 minutes.

■ Add the stock, still whisking. Increase heat to medium-high, and bring to a boil. Add garlic, carrots and onions. Reduce to low heat. Cook until vegetables are softened, about 5 minutes. Add turkey, mushrooms, artichoke hearts, peas, tomato, dill and basil. Cover and simmer until turkey is opaque, about 10 minutes. Add sour cream and 1 tsp. salt and pepper. Place in a 9-by-13-inch baking dish and set aside.

■ Preheat oven to 425 F.

■ In a bowl, combine cornmeal, ½ c. flour, baking powder and ½ tsp. salt. In another bowl, mix soy milk, 2 tbsp. olive oil and honey. Stir in dry ingredients

■ Pour batter over turkey mixture. Bake, uncovered, about 40 minutes. Let stand 10 minutes. Serve.

This recipe is one of 150 recipes collected in "The New Mayo Clinic Cookbook," published by Mayo Clinic Health Information and Oxmoor House and available in bookstores.

WEEK 3

DAY 7 MENU

Breakfast
1 egg fried in nonstick pan *P/D* ●
1 slice whole-grain bread *Carbohydrates* ●
1 tsp. margarine *Fat* ●
* 1 small banana *Fruit* ●
Calorie-free beverage

Lunch
Tuna salad *Vegetables* ●, *P/D* ●, *Fat* ●
Combine 1 c. mixed greens with ½ c. sliced tomatoes, cucumbers, zucchini, bell peppers and onions. Top with 3 oz. tuna mixed with 1 tbsp. reduced-calorie mayonnaise.
* 1 medium apple *Fruit* ●
Calorie-free beverage

Dinner
1 serving hearty grain-filled peppers
Vegetables ● ● ●, *Carbohydrates* ● ● ●
(See recipe on page A12.)
* 1 c. grapes *Fruit* ●
½ c. fat-free frozen yogurt *P/D* ●
Calorie-free beverage

Snack
9 large olives *Fat* ●

* The serving size stated is the minimum amount. Eat as much as you wish.

strategies

How to use a pedometer

A pedometer is a device that tracks the number of steps you take. The small device is designed to be worn at the waist, directly over the hipbone, in order to sense your body's movement. More sophisticated models convert steps into miles or estimate the number of calories you burn.

Before you can use your pedometer, you may need to determine what's called your stride length, which varies greatly from person to person. Stride length is the distance from the heel of your back foot to the heel of your front foot in a typical step.

One way to calculate stride length is to mark off a 10-foot distance on a floor or sidewalk. Count the number of steps it takes for you to cover that distance at your normal pace. Divide 10 feet by the number of steps you've counted, and that's your stride length. For example, if it took four steps for you to cover 10 feet, your stride length would be approximately 2½ feet. Program your stride length into the pedometer.

Use the pedometer each day for about one week to establish a baseline for your activity level. Attach the pedometer to your clothing at about waist level when you get dressed in the morning and, if possible, leave it there for the entire day. At night, record the number of steps you've taken.

Experts recommend that you aim for 10,000 steps a day. That's about five miles if 2,000 steps equals one mile. If 10,000 steps seem too much for you, it's OK to set a lower goal. Everyone's ability and situation is different. One option might be to add 2,000 or 3,000 extra steps to your average daily total. For example, if 5,000 steps is currently your average daily total, aim to make 7,000 steps your daily goal.

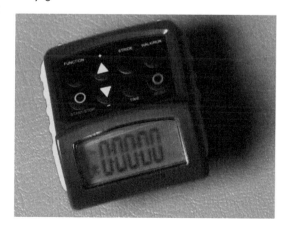

Week 4

Eating healthy

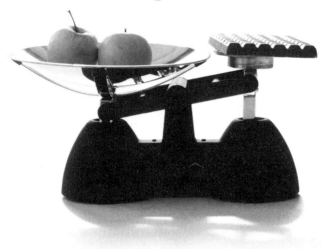

Three distinct but closely related concepts underlie a healthy diet: variety, balance and moderation. A diet that includes a variety of foods is a source for all of the approximately 40 nutrients your body needs to develop and function properly. A diet that's balanced ensures that you get adequate amounts of these nutrients. Eating in moderation means you're not overeating and contributing to weight gain.

Important steps that you can take to help make sure you get a varied, balanced and moderate diet include:

- Eating plenty of fruits, vegetables and whole grains
- Including fish on a regular basis
- Reducing saturated fat and cholesterol
- Limiting sugar and salt
- Drinking alcoholic beverages in moderation, if at all
- Eating moderate-sized portions

The Mayo Clinic Healthy Weight Pyramid offers nutritional guidelines for a healthy diet, based on the principles of variety, balance and moderation (see page A2 of the Visual Guide). The sections of the pyramid represent six food groups: vegetables, fruits, carbohydrates, protein and dairy, fats, and sweets. The bigger the pyramid section, the more servings of foods from that group you'll want to include in your meals.

To plan a menu, start at the pyramid's wide base with ample servings of vegetables and fruits. Moving up the pyramid, include plenty of whole-grain carbohydrates, then add smaller portions of lean protein, low-fat dairy and fats. The small block at the tip of the pyramid represents sweets, which you should eat sparingly. And remember to include daily physical activity, as indicated on the pyramid.

Are you eating well?

Are your current food choices providing you with a varied, balanced and moderate diet? Answer the 10 questions below and note your responses.

1. How many servings of vegetables do you eat in a typical day?
   (A serving is, for example, 2 cups of leafy greens or 1 cup of broccoli florets.)
   a. Four or more
   b. Two or three
   c. One or none

2. How many servings of fruit do you eat in a typical day?
   (A serving is typically one small piece of fruit.)
   a. Three or more
   b. Two
   c. One

3. How often does fish appear on your weekly menu?
   a. Two or more times
   b. Once
   c. Rarely or never

4. When you shop for bread, pasta and rice, how often do you buy the whole-grain versions?
   a. Always
   b. Sometimes
   c. Rarely or never

5. Which of the following are you most likely to use?
   a. Canola or olive oil
   b. Corn oil
   c. Butter or margarine

6. How often in a typical week do you eat hamburgers, cheese-rich pizzas, or sandwiches with lots of meat and cheese?
   a. Not more than once
   b. Two or three times
   c. Four or more times

7. Two cups of cooked pasta is how many carbohydrate servings?
   a. Four
   b. Not sure
   c. One

8. What kind of milk do you usually drink?
   a. Fat-free milk or soy milk
   b. 1 percent or 2 percent
   c. Whole milk or none

9. What are you most likely to reach for when you're thirsty?
   a. Water
   b. Fruit juice
   c. Regular sweetened soda

10. What's your usual snack?
    a. Nuts, fruit, or carrot or celery sticks
    b. Energy bars or other "healthy" sweets
    c. Potato chips, pretzels or cookies

Evaluating your eating habits

- If you count mostly **a's** among your answers, congratulations! You're well on your way to healthy eating.

- If you count mostly **b's** and **c's,** your menu could use a tuneup. You'll find plenty of tips and menu ideas in this book.

- If you answered with mostly **c's,** it's time for some fresh ideas about good food.

WEEK 4

Week 4 shopping list

This shopping list includes many of the fresh ingredients and general grocery items you'll need on hand for the Week 4 menus. It does not include the kitchen staples listed on page 187 — make sure you have them in stock. If you replace any of the recipes with a selection of your own, you'll need to adjust the shopping list.

Fresh vegetables	QTY
❑ bell peppers, green	_____
❑ broccoli	_____
❑ celery	_____
❑ cucumbers	_____
❑ green beans	_____
❑ green peas	_____
❑ jalapeno pepper	_____
❑ lettuce or mixed greens	_____
❑ onions, green, red and yellow	_____
❑ spinach, raw	_____

	QTY
❑ summer squash	_____
❑ tomatoes	_____
❑ tomatoes, cherry	_____
❑ zucchini	_____
❑ favorite or seasonal vegetables	_____

Fresh herbs

❑ cilantro	_____
❑ garlic	_____
❑ parsley	_____
❑ thyme	_____

Fresh fruits	
❑ apples	_____
❑ bananas	_____
❑ berries	_____
❑ cantaloupe	_____
❑ grapefruit	_____

❑ grapes	_____
❑ lemons	_____
❑ oranges	_____
❑ pears	_____
❑ favorite or seasonal fruits	_____

Carbohydrates	
❑ bagels, whole-grain	_____
❑ bread, whole-grain	_____
❑ pita bread, whole-grain	_____

❑ potatoes, baby, red-skinned	_____
❑ potatoes, baking	_____
❑ roll, whole-grain	_____

Protein & dairy	
❑ chicken breast, boneless, skinless	_____
❑ egg	_____
❑ egg substitute	_____
❑ flank steak	_____
❑ pork roast, lean	_____

❑ roast beef, lean, sliced	_____
❑ trout or other fish fillet	_____
❑ turkey, smoked, shredded	_____
❑ milk, skim	_____
❑ yogurt, fat-free, reduced-calorie	_____

Fats	
❑ avocado	_____
❑ cream cheese, fat-free	_____

❑ sour cream, fat-free	_____
❑ whipped topping, nondairy	_____

General groceries	
❑ corn, frozen	_____
❑ green peas, frozen	_____
❑ mandarin oranges	_____
❑ orange juice	_____
❑ pickles	_____
❑ pinto beans or black beans	_____

❑ popcorn, low-fat, microwave	_____
❑ salsa	_____
❑ soup, vegetable	_____
❑ tuna, water-packed	_____
❑ water chestnuts	_____

DAY 1 MENU

Breakfast
1 whole-grain bagel *Carbohydrates* ● ●
3 tbsp. fat-free cream cheese *Fat* ●
* 1 medium orange *Fruit* ●
Calorie-free beverage

Lunch
Smoked turkey wrap *Carbohydrates* ●, *P/D* ●,
Fat ●
Top 6-inch tortilla with 3 oz. thin-sliced smoked turkey, shredded lettuce, sliced tomato and onion. Top with 2 tbsp. reduced-calorie Western dressing and roll up.
* Cucumber and tomato salad *Vegetables* ● ●
Combine 1 c. thinly sliced cucumber and 8 cherry tomatoes, halved. Add balsamic, rice wine or herb-flavored vinegar to taste.

* 1 small apple *Fruit* ●
Calorie-free beverage

Dinner
3 oz. marinated, broiled flank steak *P/D* ● ●
Marinate in salsa or other tomato-style sauce.
1/2 medium baked potato *Carbohydrates* ●
3 tbsp. fat-free sour cream *Fat* ●
* 1 1/2 c. green beans *Vegetables* ● ●
* 1/4 small cantaloupe *Fruit* ●
Calorie-free beverage

Snack
* 1 serving favorite vegetable *Vegetables* ●

* The serving size stated is the minimum amount. Eat as much as you wish.

goals

Week 4

You can adapt this week's goals or substitute different goals that are more to your liking. When you meet a goal, check the corresponding box.

❏ **Follow pyramid recommendations.** Try to meet the number of food servings recommended by the Mayo Clinic Healthy Weight Pyramid for your daily calorie goal (see page A3 of the Visual Guide). Remember that the servings indicated for fresh vegetables and fruits are minimums — include more if you still feel hungry. A critical self-evaluation of your current diet — and the number of servings from each food group — may alert you to eating patterns that need adjustment.
❏ **Choose healthy strategies.** Try to incorporate one or more healthy-eating strategies into your daily routine. Use strategies in this unit or create some of your own. Many small changes can sometimes provide the most lasting benefits.
❏ **Update your weight record.** Weigh in and record the number of pounds gained or lost on the weight record. Remember that gradual weight loss of 1 or 2 pounds a week is the healthiest weight loss.

❏ **Use Week 4's Healthy Weight menu.** Try to follow the suggested menu in this week's unit. These menus are devised for a 1,200-calorie-a-day diet. At this calorie level, you'll eat a minimum of four servings each of vegetables and carbohydrates, and three servings each of fruits, protein and dairy, and fats. If your calorie goal varies from the 1,200-calorie level, you'll need to adjust the menus accordingly. See page 185.

Daily recommended servings

Vegetables (no limit)	● ● ● ●
Fruits (no limit)	● ● ●
Carbohydrates	● ● ● ●
Protein & Dairy (P/D)	● ● ●
Fats	● ● ●

DAY 2 MENU

Breakfast
   1 whole-grain bagel *Carbohydrates* ● ●
   3 tbsp. fat-free cream cheese *Fat* ●
* 1 small apple *Fruit* ●
   1 c. skim milk *P/D* ●
   Calorie-free beverage

Lunch
   1 c. vegetable soup *Vegetables* ●
* 2 c. lettuce *Vegetables* ●
   1 tbsp. reduced-calorie salad dressing *Fat* ●
   1 c. reduced-calorie, fat-free yogurt mixed with
      1 c. berries *P/D* ●, *Fruit* ●
   Calorie-free beverage

Dinner
   2½ oz. chicken breast, boneless, skinless
      P/D ●
   3 red-skinned baby potatoes with fresh parsley
      Carbohydrates ●
* 2 c. steamed broccoli *Vegetables* ● ●
   1 tsp. margarine *Fat* ●
* 1 small pear *Fruit* ●
   Calorie-free beverage

Snack
   2 c. low-fat microwave popcorn *Carbohydrates* ●

* The serving size stated is the minimum amount.
   Eat as much as you wish.

Dietitian's tips

- Vary your salad greens to take advantage of the multitude of flavors and textures. There are four basic types. Head lettuce (iceberg) has a crisp texture and mild flavor. Butterhead (Boston or bibb) lettuce is delicate in texture and flavor. Loose-leaf lettuce (oak-leaf, red-leaf or green-leaf) has easily separated leaves that are flavorful and crisp. Romaine (cos) lettuce has a crunchy texture and somewhat bitter taste. Purchase a different variety each week.

- Don't be fooled into thinking "low-calorie" dressings are really low in calories. Most aren't. According to labeling laws, a "low-calorie" salad dressing may have up to 40 calories per serving. When possible, choose "fat-free" salad dressings. They generally have 25 calories or less per serving.

- "Salsa" is the Spanish word for "sauce." Salsas can be mild, fruity or scorching, smooth or chunky. Salsa isn't only for chips. Try it on potatoes, vegetables, and as a topping for fish, chicken or meats.

- Peppers — there are hundreds of varieties — vary from mild and sweet to mouth-blistering. The heat comes from the pepper's capsaicin, which is found in its seeds and membranes. Here's the order of peppers from mild to hot: bell peppers (mild and sweet), Anaheim, poblano, jalapeno, serrano, Tabasco, habanero (fire). Chipotle peppers are smoked jalapeno peppers.

- Marinades are seasoned liquids used to add flavor and to tenderize foods. Because most marinades contain an acidic ingredient (juice, vinegar, wine), it's important to not marinate foods too long. The acid can break down the food and make it mushy. Most vegetables and fish require shorter amounts of marinade time — 30 minutes to an hour — whereas large cuts of meat can be marinated up to 8 hours.

Getting enough calcium
The Mayo Clinic Healthy Weight Program should provide you with adequate intake of calcium. However, if you're worried that you're not getting enough, or if you have a health condition that requires optimal levels of calcium, you might want to take a daily calcium supplement. If you're unsure whether you're getting adequate calcium, talk with your doctor or a dietitian.

DAY 3 MENU

Breakfast
1 c. reduced-calorie, fat-free yogurt *P/D* ●
* 1 small banana *Fruit* ●
Calorie-free beverage

Lunch
Mixed green salad *Vegetables* ● ●
*Combine 2 c. spring mix greens with 1/2 sliced
tomato, 1/2 sliced cucumber and red onion.*
2 tbsp. reduced-calorie French dressing *Fat* ●
* 1 small apple *Fruit* ●
1 c. skim milk *P/D* ●
Calorie-free beverage

Dinner
1 serving soft taco with Southwestern vegetables
Vegetables ● ●, *Carbohydrates* ● ● ● ●, *P/D* ●,
Fat ●
* 1 c. berries *Fruit* ●
Calorie-free beverage

Snack
7 smokey almonds *Fat* ●

* The serving size stated is the minimum amount.
Eat as much as you wish.

recipe serves 4

Soft taco with Southwestern vegetables

1 tbsp. olive oil
1 medium red onion, chopped
1 c. diced yellow summer squash
1 c. diced green zucchini
3 large garlic cloves, minced
4 medium tomatoes, seeded and chopped
1 jalapeno pepper, seeded and chopped
1 c. corn, frozen
1/2 c. fresh cilantro, chopped
1 c. canned pinto or black beans, rinsed
4 8-in. fat-free tortillas
1/2 c. salsa

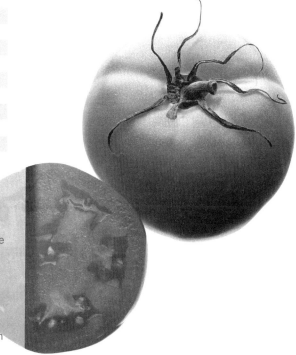

- Heat oil in large skillet; add onion and cook
until tender. Add squash and zucchini, stir and
continue cooking about 5 minutes. Add garlic,
half of the tomatoes and all of the pepper. Reduce
heat to medium-low and cook until flavorful.
Add corn kernels; stir and cook until kernels are
tender-crisp. Add the cilantro, the remaining
tomatoes and beans. Stir together and remove
from heat.
- Warm the tortillas on a hot, dry skillet. Fill each with
the vegetable mixture. Top with salsa and serve.

DAY 4 MENU

Breakfast

1 c. whole-grain breakfast cereal
  Carbohydrates ● ●
1 c. skim milk *P/D* ●
* 1 medium orange *Fruit* ●
Calorie-free beverage

Lunch

Grilled chicken salad *Vegetables* ● ●, *P/D* ●,
  Fat ●

Combine 2 c. mixed greens with 2½ oz. grilled boneless, skinless chicken breast and 1 c. sliced tomatoes,
bell peppers and chopped green onions. Top with 1
tsp. extra-virgin olive oil mixed with 2 tbsp. red wine
vinegar. Sprinkle with cracked black pepper.
* 1 small pear *Fruit* ●
Calorie-free beverage

Dinner

3 oz. grilled tuna or other fish *P/D* ●
  Sprinkle with lemon juice and basil.
2/3 c. cooked brown rice *Carbohydrates* ● ●
* 1½ c. steamed summer squash and zucchini
  Vegetables ● ●
1 tsp. margarine *Fat* ●
* 1 c. grapes *Fruit* ●
Calorie-free beverage

Snack

8 whole peanuts *Fat* ●

* The serving size stated is the minimum amount.
  Eat as much as you wish.

strategies

10 practical steps to healthier eating

*You don't need to turn your life upside down to eat for
better health. A few simple changes can make a big
difference in the nutritional value of your daily meals.*

1. Have at least one serving of fruit at each meal
   or one as a snack during the day.
2. Try to include at least two servings of vegetables
   at lunch and at dinner.
3. Switch from low-fiber breakfast cereal to lower
   sugar, higher fiber alternatives.
4. Choose coarse whole-grain breads, switch to
   brown rice instead of white, and when baking,
   experiment with whole-wheat flour.
5. Lighten your milk by moving down one step in
   fat content — from whole to 2 percent, for
   instance, or from 1 percent to fat-free.
6. Whenever you can, cook with olive, canola
   or another vegetable oil instead of butter or
   margarine.
7. Flavor foods with herbs and spices rather than
   sauces and gravies.
8. Have fish at least twice a week.
9. Serve fresh fruit for dessert.
10. Limit high-calorie sweetened beverages.

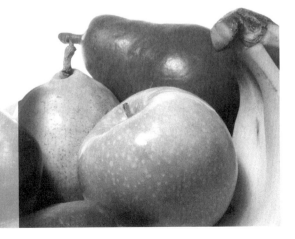

WEEK 4

DAY 5 MENU

Breakfast

1 c. whole-grain breakfast cereal
  Carbohydrates ● ●
1 c. skim milk *P/D* ●
* ½ large grapefruit *Fruit* ●
Calorie-free beverage

Lunch

Spinach fruit salad *Fruit* ●, *Vegetables* ● ●
*Top 2 c. baby spinach leaves with ½ c. green
pepper strips and water chestnuts and ½ c. mandarin
orange sections.*
2 tbsp. reduced-calorie French dressing *Fat* ●
6 whole-grain crackers *Carbohydrates* ●
1 c. skim milk *P/D* ●
Calorie-free beverage

Dinner

2 oz. lean pork *P/D* ●
½ c. wild rice *Carbohydrates* ●
* ½ c. green peas *Vegetables* ● ●
1 tsp. margarine *Fat* ●
Calorie-free beverage

Snack

* 1 c. berries *Fruit* ●
½ c. nondairy whipped topping *Fat* ●

* The serving size stated is the minimum amount.
  Eat as much as you wish.

strategies

Adjusting your daily calorie goal

The Mayo Clinic Healthy Weight Pyramid is not a
rigid program that dictates what people must eat
every day. The pyramid is a flexible tool that you
use to personalize a weight program and to guide
your food choices. It can assist people with different
physical characteristics, activity levels, health risks
and calorie goals to eat healthier.

To maintain a healthy weight, most adults typically
eat between 1,600 and 2,400 calories a day. To
lose weight at a healthy rate, it's recommended that
most women start with a 1,200 daily calorie goal
and most men start with a 1,400 daily calorie goal.
The table on page 185 indicates how many servings you'll need from each food group in order to
meet a specific calorie goal.

The daily menus of the Healthy Weight Program
are based on 1,200 calories. They'll provide you
with minimums of 4 vegetable servings and 3 fruit
servings, along with 4 carbohydrate servings, 3 protein and dairy servings, and 3 fat servings every
day. Your calorie goal won't be affected when you
substitute other foods or recipes into the suggested
menus, so long as you meet the overall servings total
from each food group. If you're at a higher calorie

level, adjust the menus to match the servings totals
indicated on the table. Don't hesitate to experiment
and to personalize the menus to suit your tastes.

You also have some flexibility to adjust the servings totals from day to day. For example, there's no
limit on the number of servings you can eat from
vegetables and fruits (but not fruit juice and dried
fruits). Rather than restricting sweets consumption to
only a small amount each day, you can eat a
dessert on one day and then skip sweets entirely for
several following days. Use good discretion and
don't get too hung up on the daily totals.

Of course, your servings totals may also be affected by how active you are from day to day. An afternoon of strenuous exercise obviously burns more
calories than the same amount of time spent sitting
in an office chair. You can slightly adjust the daily
servings, depending on whether you're meeting your
weight goals and on how full you feel — although
it's best if the extra servings come from the vegetable and fruit groups. Remember that if you're feeling too hungry or you've reached your target
weight, you can adjust your calorie goal up to the
next higher level.

DAY 6 MENU

Breakfast
1 egg, fried in nonstick pan *P/D* ●
1 slice whole-grain toast *Carbohydrates* ●
1 tsp. margarine *Fat* ●
1/2 c. orange juice *Fruit* ●
Calorie-free beverage

Lunch
Roast beef sandwich *Carbohydrates* ● ●, *P/D* ●,
   Vegetables ●
*Fill 1 whole-grain roll with 1 1/2 oz. sliced lean roast
beef, Dijon mustard, lettuce, tomato and red
onion slices.*
* 1 c. grapes *Fruit* ●
Calorie-free beverage

Dinner
1 serving broiled trout with tomato and red
   onion relish *Vegetables* ● ●, *P/D* ●
1/2 medium baked potato *Carbohydrates* ●
1 tsp. margarine *Fat* ●
* 2 c. mixed greens *Vegetables* ●
2 tbsp. reduced-calorie salad dressing *Fat* ●
Calorie-free beverage

Snack
* 1 serving favorite fruit *Fruit* ●

* The serving size stated is the minimum amount.
  Eat as much as you wish.

recipe *serves 4*

Broiled trout with tomato and red onion relish

3 c. cherry tomatoes, halved
1 tsp. olive oil
1/4 c. red onion, chopped
1/4 c. balsamic vinegar
1 tsp. light molasses
1 tbsp. grated lemon zest
1 tbsp. chopped fresh flat-leaf (Italian) parsley
1/2 tsp. salt
1/4 tsp. freshly ground pepper
1 tsp. fresh thyme, chopped
4 trout fillets, 5 oz. each

- Preheat the broiler. Position the rack 4 inches from the heat source.
- Arrange the tomatoes cut-side down on a baking sheet lined with aluminum foil or parchment (baking) paper. Broil until the skins wrinkle and begin to brown, about 5 minutes. Set aside and leave the broiler on.
- In a frying pan, heat the olive oil over medium-high heat. Add the onion and sauté until soft and translucent, about 4 minutes. Add the vinegar and molasses and bring to a boil. Reduce the heat to medium and simmer until slightly reduced, about

2 minutes. Add the broiled tomatoes, lemon zest, parsley, 1/4 tsp. of the salt, and the pepper. Stir to combine. Remove from heat, set aside and keep warm.

- Lightly coat a broiler pan with olive oil cooking spray. Sprinkle the thyme and the remaining 1/4 tsp. salt over the fillets and place on the prepared pan. Broil until the fish is opaque throughout when tested with the tip of a knife, about 5 minutes. Transfer to warmed individual plates and serve topped with warm tomato relish.

This recipe is one of 150 recipes collected in "The New Mayo Clinic Cookbook," published by Mayo Clinic Health Information and Oxmoor House and available in bookstores in the United states and Canada.

DAY 7 MENU

Breakfast

1 breakfast burrito *Vegetables* ●,
  Carbohydrates ● ●, *P/D* ●
Sauté ½ c. chopped tomato, 2 tbsp. chopped onion, ¼ c. canned corn and some of its liquid. Add ¼ c. egg substitute and scramble with vegetables. Spread on a fat-free tortilla, roll up, top with 2 tbsp. salsa.
* 1 medium orange *Fruit* ●
Calorie-free beverage

Lunch

Turkey pita sandwich *Carbohydrates* ●, *P/D* ●,
  Vegetables ●, *Fat* ●
Top ½ whole-grain pita with 3 oz. shredded turkey, ⅙ avocado, chopped lettuce, tomato and onion.
* 1 small apple *Fruit* ●
Calorie-free beverage

review

Week 4

You're now completing the fourth week of your Healthy Weight Program. How is it going so far? As you work through the program, it's good to step back and assess how you're doing.

- **Evaluating your progress.** Review your weight record over the first four weeks of the Healthy Weight Program. Have you been able to establish a regular schedule for weigh-ins? Do you look forward to the weigh-ins or regard them with just a little anxiety? Remember that the scale is not your enemy — it's a tool to help control your weight. It's best to focus on long-term trends and not on the day-to-day weight fluctuations. With the Healthy Weight Program, you should expect to lose between 4 and 8 pounds after four weeks. The fact that you've stayed with the program this long is an important achievement in itself.
- **Bringing it all together.** Topics covered in the previous three weeks are important elements for your understanding and use of the Mayo Clinic Healthy Weight Pyramid in your weight program. Take time to review what you've learned so far and consider how the information interrelates.

Dinner

Tuna-stuffed tomato *P/D* ●, *Vegetables* ●, *Fat* ● ●
Mix 3 oz. water-packed tuna (drained) with 2 tsp. reduced-calorie mayonnaise. Season with black pepper and a bit of chopped pickle, if desired. Core and partially quarter a tomato. Stuff it with tuna mixture.
* 4 medium celery sticks *Vegetables* ●
6 wheat crackers *Carbohydrates* ●
Calorie-free beverage

Snack

* 1 serving favorite fruit *Fruit* ●

* The serving size stated is the minimum amount. Eat as much as you wish.

Knowledge of serving sizes guides your choices from the six food groups and helps you meet your daily calorie goal. Record keeping allows you to compare and analyze eating behaviors based on the pyramid and to identify problem situations. Weighing in can indicate how well you're following the pyramid guidelines, along with tracking your progress to your weight goal.

- **Looking forward.** The weekly topics so far may have emphasized diet more than physical activity. But note that a location for physical activity is placed in the center of the Healthy Weight Pyramid — indicating the central role it plays in weight control. Already in Week 1 you were instructed to get more active and to start walking regularly. Hopefully, over these past weeks, you've been able to move more and gradually increase the intensity of your walks. Week 5 will focus on adding more physical activity to your day.

Week 5

Physical activity

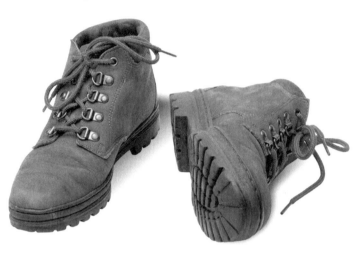

Being physically active is one of the most important steps you can take to maintain your weight, health and independence, regardless of your age or size. Regular physical activity is what helps you reach your weight goal and then keep off the pounds you lose. The best thing is, being active can be simple and convenient — not something you have to prepare, wait or pay for. You can be physically active anytime and anywhere.

Physical activity refers to any movement of your body that burns calories. Cleaning the house, making the bed, shopping, mowing the lawn, walking, gardening, swimming, dancing and playing a pickup game of basketball — these are all forms of physical activity. Experts recommend that you include at least 30 to 60 minutes of moderately intense physical activity into your routine every day.

The term *intensity* refers to how hard your body is working. You benefit most from physical activity that's performed at a moderately intense level.

So, what's moderate intensity? It's not easy to define in absolute terms. For an activity to be of moderate intensity you should be able to feel the exertion on your body, for example, an increased heart rate and breathing rate, and slight perspiration. But you shouldn't feel pain or discomfort. However, what's moderately intense for you might be too intense or not intense enough for the next person, depending on his or her level of fitness, physical health and commitment.

To learn more about gauging the intensity of physical activity, read Chapter 6. If you haven't been physically active, start at a low intensity level and gradually work your way up to a moderate level.

How active is your day?

Doctors recommend that you try to move and be physically active every day to stay healthy and control your weight. The questions below can help you assess your overall activity level.

1. How many days a week do you perform at least 15 minutes of physical work, such as housecleaning, yardwork, animal care or manual labor on the job?
   a. Five to seven days
   b. Three to four days
   c. One to two days
   d. None

2. How many days a week do you participate in at least 15 minutes of exercise, such as brisk walking, jogging, swimming, biking, stretching exercises, strength training and team sports?
   a. Five to seven days
   b. Three to four days
   c. One to two days
   d. None

3. Approximately how many minutes each day do you walk? This would include doing neighborhood errands, walking from your car to the store or office, exercising the dog, and going up and down stairs.
   a. More than 30 minutes
   b. 16 to 30 minutes
   c. 10 to 15 minutes
   d. Less than 10 minutes

4. Do you generally get up to stretch your legs and move around after you've been seated for an hour or more while at work or at leisure?
   a. Yes
   b. No

5. Do you have a medical condition that prevents you from being active or interferes in your enjoyment of exercise?
   a. No
   b. Yes

Evaluating your activity level

- If your responses to questions 1 to 3 were mainly **a** or **b** and you answered **a** to questions 4 and 5, you're already at a good activity level. Way to go!

- If your responses to questions 1 to 3 were mainly **c** or **d** and you answered **b** to questions 4 and 5, you'll need to work on increasing your activity level. Think about ways you can move just a few minutes more each day.

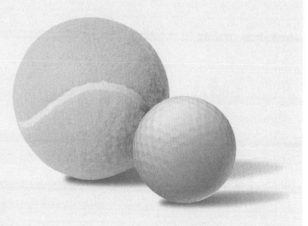

Week 5 shopping list

This shopping list includes many of the fresh ingredients and general grocery items you'll need on hand for the Week 5 menus. It does not include the kitchen staples listed on page 187 — make sure you have them in stock. If you replace any of the recipes with a selection of your own, you'll need to adjust the shopping list.

Fresh vegetables	QTY		QTY
❏ asparagus spears	_____	❏ onions, green	_____
❏ bell peppers	_____	❏ onions, pearl, red and yellow	_____
❏ broccoli	_____	❏ pepperoncini peppers	_____
❏ carrots	_____	❏ shallots	_____
❏ carrots, baby	_____	❏ tomatoes, regular and cherry	_____
❏ cauliflower	_____	❏ favorite or seasonal vegetables	_____
❏ cucumbers	_____		
❏ green beans	_____	*Fresh herbs*	
❏ lettuce or mixed greens	_____	❏ chives	_____
❏ mushrooms	_____	❏ garlic	_____
		❏ thyme	_____

Fresh fruits	QTY		QTY
❏ apples	_____	❏ grapefruit	_____
❏ bananas	_____	❏ pears	_____
❏ blueberries	_____	❏ favorite or seasonal fruit	_____

Carbohydrates	QTY		QTY
❏ bagels, whole-grain	_____	❏ muffin, small, any flavor	_____
❏ bread, whole-grain	_____	❏ potatoes, Yukon gold, baking	_____
❏ hamburger buns, whole-grain	_____	❏ potatoes, red-skinned, baby	_____

Protein & dairy	QTY		QTY
❏ chicken breast, boneless, skinless	_____	❏ shrimp, large or other fish fillet	_____
❏ chicken legs	_____	❏ turkey, smoked, sliced	_____
❏ chicken thighs, skinless	_____	❏ cheese, feta, crumbled	_____
❏ ground beef, extra-lean	_____	❏ cheese, Parmesan, grated	_____
❏ ham, lean, sliced	_____	❏ cottage cheese, low-fat	_____
❏ round steak	_____	❏ milk, skim	_____
❏ sea scallops	_____	❏ yogurt, reduced-calorie, fat-free	_____

Fats	QTY		QTY
❏ olives, kalamata	_____	❏ vegetable dip, reduced-calorie	_____
❏ sour cream, fat-free	_____		

General groceries	QTY		QTY
❏ anchovy paste	_____	❏ mandarin orange sections	_____
❏ cranberry sauce	_____	❏ pineapple rings	_____
❏ lemon juice	_____	❏ tofu, silken or soft	_____
❏ lemon zest	_____		

WEEK 5

DAY 1 MENU

Breakfast

Blueberry pancake *Fruit ●, Carbohydrates ●*
*Top a 4-inch-diameter pancake with ³/₄ c. blueberries
and 1¹/₂ tbsp. syrup.*
1 c. skim milk *P/D ●*
Calorie-free beverage

Lunch

1 serving dilled pasta salad with spring
vegetables *Vegetables ●, Carbohydrates ● ●,
Fat ●* (See the recipe on page 196.)
* 1 small apple *Fruit ●*
Calorie-free beverage

Dinner

Rosemary chicken *P/D ● ●, Fat ●*
*Brush 5 oz. boneless, skinless chicken breast with
1 tsp. each olive oil, lemon juice and rosemary. Grill
or bake.*
¹/₂ medium baked potato *Carbohydrates ●*
3 tbsp. fat-free sour cream *Fat ●*
* 2 c. steamed cauliflower *Vegetables ● ●*
* 2 pineapple rings *Fruit ●*
Calorie-free beverage

Snack

* 1 serving favorite vegetable *Vegetables ●*

* The serving size stated is the minimum amount.
Eat as much as you wish.

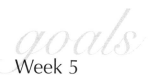

Week 5

*You can adapt this week's goals or substitute differ-
ent goals that are more to your liking. When you
meet a goal, check the corresponding box.*

❏ **Plan a walking program.** Devise a week-by-week
program that gradually increases the frequency,
duration and intensity of your walks over several
months. The example of a 12-week walking program on page 61 may help you. With a good
plan, you'll reach your goal of at least 30 minutes
of walking each day before you know it.
❏ **Gauge the intensity level of your activity.** Try to
apply the principles of the perceived exertion
scale (see pages 60-61) while you're involved in
various activities. Determine a level of intensity
that you consider moderate, based on a combination of the physical sensations you experience,
including heart rate, breathing rate, perspiration
and muscle fatigue.
❏ **Get more physically active.** Choose one or more
strategies to get more active — either from the
lists provided on pages 198 and 238 or from a
strategy of your own — and work at further
increasing the amount of activity in your day.

❏ **Update your Weight Record.** Weigh in and record
the number of pounds gained or lost on the
Weight Record. Remember that gradual weight
loss of 1 or 2 pounds a week is the healthiest.
❏ **Use Week 5's Healthy Weight menu.** Try to follow
the suggested menus in this week's unit. These
menus are devised for a 1,200-calorie-a-day diet.
Remember that there are no restrictions on your
vegetables and fruits servings. If your calorie goal
varies from the 1,200-calorie level, you'll need to
adjust the menus accordingly. See page 185.

Daily recommended servings

Vegetables (no limit)	● ● ● ●
Fruits (no limit)	● ● ●
Carbohydrates	● ● ● ●
Protein & Dairy (P/D)	● ● ●
Fats	● ● ●

DAY 2 MENU

Breakfast

1 slice whole-grain toast *Carbohydrates* ●
1½ tbsp. jam
* 1 large grapefruit *Fruit* ●●
Calorie-free beverage

Lunch

California burger *Vegetables* ●, *Carbohydrates* ●●,
P/D ●●, *Fat* ●

Top 3 oz. cooked extra-lean ground beef patty with ½
grilled onion, lettuce and tomato slices. Serve on a
small whole-grain bun spread with 1 tbsp. reduced-
calorie mayonnaise.
* 1 small apple *Fruit* ●
Calorie-free beverage

Dinner

1 serving Greek salad *Vegetables* ●●, *P/D* ●,
Fat ●
6 whole-grain crackers *Carbohydrates* ●
Calorie-free beverage

Snack

1 serving favorite vegetable dipped in 3 tbsp.
fat-free sour cream *Vegetables* ●, *Fat* ●

* The serving size stated is the minimum amount.
Eat as much as you wish.

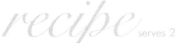 *recipe* serves 2

Greek salad

4 c. red and green leaf lettuce
½ c. diced cucumber
½ c. diced sweet (bell) pepper
½ c. diced carrots
½ c. crumbled feta cheese
2 slices red onion
4 pitted kalamata olives
4 pepperoncini peppers

- Place 2 c. of the mixed lettuce on separate plates.
- Dice the cucumber, sweet pepper and carrots.
  Toss each plate of greens with ¼ c. of the diced
  cucumber, sweet pepper and carrots. Top with
  ¼ c. of feta cheese.
- Slice red onions into ⅛-in. slices. Separate the
  slices into rings and place on each salad.
- Garnish with two pitted kalamata olives and two
  pepperoncini peppers. Drizzle 1 tbsp. of balsamic
  vinegar dressing on each salad. Serve immediately.

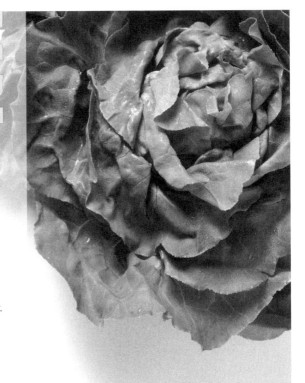

DAY 3 MENU

Breakfast

Fruit yogurt parfait *Fruit* ●, *P/D* ●
Combine 1 c. reduced-calorie, fat-free vanilla yogurt
with 1 serving fruit.
1 small muffin, any flavor *Carbohydrates* ●
Calorie-free beverage

Lunch

2/3 c. low-fat cottage cheese mixed with 2 small
  pear halves *P/D* ●, *Fruit* ●
1 slice whole-grain toast *Carbohydrates* ●
1 1/2 tsp. peanut butter *Fat* ●
* 1 c. raw broccoli *Vegetables* ●
2 tbsp. reduced-calorie vegetable dip *Fat* ●
Calorie-free beverage

Dinner

3 oz. large shrimp *P/D* ●
Steam and sprinkle with lemon juice or seafood
seasoning.
2/3 c. cooked brown rice *Carbohydrates* ● ●
* 12 steamed asparagus spears *Vegetables* ● ●
* 2 c. lettuce *Vegetables* ●
2 tbsp. reduced-calorie French dressing *Fat* ●
* 1/2 c. mandarin orange sections *Fruit* ●
Calorie-free beverage

Snack

* 1 serving favorite fruit *Fruit* ●

* The serving size stated is the minimum amount.
Eat as much as you wish.

Dietitian's tips

- Don't be fooled by the instant packages of oatmeal. They're often loaded with sugar and dried
  fruit, which drive up calories. A packet of "plain"
  instant oatmeal makes a serving size that has
  about 1 1/2 times the calories of a half-cup of
  quick-cooked oatmeal.

- The menu for Day 5 calls for 3 tbsp. of cranberry
  sauce. How long cranberry sauce stays fresh after
  opening is variable. Be sure to purchase it in the
  smallest amount you can. And after opening,
  cover the container tightly and store it in the cold-
  est part of the refrigerator — at the back on the
  lowest shelf (not in the door).

- Snacks can be healthy and help curb your hunger,
  or they can undermine your weight-control efforts.
  The best snacks are ones that are planned and that
  include fruits, vegetables, whole grains or low-fat
  dairy products. Choose snacks from the food lists
  on A7-A10 of the Visual Guide, and make sure
  they're a part of your overall meal plan. See also
  page 306 for suggestions on healthy snacks.

- Fish is a staple in many diets because it offers
  specific health benefits. Certain types of fish are
  rich in omega-3 fatty acids. These fatty acids can
  help protect you against coronary artery disease
  by improving your high-density lipoprotein (HDL or
  "good") cholesterol and by lowering your triglyceride levels. Triglycerides are another type of
  blood fat. Examples of fish high in omega-3s
  include anchovies, bass, bluefish, herring, mackerel, salmon, sardines, shark, swordfish, trout (rain-
  bow and lake) and tuna (especially white, alba-
  core and bluefin). Omega 3s are also found in
  some plants. Good plant sources include canola
  oil, flaxseed (ground and oil), soybeans (whole
  and oil), tofu and walnuts (whole and oil).

Note: Although fish and other seafood provide important health
benefits, the Food and Drug Administration advises pregnant
women, nursing mothers and children not to eat king mackerel,
shark, swordfish and tilefish because they contain higher amounts
of mercury. Pregnant women also shouldn't eat more than 12
ounces of fish a week.

DAY 4 MENU

Breakfast
1 c. reduced-calorie, fat-free yogurt *P/D* ●
* 1 large banana *Fruit* ●●
Calorie-free beverage

Lunch
Turkey sandwich *Carbohydrates* ●●, *P/D* ●
Top 2 slices whole-grain bread with 3 oz. smoked turkey, Dijon mustard, lettuce and tomato slices.
* 2 c. mixed greens *Vegetables* ●
2 tbsp. reduced-calorie Western dressing *Fat* ●
Calorie-free beverage

Dinner
Pasta primavera *Carbohydrates* ●●, *P/D* ●,
   Vegetables ●●, *Fat* ●
Top 1 c. cooked whole-grain pasta with 1 c. steamed carrots, broccoli and cauliflower. Sprinkle with 1 tsp. olive oil and 4 tbsp. shredded Parmesan cheese.
* 1 small apple *Fruit* ●
Calorie-free beverage

Snack
* 1 serving favorite vegetable *Vegetables* ●
2 tbsp. reduced-calorie vegetable dip *Fat* ●

* The serving size stated is the minimum amount. Eat as much as you wish.

strategies
10 more ways to add physical activity to your day

OK. You're told you need to include more physical activity in your daily routine. So how do you go about doing it? Week 1 gave you a list of ways to get more active and jump-start your weight program. Here are 10 more strategies for you to try:

- Go for a short walk before breakfast and after dinner.
- Several times a day, take a few moments to move around and stretch your legs, regardless of what you're doing.
- If you have a cordless phone, walk around the house while you talk, or at least stand rather than sit.
- Participate in your kids' activities at a playground or park.
- Spend time in your yard planting flowers, pulling weeds, mowing or raking.
- Put aside kitchen appliances or power tools whenever you can. Instead of using an electric mixer, mix ingredients by hand. Instead of a power saw, use a handsaw.
- Clean up the garage or organize your closets or kitchen cupboards.
- Avoid restaurant drive-throughs. Park the car and walk inside.
- Go shopping. You don't have to buy anything, just walk the aisles and look at the items.
- Walk from hole to hole at the golf course instead of using a motorized cart.

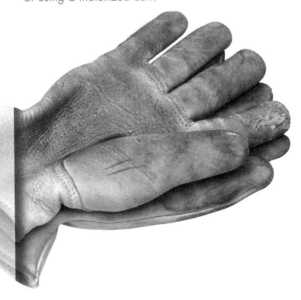

DAY 5 MENU

Breakfast

2 small muffins, any flavor *Carbohydrates* ● ●

2 tsp. margarine *Fat* ● ●

* 2 pear halves *Fruit* ●

Calorie-free beverage

Lunch

Chicken wrap *P/D* ●, *Fruit* ●, *Carbohydrates* ●
Combine 2 1/2 oz. shredded cooked chicken, 2 tbsp.
raisins, 3 tbsp. cranberry sauce and shredded lettuce.
Wrap in a fat-free tortilla.

1 sliced tomato *Vegetables* ●, *Fat* ●
Drizzle tomato with 1 tsp. extra-virgin olive oil and
balsamic vinegar to taste.

Calorie-free beverage

Dinner

Beef kebabs *P/D* ● ●, *Vegetables* ● ●
Place 3 oz. marinated cubed round steak and a total
of 2 c. diced fresh mushrooms, tomatoes, green peppers and onions on skewers. Broil or grill.

3 baby, red-skinned potatoes *Carbohydrates* ●

* 2 pineapple rings *Fruit* ●

Calorie-free beverage

Snack

* 1 serving favorite vegetable *Vegetables* ●

* The serving size stated is the minimum amount.
Eat as much as you wish.

strategies

How to intensify your walking routine

In the first week of the Mayo Clinic Healthy Weight
Program, your walk may have been just one time
around the block. If that's one block more than you
were doing before you started the program, you're
on the right track. But greater benefits will come as
you gradually increase the duration and intensity of
your walk. Increased duration and intensity improves
your cardiovascular health, gives you more endurance and vitality, and burns more calories.

Your eventual goal is to walk at least 30 minutes
a day at a moderately brisk pace — equalling a
total of about three to four hours a week of walking.
Refer to the example of a walking program shown
on page 61. Notice how a four-hour goal is
reached by gradually adjusting the duration and frequency of the walks over a period of 12 weeks.

It's important, however, to build up to that four-
hour goal at a pace that you're comfortable with.
Don't feel bound to a 12-week timetable if you think
that it's too aggressive for you. Adjust your walking
program to your level of fitness and your daily
schedule. It really doesn't matter how long it takes
you to reach your goal, so long as you continue to
work at it.

If you've been walking regularly and you feel
comfortable with your walking routine, now may be
the time for you to add more structure and intensity
to your exercise. Consider developing a walking
program. Establish your own pace, based on your
own determination of exercise intensity. What's
important is that from week to week, you challenge
yourself to slightly increase one aspect of your walking routine:

■ How long you walk
■ How often you walk
■ How fast you walk

Most important, though, make the program enjoyable, not demanding. If you've been walking for a
while, plan a hike at a nearby park or participate in
a charity walk. These activities can help boost your
motivation. You might also look for a walking partner, someone whose company you enjoy. Walking
with a partner can be a great source of motivation
and support.

DAY 6 MENU

Breakfast
½ c. cooked oatmeal *Carbohydrates* ●
2 tbsp. raisins *Fruit* ●
1 c. skim milk *P/D* ●
Calorie-free beverage

Lunch
Banana and peanut butter bagel *Fruit* ●,
  Carbohydrates ● ●, *Fat* ● ●
*Spread 1 tbsp. of peanut butter onto a whole-grain
bagel. Top with a small, sliced banana.*
* 1 small apple *Fruit* ●
Calorie-free beverage

Dinner
1 serving braised chicken with mushrooms and
  pearl onions *Vegetables* ●, *P/D* ● ●, *Fat* ●
½ c. wild rice *Carbohydrates* ●
* 1½ c. green beans *Vegetables* ● ●
Calorie-free beverage

Snack
* 1 serving favorite vegetable *Vegetables* ●

* The serving size stated is the minimum amount.
  Eat as much as you wish.

recipe serves 4

Braised chicken with mushrooms and pearl onions

¼ c. all-purpose (plain) flour
1 tsp. salt
½ tsp. freshly ground pepper
2 skinless, bone-in chicken breast halves, about ¾
lb. total weight, each cut in half crosswise
2 skinless, bone-in chicken thighs
2 chicken legs
1½ tbsp. olive oil or canola oil
1 shallot, chopped
1 lb. small white button mushrooms, brushed clean
½ lb. peeled pearl onions
¾ c. vegetable stock, chicken stock or broth
½ c. port or dry red wine
2 tbsp. balsamic vinegar
2 tbsp. chopped fresh thyme, plus sprigs for garnish

- In a shallow dish, stir together the flour, ½ tsp. of
  the salt, and ¼ tsp. of the pepper. Dredge the
  chicken pieces in the seasoned flour.
- In a large, heavy saucepan or Dutch oven, heat
  the oil over medium-high heat. Add the chicken
  and cook, turning to brown on both sides, about
  5 minutes total. Transfer to a platter. Add the shallot to the pan and sauté until softened, about a

minute. Add the mushrooms and sauté until lightly
browned, 3 to 4 minutes. Stir in the onions and
sauté until they begin to pick up some brown
color, 2 to 3 minutes.
- Stir in the stock and wine and deglaze the pan,
  stirring to scrape up any browned bits. Return the
  chicken pieces to the pan, and bring to a boil.
  Cover, reduce the heat to low, and simmer, stirring occasionally, until the chicken and vegetables
  are tender, 45 to 50 minutes. Stir in the vinegar,
  the chopped thyme, and the remaining ½ tsp.
  salt and ¼ tsp. pepper.
- To serve, divide the vegetables among shallow
  individual bowls. Top each portion with two pieces
  of chicken, one light meat and one dark. Garnish
  with thyme sprigs and serve.

*This recipe is one of 150 recipes collected in "The New Mayo
Clinic Cookbook," published by Mayo Clinic Health Information
and Oxmoor House and available in bookstores in the United
States and Canada.*

DAY 7 MENU

Breakfast
1 slice whole-grain toast *Carbohydrates* ●
1 tsp. margarine *Fat* ●
* 1 large grapefruit *Fruit* ● ●
Calorie-free beverage

Lunch
Ham sandwich *P/D* ●, *Carbohydrates* ● ●,
Vegetables ●
2 oz. lean ham on two slices whole-grain bread,
topped with lettuce, tomato slices and Dijon mustard
* ½ c. raw baby carrots *Vegetables* ●
2 tbsp. reduced-calorie ranch dressing *Fat* ●
Calorie-free beverage

Dinner
1 serving seared scallops with new
potatoes and field greens *P/D* ● ●,
Vegetables ●, *Carbohydrates* ●, *Fat* ● (See
recipe on page A13.)
* 1 small apple, sliced *Fruit* ●
Calorie-free beverage

Snack
* 1 serving favorite vegetable *Vegetables* ●

* The serving size stated is the minimum amount.
Eat as much as you wish.

strategies

Reducing the risks of exercise

*Most injuries associated with physical activity stem
from doing too much, too vigorously, with too little
previous activity. To reduce your risk of injury:*

■ **Begin gradually.** Don't overdo it. If you have trouble talking to a companion during your workout,
you're probably pushing too hard.
■ **Stretch.** Proper stretching lengthens the muscle tissue, making it less tight and therefore less prone to
trauma and tears. Start slowly and hold your stretch
at least 15 to 30 seconds, with a minimum of three
repetitions for each stretch. Don't bounce. And
don't stretch cold muscles — it can strain and irri-
tate the tissue. Warm up first. Walk before you jog,
and jog before you run. It's actually best to stretch
after you exercise when your muscles are heated
by increased blood flow and are more flexible.
■ **Exercise at moderate level of intensity.** Never exercise to the point of nausea, dizziness or severe
shortness of breath. Other exercise red flags are
listed on page 62. They may indicate a more serious medical problem. If you experience any of
these signs or symptoms, stop exercising and get
immediate medical care.

■ **Drink water to prevent dehydration.** Drink two
cups of water about two hours before exercising
and about one-half cup (a large sip) every 15 to
20 minutes while exercising. Don't rely on your
thirst to tell you when you need a drink. When
you exercise, your thirst mechanism is suppressed.
■ **Consider low-impact exercises.** If you're worried
about injury, try low-impact activities such as
swimming and water aerobics.
■ **Always cool down.** Reduce the intensity of your
activity before you stop and then finish with
stretching. This reduces stress on your heart as
well as on your muscles.

Week 6

Changing behaviors

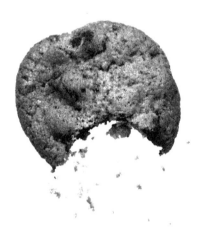

Weight control is a lifelong commitment. You can't simply "diet" or "watch your weight" for a few months and then return to your old ways of doing things. To be successful at weight control, you may need to learn new, healthy behaviors and abandon the old, familiar but unhealthy behaviors for good.

What's a behavior? A behavior is how you respond to a specific stimulus or situation. For example, whenever you get ready to eat dinner, you may fill your plate with helpings of everything on the table. You do this, whether you're hungry or not, because that's the way you've always done it. Your mother filled your plate as a kid — because you were a growing boy or growing girl — and you've continued the tradition ever since. You may also be a charter member of the "clean plate club," feeling obliged to eat everything on your plate, even when you feel full, so that nothing goes to waste.

Unfortunately, behaviors such as these can cause you to eat much more than you should. To change them, you need to consciously think about how you respond to an empty plate. And you have to be willing to try alternative responses. Instead of always taking generous portions of everything, think about what you're doing and the foods you're selecting as you place the food on your plate — you want to choose appropriate portions of the appropriate foods.

It's also important that you learn to stop eating when you feel full, even if there's food on your plate. To prevent yourself from continuing to eat, remove your plate immediately once you determine that you're full. If the plate sits there, the temptation to eat more is too great.

What's your meal routine?

As you examine your eating behaviors and try to identify unhealthy habits, it's important to reflect on your mealtimes. Just as important as what you eat is the manner in which you eat. The following questions can help you assess if your meal routine is helping or hurting your efforts to lose weight.

For this assessment, a *meal* means the food you typically eat for nourishment at regular intervals of the day. Snacking isn't considered a meal.

1. How many meals do you eat in a day?
   a. Two or less
   b. Three
   c. Four
   d. Five more

   Having just one or two meals a day generally isn't the best approach to eating, especially if you're skipping breakfast or snacking throughout the day. When snacking, you often don't pay attention to how much you eat, and you end up overeating. Aim for three planned, balanced meals each day.

2. How many between-meal snacks do you have each day?
   a. One or none
   b. Two
   c. Three
   d. Four or more

   Snacking between meals to relieve hunger is OK as long as you're nibbling on something healthy. Remember, you can eat unlimited amounts of vegetables and fruits. However, you don't want snacking to take the place of meals.

3. Where do you most often eat your meals?
   a. At the kitchen table
   b. At the kitchen counter
   c. In another room in the house
   d. On the go, such as in your car or office

   Mealtime should be a time to relax and enjoy your food without distraction. Get in the habit of eating meals at the kitchen table without watching television or doing other activities.

4. How long does it generally take you to eat a meal?
   a. Less than five minutes
   b. Five to 10 minutes
   c. 10 to 20 minutes
   d. 20 or more minutes

   The longer it takes you to eat, the more time your brain has to register how much food is in your stomach. Eating too fast creates a time lag between when you stop eating and when your brain registers that you're full. You overeat before you begin to feel full.

5. How often do you eat alone?
   a. Never or only on occasion
   b. A few meals a week
   c. At least one meal a day
   d. Always

   Eating is generally more enjoyable when done with someone else. When eating alone, you may eat too fast or be distracted by other things, which can lead to mindless eating. If you live alone, brainstorm ways to make mealtime more social.

Week 6 shopping list

This shopping list includes many of the fresh ingredients and general grocery items you'll need on hand for the Week 6 menus. It does not include the kitchen staples listed on page 187 — make sure you have them in stock. If you replace any of the recipes with a selection of your own, you'll need to adjust the shopping list.

Fresh vegetables   QTY

- ❏ asparagus spears _____
- ❏ bell peppers, green _____
- ❏ broccoli _____
- ❏ brussels sprouts _____
- ❏ carrots _____
- ❏ cucumbers _____
- ❏ green beans _____
- ❏ lettuce or mixed greens _____
- ❏ mushrooms _____
- ❏ onions, green, red and yellow _____

QTY

- ❏ shallots _____
- ❏ tomatoes, medium _____
- ❏ tomatoes, cherry _____
- ❏ zucchini _____
- ❏ favorite or seasonal vegetables _____

Fresh herbs

- ❏ garlic _____
- ❏ parsley _____

Fresh fruits

- ❏ apples _____
- ❏ bananas _____
- ❏ grapefruit _____
- ❏ grapes _____
- ❏ lemons

- ❏ oranges _____
- ❏ pears _____
- ❏ strawberries _____
- ❏ favorite or seasonal fruit _____

Carbohydrates

- ❏ bagels, whole-grain _____
- ❏ bread, whole-grain _____
- ❏ bun, whole-grain _____

- ❏ English muffins, whole-grain _____
- ❏ pita bread, whole-grain _____
- ❏ potatoes, baking _____

Protein & dairy

- ❏ chicken breast, boneless, skinless _____
- ❏ New York strip steak _____
- ❏ orange roughy or other fish fillet _____
- ❏ pork tenderloin _____
- ❏ salmon or other fish fillet _____
- ❏ turkey _____
- ❏ cheese, cheddar, low-fat _____

- ❏ cheese, mozzarella, low-fat _____
- ❏ cheese, Parmesan _____
- ❏ eggs _____
- ❏ milk, skim _____
- ❏ yogurt, frozen, fat-free _____
- ❏ yogurt, reduced-calorie, fat-free _____

Fats

- ❏ avocado _____

- ❏ vegetable dip, reduced-calorie _____

General groceries

- ❏ allspice _____
- ❏ garbanzos, canned _____
- ❏ pineapple, crushed _____
- ❏ pizza, cheese, thin-crust _____
- ❏ popcorn, low-fat, microwave _____

- ❏ spaghetti sauce, meatless _____
- ❏ soup, chicken noodle, canned _____
- ❏ soup, tomato, canned _____
- ❏ tuna, water-packed, canned _____

DAY 1 MENU

Breakfast
- ½ whole-grain English muffin *Carbohydrates* ●
- 1 tbsp. honey
- * ½ large grapefruit *Fruit* ●
- 1 c. skim milk *P/D* ●
- Calorie-free beverage

Lunch
- Southwestern salad *Fruit* ●, *Vegetables* ●●, *P/D* ●, *Fat* ●●

Top 2 c. shredded lettuce with 2½ oz. shredded cooked chicken, 1 c. chopped green peppers and onions, ½ c. crushed pineapple, ⅙ avocado, and 2 tbsp. reduced-calorie Western-style salad dressing.
- ½ whole-grain pita bread *Carbohydrates* ●
- Calorie-free beverage

Dinner
- Spaghetti with tomato sauce *Carbohydrates* ●●, *P/D* ●, *Vegetables* ●

Top 1 c. cooked whole-grain spaghetti with ¼ c. meatless spaghetti sauce from a jar and 4 tbsp. Parmesan cheese
- * ¾ c. steamed zucchini *Vegetables* ●
- * 1 c. grapes *Fruit* ●
- Calorie-free beverage

Snack
- 8 whole peanuts *Fat* ●

* The serving size stated is the minimum amount. Eat as much as you wish.

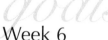

Week 6

You can adapt this week's goals or substitute different goals that are more to your liking. When you meet a goal, check the corresponding box.

❑ **Identify an unhealthy behavior.** Take some time to think about your eating behaviors. Identify a specific behavior that you feel hampers your efforts to lose weight. Think about ways that you might change it to a more healthy behavior. Be specific on how you're going to make the change.

❑ **Identify a problem situation.** As you work on improving your eating and exercise behaviors, try to identify situations — specific locations or circumstances or times of day — that stimulate an unhealthy behavior. When you feel lonely, do you turn to food for comfort? When you get ready for bed, do you have an urge to snack? When you're with friends, do you tend to overeat? Identify one problem situation and think of ways to make that situation less of a difficulty for you.

❑ **Go for whole grain.** This week, swap one of your favorite carbohydrate foods for a similar whole-grain product. For example, if you normally eat white bread, try whole-wheat bread.

❑ **Update your Weight Record.** Weigh in at your regular time and record the number of pounds gained or lost on the Weight Record. If you're struggling to lose weight in the sixth week of this program, take some time to reassess your barriers to weight loss.

❑ **Use Week 6's Healthy Weight menu.** Try to follow the suggested menus in this unit. These menus are devised for a 1,200 daily calorie goal. If your calorie goal varies from the 1,200-calorie level, you'll need to adjust the menus accordingly. See page 185.

Daily recommended servings

Vegetables (no limit)	●●●●
Fruits (no limit)	●●●
Carbohydrates	●●●●
Protein & Dairy (P/D)	●●●
Fats	●●●

DAY 2 MENU

Breakfast
- 1 medium hard-boiled egg *P/D* ●
- 1 slice whole-grain toast *Carbohydrates* ●
- 1 tsp. margarine *Fats* ●
- * 1 medium orange *Fruit* ●
- Calorie-free beverage

Lunch
- 1 whole-grain pita bread with hummus
  Carbohydrates ● ●, *P/D* ●, *Fat* ●
  Combine 1/3 c. mashed garbanzos with 1 tsp. extra-virgin olive oil. Add garlic, cumin, lemon and parsley to taste.
- * Cucumber and tomato salad *Vegetables* ●
  Combine 1/2 c. thinly sliced cucumber and 4 cherry tomatoes, halved. Add rice wine or herb-flavored vinegar to taste.

- * 1 small banana *Fruit* ●
- Calorie-free beverage

Dinner
- 3 oz. orange roughy or other fish *P/D* ●
  Sprinkle with seafood seasoning.
- 1/3 c. brown rice *Carbohydrates* ●
- 1 serving brussels sprouts with shallots and lemon *Vegetables* ● ● ●, *Fat* ●
- Calorie-free beverage

Snack
- * 1 serving favorite fruit *Fruit* ●

* The serving size stated is the minimum amount. Eat as much as you wish.

recipe *serves 4*

Brussels sprouts with shallots and lemon

1 tbsp. extra-virgin olive oil
3 shallots, thinly sliced
1/4 tsp. plus 1/8 tsp. salt
1 pound brussels sprouts, trimmed and cut into quarters
1/2 c. vegetable stock or broth
1/4 tsp. finely grated lemon zest
1 tbsp. fresh lemon juice
1/4 tsp. freshly ground pepper

- In a large, nonstick frying pan, heat 2 tsp. of the olive oil over medium heat. Sauté the shallots until soft and lightly golden, about 6 minutes. Stir in the 1/8 tsp. salt. Transfer to a bowl and set aside.
- In the same frying pan, heat the remaining 1 tsp. olive oil. Sauté the brussels sprouts until they begin to brown, 3 to 4 minutes. Add the vegetable stock and simmer. Cook, uncovered, until the brussels sprouts are tender, 5 to 6 minutes. Return the shallots to the pan. Stir in the lemon zest and juice, the 1/4 tsp. salt and the pepper. Serve immediately.

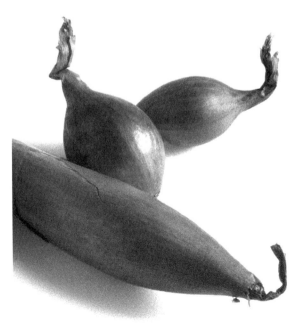

This recipe is one of 150 recipes collected in "The New Mayo Clinic Cookbook," published by Mayo Clinic Health Information and Oxmoor House and available in bookstores.

WEEK 6

DAY 3 MENU

Breakfast

1 whole-grain English muffin *Carbohydrates* ● ●
1 ½ tsp. peanut butter
* ½ large grapefruit *Fruit* ●
Calorie-free beverage

Lunch

Chef salad *Vegetables* ● ●, *P/D* ●
Top 2 c. mixed greens with 1 oz. low-fat cheddar
cheese strips, 1 ½ oz. turkey strips, and 1 c. sliced
tomatoes, cucumbers, green peppers, broccoli florets
and red onion.
2 tbsp. reduced-calorie French dressing *Fat* ●
6 wheat crackers *Carbohydrates* ●
* 1 small banana *Fruit* ●
Calorie-free beverage

Dinner

Chicken kebabs *Protein* ●, *Vegetables* ● ●, *Fat* ●
Place on skewers 2 ½ oz. cubed boneless, skinless
chicken marinated in fat-free Italian salad dressing and
a total of 2 c. of diced mushrooms, green pepper and
onion chunks, and cherry tomatoes. Broil or grill.
⅓ c. brown rice with chopped green onions
     Carbohydrates ●
1 tsp. margarine *Fat* ●
* 1 small apple *Fruit* ●
Calorie-free beverage

Snack

½ c. fat-free frozen yogurt *Protein* ●

* The serving size stated is the minimum amount.
Eat as much as you wish.

Dietitian's tips

- Regarding the cheese pizza from Day 4 of this week's menu, you can purchase a frozen cheese pizza or make your own. If you purchase a pizza, look for a brand that contains 300 to 350 calories and 3 to 5 grams of fat per serving. For an easy way to make your own cheese pizza, see the dinner recipe from Week 1 on page 197.
- As you follow these weekly menus, it's OK on occasion to substitute a convenience food for a conventional dinner, especially on those days when you have little time to cook. Convenience foods, such as pizza or frozen entrees, can be healthy, provided you choose wisely. Read the nutrition label on the packages. Look for dishes that have no more than 300 to 450 calories and 5 to 10 grams of fat for the whole meal. Some healthy frozen entrees include chicken chow mein with rice, salisbury steak, vegetarian chili, shrimp primavera and chicken cacciatore.
- For dinner on Day 7 of this week, the menu calls for Jamaican barbecued pork tenderloin. To save yourself time, you can combine all of the dry spices earlier in the day or even the day before. Store the spice mixture in an airtight container.

When it's time to begin preparing the meal, rub the spice mixture on the pork tenderloin.
- If you prefer not to use whiskey in the Day 6 dinner recipe, you can sauté the mushrooms in one teaspoon of olive oil and one tablespoon of Worcestershire sauce. Top the steak with the sautéed mushrooms. Or sauté the mushrooms in one-half cup of beef broth seasoned with a half-teaspoon mixture of black pepper and oregano. Another option is to marinate the steak in one-half cup of red wine, one teaspoon of olive oil, one-half teaspoon mixture of oregano and thyme and a generous amount of cracked black pepper. Remove the steak from the marinade and grill. While the steak is cooking, boil the marinade. Sauté the mushrooms in one teaspoon of olive oil in a separate pan. Top the steak with the mushrooms and spoon the boiled marinade over the steak.

DAY 4 MENU

Breakfast

Fruit yogurt parfait *P/D* ●, *Fruit* ●
*1 c. reduced-calorie, fat-free yogurt mixed with
1 serving fruit.*
Calorie-free beverage

Lunch

¼ recipe of tuna and pasta salad
  Carbohydrates ● ●, *Vegetables* ●, *P/D* ●, *Fat* ●
*Combine 1 can tuna in spring water, 4 c. cooked shell
pasta, 2 c. diced carrots and zucchini, and 4 tbsp.
reduced-calorie mayonnaise*
* 1 small orange *Fruit* ●
Calorie-free beverage

Dinner

½ 10-inch, thin-crust cheese pizza
  Carbohydrates ● ●, *Vegetables* ●, *P/D* ●
* 2 c. lettuce with ½ c. sliced tomatoes, red
  onions and mushrooms *Vegetables* ● ●
  2 tbsp. reduced-calorie salad dressing *Fat* ●
  Calorie-free beverage

Snack

* 1 small apple, sliced *Fruit* ●
  1½ tsp. peanut butter *Fat* ●

* The serving size stated is the minimum amount.
  Eat as much as you wish.

strategies

How to change behavior

Behavior change doesn't happen by accident. If you want to make lasting changes to your eating habits or increase your activity level, you need a plan.

There are many strategies for how to change an unhealthy behavior. Everyone has his or her own approach and his or her own pace for making the change. And it's likely that you won't follow the same plan for every problem you face. What's important is that you clearly identify and examine the behaviors that interfere with your ability to lose weight and find healthy ways to deal with them.

Following is a list of steps that you may take to change an unhealthy behavior into a healthy one:

1. List those behaviors that you feel are unhealthy. Common examples include eating too quickly, snacking throughout the day instead of eating regular meals, eating whenever you're under stress, and skipping your walk when the weather's not perfect or if the television beckons.
2. Select one behavior that you would like to change. Trying to change all the behaviors on your list at once can feel overwhelming and increase the chance that you won't be successful. Focus on one behavior at a time.

3. As you think of strategies for change, consider how you developed the behavior. Are there underlying causes for the behavior that also need to be addressed? For example, is your all-day snacking related to constant stress?
4. Brainstorm ways to change this behavior. Think of five to seven possible solutions, then decide on one strategy that you feel is practical and doable. Locking yourself out of the kitchen and carrying no money with you are two ways to prevent snacking, but they aren't realistic. Taking time over your noon hour to eat a healthy lunch and exercise is more realistic. Retain your other strategies as backups.
5. Devise a plan to promote this strategy. How will you go about making sure that you have the time to eat and exercise during the day? One option might be to reserve 30 minutes to an hour every day over the lunch hour for yourself — a time when nothing else is scheduled.
6. Identify obstacles that might hinder you. Look for any potential conflicts that might interfere with your strategy and make contingency plans. For example, exercising in the morning before work.

DAY 5 MENU

Breakfast
½ English muffin *Carbohydrates* ●
1 tsp. margarine *Fat* ●
* 1 small banana *Fruit* ●
1 c. skim milk *P/D* ●
Calorie-free beverage

Lunch
Chicken sandwich *Carbohydrates* ● ●, *P/D* ●
*Spread a whole-grain bun with honey mustard. Add
2½ oz. grilled boneless, skinless chicken breast, lettuce
and tomato slices.*
* 2 c. mixed greens *Vegetables* ●
2 tbsp. reduced-calorie ranch dressing *Fat* ●
* 1 orange *Fruit* ●
Calorie-free beverage

Dinner
3 oz. salmon or other fish *P/D* ●
½ c. linguine topped with 1 tsp. olive oil and
1 c. steamed broccoli *Carbohydrates* ●
Vegetables ●, *Fat* ●
* 8 cherry tomatoes *Vegetables* ●
* 1 small pear *Fruit* ●
Calorie-free beverage

Snack
* 1 serving favorite vegetable *Vegetables* ●

* The serving size stated is the minimum amount.
Eat as much as you wish.

7. Set a date for when you want to achieve your goal — making the changed behavior routine. Establish a comfortable pace to attempt change. Depending on what kind of behavior you're trying to change, it may take you only a few days, or it may take you several weeks or months.

8. When you reach the goal date, evaluate your success. What worked and what didn't? What would you do differently? If you didn't reach your goal, why not? What got in your way?

9. Consider what you need to do to maintain this change. Reaching your goal doesn't mean that now you can stop doing what you've been working so hard at. If you start letting work responsibilities erode your lunch hour, you'll be back to your old habit of skipping lunch and snacking all day. Think about what you need to do to make your healthy behavior a permanent one.

10. When ready, select another unhealthy behavior and restart the process. Use the insight you gained from previous behavior change to help you be successful in future attempts.

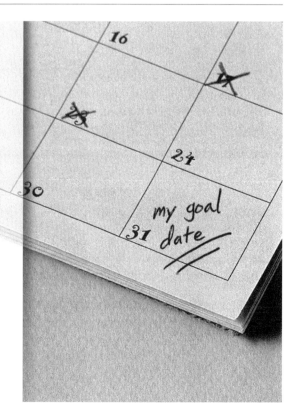

DAY 6 MENU

Breakfast
1 c. reduced-calorie, fat-free yogurt *P/D* ●
* 1 large grapefruit *Fruit* ● ●
Calorie-free beverage

Lunch
1 c. cream of tomato soup *Vegetables* ●
6 saltine crackers *Carbohydrates* ●
* 1 c. raw mixed vegetables *Vegetables* ●
Calorie-free beverage

Dinner
1/2 New York strip steak with whiskey-mushroom sauce *P/D* ● ●, *Vegetables* ●
* 1/2 c. asparagus *Vegetables* ●
1 baked potato *Carbohydrates* ● ●
1 tsp. margarine *Fat* ●
* 1 1/2 c. strawberries *Fruit* ●
Calorie-free beverage

Snack
2 c. low-fat microwave popcorn *Carbohydrates* ●

* The serving size stated is the minimum amount. Eat as much as you wish.

recipe serves 2

New York strip steak with whiskey-mushroom sauce

6 oz. New York strip steak
1 tsp. margarine
3 chopped garlic cloves
1/2 c. sliced shitake mushrooms
1/2 c. button mushrooms
1/4 tsp. thyme
1/4 tsp. rosemary
2 oz. whiskey

- Grill steak to desired doneness.
- In the meantime, in a sauté pan, heat the margarine and add the garlic. Then add the mushrooms and herbs. Sauté lightly over medium heat for about 1 to 2 minutes. Remove the pan from heat and carefully add the whiskey. (Be careful not to flame.) Cook for another minute and top steak with sauce.

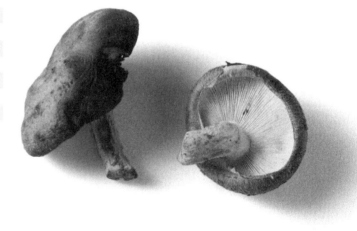

WEEK 6

DAY 7 MENU

Breakfast

1 slice whole-grain toast *Carbohydrates* ●
1 tsp. margarine *Fat* ●
* 1 large grapefruit *Fruit* ● ●
Calorie-free beverage

Lunch

Cheese sandwich *Carbohydrates* ●, *P/D* ●
Top ½ whole-grain bagel with a tomato slice and 1½
oz. mozzarella cheese. Broil until cheese melts.
1 c. canned chicken noodle soup *Carbohydrates* ●
* 1 medium orange *Fruit* ●
Calorie-free beverage

Dinner

1 serving Jamaican barbecued pork tenderloin
P/D ● ● (See recipe on page A14.)
⅓ c. cooked brown rice *Carbohydrates* ●
* 1½ c. green beans *Vegetables* ● ●
1 sliced tomato *Vegetables* ●, *Fat* ●
Drizzle tomato with 1 tsp. extra-virgin olive oil and
balsamic vinegar to taste.
Calorie-free beverage

Snack

* 1 serving favorite vegetable *Vegetables* ●
2 tbsp. low-calorie vegetable dip *Fat* ●

* The serving size stated is the minimum amount.
Eat as much as you wish.

strategies

Out of sight, out of mind

You bought a bag of chocolate chips to have on hand in case you need to bake something quick for a social event or a family potluck. But every time you open the pantry to gather ingredients for dinner, there's that bag staring you in the face. How long before you can no longer resist your craving for chocolate and you tear the bag open?

An important strategy for weight control is keeping certain foods that you crave out of the house or, at least, out of your sight. For example, if you feel that you must have chocolate chips in the house, hide them at the back of the cupboard. Then, chances are greater they'll stay out of your mouth!

Where and how you store high-calorie foods can influence how much of them you eat. The foods that you eat on impulse should be placed where you can't see them. For example, don't keep cookies in a cookie jar on the kitchen counter. They're too visible and too accessible. Tuck them in the back of a drawer. If you have ice cream in the house, hide it in the freezer behind the frozen vegetables. Put the can of peanuts or the bag of potato chips on a high shelf in the broom closet, and move the chip dip to the back of the refrigerator.

Of course, you know where these foods are stored, and on a day when you're super stressed, you may have difficulty resisting them. But on other days, the "out of sight, out of mind" strategy can work in your favor. If you don't see high-calorie foods, you may not be tempted to eat them. Keeping such foods hidden also helps avoid the automatic hand response — grabbing for accessible food, such as a cookie, without even realizing what you're doing. You eat the cookie because it's there, not because you're hungry.

This doesn't mean that your kitchen shelves and countertops need to be bare. In place of the cookie jar, put a bowl of fruit on your counter and fill it with apples, pears and bananas. In your pantry, keep healthy snacks such as raisins, pretzels and whole-grain crackers within easy view. Line the front of the refrigerator with low-fat, reduced-calorie yogurt and fresh grapes. These are the items you want to reach for when you experience an urge to eat.

Week 7

Exercising

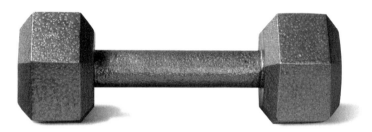

Your body is always burning calories. Even while you're sitting or lying still, certain body systems demand energy, for example, to breathe or to digest food. But in order to burn enough calories to balance out the number of calories you consume each day, you need to engage in planned physical activity on most days of the week. The routine tasks of everyday life generally don't provide a sufficient amount of activity.

That's why regular exercise is an important part of your Healthy Weight Program. Exercise is structured and repetitive activity that you do on a regular basis. Exercise can help improve your fitness, as well as help you lose weight and deal with everyday stress. Regular exercise — at least 30 to 60 minutes on most days of the week — also helps protect against serious health problems such as diabetes.

Exercise may include regular walking at a moderate intensity, swimming laps at the community pool, taking a ballroom dance class, enjoying weekly tennis workouts or lifting weights at the gym.

Most adults can safely do some form of regular exercise. And it's never too late to start, no matter what your age.

The focus of this week's unit is on increasing your level of physical activity, perhaps with a type of exercise other than your walking program. This increased physical activity can bolster your weight-loss effort and help keep you motivated. Read Chapter 10 in this book for more information on expanding your exercise program. If you have a health problem, or you're over age 40 and you've been relatively inactive, it's probably a good idea to talk with your doctor before beginning a more intense level of activity.

Are you ready to exercise?

It's essential that you stay healthy while you exercise and that you enjoy the activity. Here are questions that may help you expand your exercise program and prevent injury while you're participating:

1. What factors should I consider when choosing a new exercise?

   Answers may include:

   - *Personal enjoyment or interest*
   - *Convenience*
   - *Social factors (Do you prefer to participate with others or exercise alone?)*
   - *Required skill level (Can you take a class or meet with an instructor if you need to?)*
   - *Level of physical impact (Does the activity involve high-impact movements that may not be suitable for you?)*

2. What's best, an exercise focused on a specific part of my body — for example, the waist or thighs — or several kinds of exercise that use different body parts?

   If only abdominal exercises are what you want to do, that's OK. They'll help strengthen muscle and improve posture. But the secret to weight loss — and a trimmer figure — is burning calories. Mixed training (cross-training), which alternates among various exercises, can reduce your chance of injury to a specific muscle or joint due to overuse, and it can help alleviate boredom.

3. Should an exercise cause pain in order for it to be beneficial?

   The answer is no. Exercise that causes pain isn't beneficial and can result in serious injury. It also can stamp out your motivation. Stop any activity if it hurts.

4. What steps can help prevent injury while exercising?

   - *Warm up before exercising.*
   - *Wear proper shoes and protective gear.*
   - *Take precautions in inclement weather.*
   - *Drink plenty of fluids before, during and after exercising.*
   - *Cool down after exercising.*
   - *Get adequate sleep.*

5. What do the letters in the acronym P.R.I.C.E. stand for?

   P = Protect the area from further injury

   R = Rest the injured area

   I = Ice the injured area

   C = Compress the injured area with a bandage or elastic wrap

   E = Elevate the injured area above heart level whenever possible, to limit swelling.

6. How do I respond to a common cold? Should I stop all exercising until I've recovered completely?

   Not necessarily. Generally speaking, exercising while you have a cold won't prolong it or make it worse. One guideline to use is the neck check. If your signs and symptoms are above your neck — runny nose, sneezing or sore throat — then moderate exercise is generally safe. Start at half speed. If you feel better after 10 minutes, you can increase your speed. If you feel miserable, stop. Avoid intense exercise if you have signs and symptoms below the neck.

Week 7 shopping list

This shopping list includes many of the fresh ingredients and general grocery items you'll need on hand for the Week 7 menus. It does not include the kitchen staples listed on page 187 — make sure you have them in stock. If you replace any of the recipes with a selection of your own, you'll need to adjust the shopping list.

Fresh vegetables	QTY		QTY
❑ alfalfa sprouts	_____	❑ onions, red and yellow	_____
❑ asparagus spears	_____	❑ squash, yellow	_____
❑ bell peppers, green, red and yellow	_____	❑ tomatillo	_____
❑ cabbage	_____	❑ tomatoes, regular and cherry	_____
❑ carrots, regular and baby	_____	❑ zucchini	_____
❑ celery	_____	❑ favorite or seasonal vegetables	_____
❑ cucumbers	_____		
❑ green beans	_____	*Fresh herbs*	
❑ green peas, fresh or frozen	_____	❑ basil	_____
❑ jalapeno pepper	_____	❑ dill	_____
❑ lettuce, romaine	_____	❑ garlic	_____
❑ mushrooms	_____	❑ ginger	_____
		❑ parsley, flat-leaf (Italian)	_____

Fresh fruits			
❑ apples	_____	❑ lemons	_____
❑ berries	_____	❑ oranges	_____
❑ cherries	_____	❑ pears	_____
❑ grapes	_____	❑ favorite or seasonal fruit	_____

Carbohydrates			
❑ bagels, whole-grain	_____	❑ English muffins, whole-grain	_____
❑ bread, sourdough	_____	❑ pita, whole-grain	_____
❑ bread, whole-grain	_____		

Protein & dairy			
❑ chicken breast, boneless, skinless	_____	❑ pork, lean	_____
❑ egg	_____	❑ turkey, smoked, sliced	_____
❑ egg substitute	_____	❑ cheese, Colby, low-fat	_____
❑ flank steak, lean	_____	❑ cheese, Gouda, low-fat	_____
❑ halibut or other fish fillet	_____	❑ milk, skim	_____
❑ perch or other fish fillet	_____	❑ yogurt, reduced-calorie, fat-free	_____

Fats			
❑ cream cheese, fat-free	_____	❑ walnuts	_____
❑ olives, large	_____	❑ whipped topping, nondairy	_____

General groceries			
❑ angel food cake mix	_____	❑ orange juice	_____
❑ black beans, canned	_____	❑ pineapple rings, canned	_____
❑ coleslaw dressing	_____	❑ salsa	_____
❑ garbanzos, canned	_____	❑ tofu	_____
❑ kidney beans, canned	_____	❑ tomatoes, diced, canned	_____
❑ lentil soup, canned	_____		

WEEK 7

WEEK 7

DAY 1 MENU

Breakfast

1 whole-grain bagel *Carbohydrates* ● ●
3 tbsp. fat-free cream cheese *Fat* ●
½ c. orange juice *Fruit* ●
Calorie-free beverage

Lunch

Egg salad sandwich *Carbohydrates* ● ●, *P/D* ●,
Fat ●
*Mash one hard-boiled egg with a fork. Add chopped
onion and 1 tbsp. reduced-calorie mayonnaise. Serve
on 2 slices whole-grain bread.*
* 1 small pear *Fruit* ●
1 c. skim milk *P/D* ●
Calorie-free beverage

Dinner

3 oz. halibut or other fish topped with vegetable
salsa *P/D* ●, *Vegetables* ● ●
*Combine 1 medium diced tomato, ¼ c. each diced
tomatillo and red onion, and 1 diced jalapeno pepper.*
* 1 c. sliced cucumber *Vegetables* ●
Sprinkle with cider vinegar and dill.
* 2 grilled pineapple rings *Fruit* ●
Calorie-free beverage

Snack

* 1 serving favorite vegetable *Vegetables* ●

* The serving size stated is the minimum amount.
Eat as much as you wish.

goals

Week 7

You can adapt this week's goals or substitute different goals that are more to your liking. When you
meet a goal, check the corresponding box.

❑ **Increase your aerobic activity.** Reassess the walking program you developed in Week 5. Have you
been able to stick with your program? Are you
feeling more fit and in better shape? Think of
ways you might increase your aerobic activity
by adjusting the duration, frequency or intensity
of your walks.

❑ **Try a new activity.** Choose a new activity or exercise that you've always wanted to try. Base your
decision on personal interest and appeal and not
necessarily on what you think will help you lose
weight or be more fit. After giving it a try, take
time to consider how practical it would be to pursue this activity on a regular basis. Refer to the
factors listed on page 258.

❑ **Investigate exercise facilities.** If you're not already
a member of an exercise facility, make plans to
check out at least one fitness center, gym or community center this week. Ask for a brochure with
hours of operation, a listing of classes and the

types of equipment they offer. Find out if they offer
fitness assessments and program guidance.

❑ **Update your Weight Record.** Weigh in and record
the number of pounds gained or lost on your
Weight Record. Remember that gradual weight
loss of 1 or 2 pounds a week is healthy.

❑ **Use Week 7's Healthy Weight menu.** Try to
follow the suggested menu in this week's unit.
These menus are devised for a 1,200-calorie-a-
day diet. If your calorie goal varies from the
1,200-calorie level, you'll need to adjust the
menus accordingly. See page 185.

Daily recommended servings

Vegetables (no limit)	● ● ● ●
Fruits (no limit)	● ● ●
Carbohydrates	● ● ● ●
Protein & Dairy (P/D)	● ● ●
Fats	● ● ●

DAY 2 MENU

Breakfast

1 slice whole-grain toast *Carbohydrates* ●
1 tsp. margarine *Fat* ●
* 1 medium orange *Fruit* ●
Calorie-free beverage

Lunch

Open-faced turkey sandwich *Carbohydrates* ●,
   P/D ● ●, *Fat* ●
Spread 1 tbsp. reduced-calorie mayonnaise on a slice of sourdough bread. Top with 3 oz. smoked turkey, 2 oz. low-fat Gouda cheese, 1 slice tomato and chopped basil.
*1 c. carrot and celery sticks *Vegetables* ●
Calorie-free beverage

Dinner

¼ recipe vegetarian chili *Carbohydrates* ● ●,
   P/D ● ●, *Vegetables* ● ● ●
Sauté ½ c. onion in olive oil. Add 12 oz. tofu pieces, 2 14-oz. cans diced tomatoes, 2 14-oz. cans kidney beans and 1 14-oz. can black beans (drained), 3 tbsp. chili powder, 1 tbsp. oregano. Simmer 30 minutes.
* 1 c. grapes *Fruit* ●
Calorie-free beverage

Snack

* 1 small apple, sliced *Fruit* ●
  1½ tsp. peanut butter *Fat* ●

* The serving size stated is the minimum amount.
  Eat as much as you wish.

Dietitian's tips

Dishes prepared with boneless, skinless chicken are frequent offerings in a healthy diet. Here are simple ways to vary your menu.

Seasonings to use with chicken:

■ Barbecue sauce
■ Chili sauce
■ Curry powder, salt and pepper
■ Dijon-style mustard and honey (equal parts)
■ Garlic-herb or lemon-herb blend
■ Italian seasoning
■ Pineapple (crushed) and onion (chopped)
■ Smoke (Plank the chicken onto an untreated hickory, applewood or maple plank, or use similar wood chips, and grill.)
■ Taco seasoning
■ Tarragon and lemon juice
■ Teriyaki or soy sauce

Marinades to use with chicken:

Mix the ingredients from one of the bullet points in the following list. Place the mixture along with the chicken in a covered glass dish or plastic bag and marinate for about 1 hour (turning the chicken once).

■ 1 tsp. olive oil, 2 cloves garlic (chopped), Cajun seasoning, ¼ c. lemon juice
■ 1 tsp. olive oil, juice from 1 lemon and 1 lime, 1 tsp. ground coriander
■ ¼ c. each: soy sauce, rice wine vinegar, 1 tbsp. ginger (chopped)
■ ¼ c. each: lemon juice, apple juice, 1 tbsp. dried onion flakes, 1 tsp. dried basil

Aromatic companions for chicken:

In a covered baking dish, bake skinless chicken at 325 F topped with the ingredients from one of the bullets in the following list:

■ 4 tbsp. fresh tarragon (chopped), 4 green onions (chopped), 1 c. chicken broth
■ 2 dried apricots (chopped), ½ onion (chopped), 1 tbsp. thyme, ¼ c. chicken broth
■ 1 apple (peeled and chopped), ½ tsp. sage, 1 c. chicken broth
■ 1 onion (chopped), ½ c. mushrooms (sliced), ½ tsp. thyme, ½ c. chicken broth

DAY 3 MENU

Breakfast

½ English muffin *Carbohydrates* ●
1 tsp. margarine *Fat* ●
* 1 medium orange *Fruit* ●
Calorie-free beverage

Lunch

Cheese sandwich *Carbohydrates* ● ●, *P/D* ●, *Fat* ●
Top 2 slices whole-grain bread with 2 tsp. mayonnaise, 2 oz. low-fat Colby cheese, tomato slices and alfalfa sprouts.
* ½ c. raw baby carrots *Vegetables* ●
* 1 c. cherries *Fruit* ●
Calorie-free beverage

Dinner

4 oz. lean pork *P/D* ● ●
⅓ c. cooked brown rice *Carbohydrates* ●
1 serving sesame asparagus and carrot stir-fry
    Vegetables ● ●, *Fat* ●
1 small slice angel food cake
* 1 c. berries *Fruit* ●
Calorie-free beverage

Snack

* 1 serving favorite vegetable *Vegetables* ●

* The serving size stated is the minimum amount.
Eat as much as you wish.

recipe serves 6

Sesame asparagus and carrot stir-fry

24 asparagus stalks
6 large carrots
¼ c. water
1 tbsp. grated fresh ginger
1 tbsp. reduced-sodium soy sauce
1½ tsp. sesame oil
1½ tbsp. sesame seeds, toasted

- Cut the asparagus into ½-inch-thick slices. Cut the carrots into ¼-inch-thick slices.
- Coat a nonstick wok or a large frying pan with nonstick cooking spray and place over high heat. Add the carrots and stir-fry for 4 minutes. Add the asparagus and water. Stir and toss to combine. Cover and cook until the vegetables are barely tender, about 2 minutes. Uncover and add the ginger. Stir-fry until any remaining water evaporates, about 1 to 2 minutes.
- Add the soy sauce, sesame oil and sesame seeds. Stir-fry to coat the vegetables evenly. Dish onto individual plates and serve immediately.

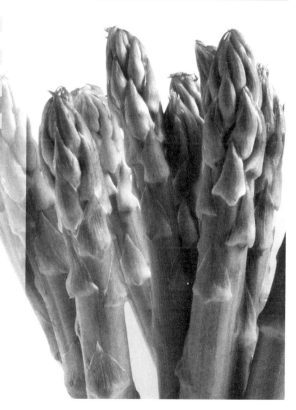

WEEK 7

DAY 4 MENU

Breakfast
* 1 small pear *Fruit* ●
  1 c. reduced-calorie, fat-free yogurt *P/D* ●
  Calorie-free beverage

Lunch
  1 c. canned lentil soup *P/D* ●
  10 baked tortilla chips *Carbohydrates* ●
* ½ c. salsa *Vegetables* ●●
  Calorie-free beverage

Dinner
  1 serving spring pasta salad *Vegetables* ●●●,
  Carbohydrates ●●, *Fat* ● (See recipe on page
  217.)

  1 slice whole-grain bread *Carbohydrates* ●
  1 tsp. margarine *Fat* ●
* 1 medium orange *Fruit* ●
  ½ c. skim milk *P/D* ●
  Calorie-free beverage

Snack
* 1 serving favorite fruit *Fruit* ●
  ½ c. nondairy whipped topping *Fat* ●

* The serving size stated is the minimum amount.
  Eat as much as you wish.

strategies
Choosing a new activity

New types of physical activity can decrease exercise boredom, boost your self-confidence and bolster your weight-loss efforts. Before adding a new activity to your routine, you may want to think about how the following factors apply:

- **Access.** Nearby facilities or playing fields make participation easier. Driving long distances, needing to reserve time, or waiting for a change of season can be a barrier to certain activities.
- **Cost.** Are there participation fees? Are there expensive equipment, clothing and shoes to consider? To minimize costs, rent equipment while trying something new.
- **Availability.** To find a club or a team, contact local recreational organizations or check the Internet.
- **Impact.** Does this activity involve jumping, jarring movements and abrupt stops and starts? If you have problems with your weight-bearing joints, look for lower impact choices.
- **Risk.** What's the basic skill level for you to start participating? For high-risk endeavors, seek out qualified instructors and use appropriate safety equipment and procedures.

- **Sociability.** Look for an activity that suits your social needs, whether it's more time alone, time with family or the chance to meet new people.

Here are ideas for new activities:

Aerobics	Jogging
Archery	Jumping rope
Badminton	Karate
Ballroom dancing	Kickboxing
Basketball	Mall walking
Bicycling, outdoor	Pilates
Bicycling, stationary	Racquetball
Bowling	Resistance bands
Canoeing or kayaking	Rowing
Cross-country skiing	Snowshoeing
Dancing	Soccer
Disc golf	Squash
Fencing	Swimming
Fitness golf (speed golf)	Tai chi
Fitness machines	Tennis
Handball	Volleyball
Hiking	Water aerobics
Indoor rock climbing	Weightlifting
In-line skating	Yoga

DAY 5 MENU

Breakfast

Omelet *Vegetables* ●, *P/D* ●
Mix ½ c. egg substitute with ½ c. diced onions, tomatoes, green peppers and mushrooms, and cook until set.
1 slice whole-grain toast *Carbohydrates* ●
1 tsp. margarine *Fat* ●
* 1 medium orange *Fruit* ●
Calorie-free beverage

Lunch

Hummus pita *P/D* ●, *Fat* ●, *Carbohydrates* ● ●
Combine ⅓ c. mashed garbanzos with 1 tsp. extra-virgin olive oil. Add garlic, cumin, lemon and parsley to taste. Place in a whole-grain pita.
* Cucumber and tomato salad *Vegetables* ● ●
Mix 1 c. sliced cucumber and 8 cherry tomatoes, halved. Add balsamic or herb-flavored vinegar.

* 1 c. grapes *Fruit* ●
Calorie-free beverage

Dinner

3 oz. perch or other fish *Protein* ●
½ c. cooked lemon-peppered pasta
   Carbohydrates ●
* ¾ c. green beans *Vegetables* ●
* 1 c. berries *Fruit* ●
Calorie-free beverage

Snack

9 large olives *Fat* ●

* The serving size stated is the minimum amount. Eat as much as you wish.

strategies

Staying mentally motivated

In addition to the types of activities you participate in, your attitude toward exercise is important to your success at losing weight. If you start saying to yourself, "Exercise is boring," "Exercise takes too much time," or "I look foolish in workout clothing," you'll lose your motivation. And when you lose motivation, it's easy to quit your exercise program.

Think about the personal benefits you gain from being physically active. Many people find that exercise gives them more energy, that it improves their mood and that it reduces daily stress. Exercise may also provide you with an opportunity to spend time with friends. Most importantly, exercise improves your health and may prevent conditions such as high blood pressure and diabetes.

To help maintain your motivation, identify and focus on the personal benefits you receive from regular exercise. Write them down and put the list in a location where you can see it.

Use this list as a personal motivator. On days when you may not feel like exercising, just seeing the list may be all that's necessary to get you off your seat and on your feet.

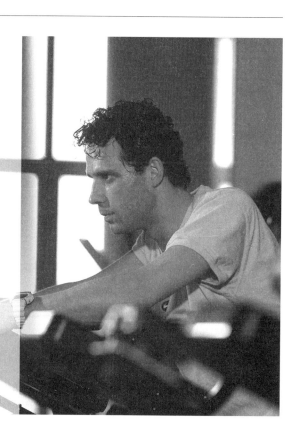

WEEK 7

DAY 6 MENU

Breakfast

1 c. reduced-calorie, fat-free yogurt *P/D* ●
* 1 c. cherries *Fruit* ●
Calorie-free beverage

Lunch

Open-faced turkey sandwich *Carbohydrates* ●,
  P/D ●●, *Fat* ●
*Spread 1 tbsp. reduced-calorie mayonnaise on 1 slice
sourdough bread. Top with 3 oz. smoked turkey, 2 oz.
low-fat Gouda cheese, 1 slice tomato and chopped basil.*
Coleslaw *Vegetables* ●●, *Fat* ●
*Combine 1 1/2 c. shredded cabbage and 1/2 c.
shredded carrots with 2 tbsp. reduced-calorie
coleslaw dressing.*
Calorie-free beverage

Dinner

1 serving spaghetti with summer squash and
  peppers *Vegetables* ●●, *Carbohydrates* ●●●,
  Fat ●●
* 1 medium orange *Fruit* ●
Calorie-free beverage

Snack

* 1 serving favorite fruit *Fruit* ●

* The serving size stated is the minimum amount.
  Eat as much as you wish.

recipe *serves 4*

Spaghetti with summer squash and peppers

1 slice day-old, whole-grain bread
2 1/2 tbsp. extra-virgin olive oil
4 cloves garlic, thinly sliced
1 1/2 tbsp. finely chopped walnuts
1/4 c. chopped fresh flat-leaf (Italian) parsley
1 tsp. salt
1 small yellow squash, cut into 2-inch julienne
1 small zucchini, cut into 2-inch julienne
1 c. shredded carrot
1 small red bell pepper, cut into julienne
1/4 c. diced yellow bell pepper
1/2 tsp. freshly ground black pepper
1/2 lb. whole-wheat spaghetti

■ In a blender or food processor, process the bread
to make fine crumbs. In a large nonstick frying
pan, heat 1 1/2 tsp. of the olive oil over medium
heat. Add the sliced garlic and sauté until lightly
golden, about 1 minute. Stir in the bread crumbs
and cook until lightly browned and crunchy, 3 to
4 minutes. Transfer to a bowl and stir in the walnuts, parsley, and 1/2 tsp. of the salt; set aside.

■ Add the remaining 2 tbsp. oil to the pan and heat
over medium heat. Add the yellow squash, zucchi-

ni and carrot, and sauté until the vegetables are
tender-crisp, about 5 minutes. Transfer to a plate
and keep warm.

■ Add the bell peppers to the pan and sauté until
they begin to soften, about 2 minutes. Stir in the
remaining 1/2 tsp. salt and the black pepper.
Return the squash mixture to the pan and toss to
mix. Set aside and keep warm.

■ Fill a large pot 3/4 full with water and bring to a
boil. Add the spaghetti and cook until al dente,
10 to 12 minutes, or according to package directions. Drain the pasta thoroughly.

■ In a warmed shallow serving bowl, combine the
spaghetti, vegetables and bread crumb mixture.
Toss gently to mix. Serve immediately.

*This recipe is one of 150 recipes collected in "The New Mayo
Clinic Cookbook," published by Mayo Clinic Health Information
and Oxmoor House and available in bookstores in the United
States and Canada.*

DAY 7 MENU

Breakfast

1 whole-grain bagel *Carbohydrates* ● ●
3 tbsp. fat-free cream cheese *Fat* ●
* 1 small pear *Fruit* ●
Calorie-free beverage

Lunch

Chicken Caesar salad *Vegetables* ●, *P/D* ●, *Fat* ●
Combine 2 c. romaine lettuce with 2½ oz. grilled
boneless, skinless chicken breast strips, 2 tbsp.
reduced-calorie Caesar dressing and 1 tbsp.
seasoned croutons.
6 wheat crackers *Carbohydrates* ●
Calorie-free beverage

Dinner

3 oz. marinated flank steak *P/D* ● ●
* ½ c. peas *Vegetables* ● ●
1 slice whole-grain bread *Carbohydrates* ●
1 tsp. margarine *Fat* ●
* 2 c. berries *Fruit* ● ●
Calorie-free beverage

Snack

* 1 serving favorite vegetable *Vegetables* ●

* The serving size stated is the minimum amount.
Eat as much as you wish.

strategies

Sticking with your program

*To make exercise a daily habit, it takes commitment.
For many people the most difficult part of exercising
isn't the activity itself, but staying committed. When
something more intriguing or demanding comes
along, it can be easy or tempting to forget about
exercising. To help prevent this from happening,
schedule daily exercise in the same way you would
any other important appointment, and look for ways
to keep your routine more interesting.*

■ **Choose activities that you enjoy.** You're more likely
to stick with activities that you think of as fun and
invigorating.

■ **Diversify.** To ensure that you'll keep exercising
year-round, choose different activities for each
season.

■ **Recruit an exercise partner.** Your spouse, a friend
or a co-worker can enliven your workouts and
motivate you when you don't feel like exercising.

■ **Set goals.** Make sure these goals are challenging
but attainable. They can be about process (such
as learning a new skill) as well as outcome (such
as walking in a charity event). When you reach a
goal, reward yourself and set another.

■ **Keep an exercise record.** If you walk, bike or
swim, record daily distances or your routes and
times. If you play a sport, write down the day's
scores. A record of your progress gives you a
sense of accomplishment and encouragement to
stay with your program.

■ **Join a group.** If basketball or soccer leagues don't
interest you, consider forming a neighborhood
walking group, or sign up for an exercise class
with friends. Group exercise can be a more powerful motivator than committing to exercise on
your own.

■ **Spread it out.** If time is limited, exercise in brief
periods throughout the day. For example, make
time for three 10-minute sessions rather than one
30-minute session.

■ **Aim for convenience.** If your workout requires a
gym, swimming pool or exercise equipment, make
sure a facility is located near home or work.
Accessibility is an important part of maintaining
an exercise program.

Week 8

Eating out

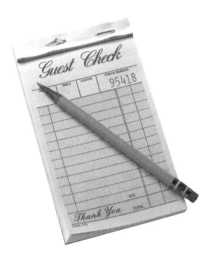

A trip to the restaurant can be a mine-field of temptations. Your best intentions may crumble when you're enjoying the company of family or friends and are bombarded with all sorts of delicious menu items. In fact, most everywhere you go these days, the sights and smells of food tantalize your senses: the supermarket deli, the bakery tray at the convenience store, the food court at the mall, the concession stand at the movie theater.

For many people, eating out is common practice. They choose to dine out because it's convenient, it's efficient and it's fun. According to the National Restaurant Association, individuals age 8 and older eat out on average more than four times a week. Eating out is also associated with weight gain. That's why dining out

deserves your full attention. To lose weight or maintain a healthy weight, you can't let down your guard just because you're at a restaurant or at a social occasion where food is present.

Does that mean if you want to eat healthy, you can't leave the house? Not at all. You can eat away from home without sabotaging your weight-loss plan. You just need to be menu savvy to healthy choices. You also need to be mindful of two common dining-out challenges: the urge to order more food than you need and the impulse to eat every bit of food on your plate — even when the portion sizes are way too large. For more strategies for eating away from home, review some of the barriers described in the Action Guide on pages 147-158 .

What are your eating-out habits?

The questions below can help you assess your habits when it comes to eating out.

1. How often do you eat out?
   a. On occasion
   b. Once or twice a week
   c. Three or four times a week
   d. Every day or almost every day

   You can eat healthy when dining out, but you need to have a plan, make wise selections and not be tempted by foods that aren't part of your plan.

2. Where do you generally eat out?
   a. Establishments that specialize in healthy foods
   b. Establishments that include a mix of foods, including healthy entrees
   c. Establishments with a few healthy items
   d. Establishments without any healthy items, except a salad

   Where you eat can make a big difference in whether you're able to eat healthy. If there's nothing healthy on the menu, it's pretty hard to stick to your meal plan.

3. What do you generally order?
   a. One of the items marked as healthy on the menu
   b. A food that appears to be somewhat healthy
   c. A favorite food prepared or served more healthfully
   d. Whatever is on special

   The special may not be the healthiest item. Items listed as healthy or that are prepared or served in a more healthy manner tend to be your best bet.

4. How often do you order an appetizer?
   a. Never
   b. Once in a while
   c. Occasionally, in place of a meal
   d. Frequently or always

   Appetizers often aren't the most healthy items on the menu, and they tend to be a source of hidden calories.

5. What do you generally drink?
   a. Water
   b. A calorie-free beverage, such as diet soda or coffee
   c. A low-calorie beverage, such as skim milk
   d. A regular soda or alcoholic drink

   Beverages such as regular sodas and alcoholic drinks contain significant amounts of calories. If you get a refill, you're getting twice the amount.

6. How do you deal with large portions?
   a. Ask for a smaller or lunch size
   b. Take half of it home in a carryout bag
   c. Split a meal with someone else
   d. Eat it all or stop eating only when you feel full

   It's better to begin with only moderate portions of food than to rely on yourself to stop eating when you think you've eaten the right amounts.

If most of your responses were *a, b,* or *c,* you've developed good habits when dining out or you're on the right track. If your responses to most of the questions were *d,* think about ways that you can improve your eating-out habits.

Week 8 shopping list

This shopping list includes many of the fresh ingredients and general grocery items you'll need on hand for the Week 8 menus. It does not include the kitchen staples listed on page 187 — make sure you have them in stock. If you replace any of the recipes with a selection of your own, you'll need to adjust the shopping list.

Fresh vegetables   QTY

❑ bell peppers, green   _____
❑ broccoli   _____
❑ celery   _____
❑ cucumbers   _____
❑ endive leaves, curly   _____
❑ green beans   _____
❑ jalapeno pepper   _____
❑ lettuce or mixed greens   _____
❑ mushrooms   _____
❑ onions, yellow and red   _____

                                      QTY
❑ squash, summer   _____
❑ tomatoes, plum   _____
❑ tomatoes, regular   _____
❑ zucchini   _____
❑ favorite or seasonal vegetables   _____

Fresh herbs

❑ basil   _____
❑ cilantro or coriander   _____
❑ garlic   _____
❑ mint leaves   _____

Fresh fruits

❑ apples, red and Granny Smith   _____
❑ bananas   _____
❑ cantaloupe   _____
❑ grapefruit, ruby red   _____

❑ lemons   _____
❑ oranges, navel   _____
❑ watermelon   _____
❑ favorite or seasonal fruit   _____

Carbohydrates

❑ bread, whole-grain   _____
❑ pita bread, whole-grain   _____

❑ potatoes, baking   _____

Protein & dairy

❑ chicken breast, boneless, skinless   _____
❑ chicken breast, precooked   _____
❑ egg   _____
❑ egg, substitute   _____
❑ flank steak   _____
❑ sole or other fish fillet   _____
❑ tuna or other fish fillet   _____

❑ turkey breast, boneless, skinless   _____
❑ turkey breast, precooked   _____
❑ cheese, cheddar, low-fat   _____
❑ cheese, mozzarella, low-fat   _____
❑ milk, skim   _____
❑ yogurt, reduced-calorie, fat-free   _____

Fats

❑ avocado   _____
❑ olives   _____

❑ sour cream, fat-free   _____
❑ walnut oil   _____

General groceries

❑ beets, canned   _____
❑ corn, canned and frozen   _____
❑ cranberries, dried   _____
❑ orange juice   _____
❑ pineapple, canned   _____
❑ pinto or black beans, canned   _____

❑ pizza crust, 12-inch   _____
❑ potatoes, canned   _____
❑ salsa, smoky   _____
❑ tuna, water-packed   _____
❑ vegetable soup, canned   _____

WEEK 8

DAY 1 MENU

Breakfast
 1 c. reduced calorie fat-free yogurt *P/D* ●
* 1 small banana *Fruit* ●
 Calorie-free beverage

Lunch
 Chef salad *Vegetables* ● ●, *P/D* ●
 *Top 2 c. mixed greens with 1 oz. low-fat cheddar
 cheese strips, 1 1/2 oz. turkey strips, and 1 c. sliced
 tomatoes, cucumbers, green peppers, broccoli florets
 and red onion.*
 2 tbsp. reduced-calorie French dressing *Fat* ●
* 1 small apple *Fruit* ●
 Calorie-free beverage

Dinner
 1 serving soft taco with Southwestern
 vegetables *Vegetables* ● ●, *P/D* ●, *Fat* ●
 Carbohydrates ● ● ● ● (See recipe on
 page 227.)
* 1 c. cubed cantaloupe *Fruit* ●
 Calorie-free beverage

Snack
 9 large olives *Fat* ●

* The serving size stated is the minimum amount.
 Eat as much as you wish.

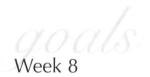

Week 8

*You can adapt this week's goals or substitute differ-
ent goals that are more to your liking. When you
meet a goal, check the corresponding box.*

❏ **Dare to experiment.** Review your eating-out habits
 and look for one area in which you might make
 an improvement — whether that be trying a different restaurant or ordering a healthier item from
 the menu at a familiar restaurant.
❏ **Test your menu skills.** The next time you're at a
 restaurant, instead of quickly glancing through the
 menu, carefully review it and look for terms that
 indicate how an item is prepared or what other
 ingredients it includes. Consider the hidden calories in sauces, dressings or seasonings. You may
 find that what you thought was a healthy choice
 really isn't, or vice versa.
❏ **Practice your salad bar skills.** Before ordering
 from the salad bar, take time to survey the ingredients and see if they meet your criteria for fresh-
 ness, taste and good nutrition. Be wary of the
 pasta salads and condiments such as croutons.
❏ **Update your Weight Record.** Weigh in and record
 the number of pounds gained or lost on your

Weight Record. Remember that gradual weight
loss of 1 or 2 pounds a week is the healthiest
weight loss.
❏ **Use Week 8's Healthy Weight menu.** Try to follow
 the suggested menu in this unit. These menus are
 devised for a 1,200-calorie-a-day diet. If your
 calorie goal varies from the 1,200-calorie level,
 you'll need to adjust the menus accordingly. See
 page 185.

Daily recommended servings

Vegetables (no limit)	● ● ● ●
Fruits (no limit)	● ● ●
Carbohydrates	● ● ● ●
Protein & Dairy (P/D)	● ● ●
Fats	● ● ●

WEEK 8

DAY 2 MENU

Breakfast
1 c. whole-grain cereal *Carbohydrates* ● ●
1 c. skim milk *P/D* ●
* 1 small apple *Fruit* ●
Calorie-free beverage

Lunch
Grilled chicken salad *Vegetables* ● ●, *P/D* ●, *Fat* ●

Combine 2 c. mixed greens with 2½ oz. grilled bone-less, skinless chicken breast strips and 1 c. sliced tomatoes, cucumbers, zucchini, bell peppers and onions. Top with 1 tsp. extra-virgin olive oil mixed with 2 tbsp. balsamic vinegar.
* 1 small banana *Fruit* ●
Calorie-free beverage

Dinner
3 oz. grilled tuna or other fish *P/D* ●
2/3 c. cooked brown rice *Carbohydrates* ● ●
* 1½ c. steamed zucchini and summer squash *Vegetables* ● ●
1 tsp. margarine *Fat* ●
* ½ c. mixed fruit *Fruit* ●
Calorie-free beverage

Snack
8 whole peanuts *Fat* ●

* The serving size stated is the minimum amount. Eat as much as you wish.

Dietitian's tips

You can enhance the flavor of food without adding fat, salt or sugar. Herbs and spices contribute bright color, savory taste and sensational aroma.

- **Basil.** An herb with a sweet, clove-like taste, best used with Italian foods, especially tomatoes, tomato sauces, pasta, chicken, fish and shellfish
- **Bay leaf.** A pungent, woodsy herb with a slight cinnamon taste, best used with bean or meat stews and soups
- **Caraway.** Seeds with a nutty, licorice flavor, best used with cooked vegetables such as beets, cabbage, carrots, potatoes, turnips and winter squash
- **Chili powder.** A commercial mix of ground chili peppers, cumin, oregano, and other herbs and spices, best used with bean or meat soups
- **Chives.** A member of the onion family, with long, hollow green stems and a mild onion flavor, best used with sauces, soups, baked potatoes, salads, omelets, pasta, seafood and meat
- **Cilantro.** An herb with a lively, citrusy, evergreen-like flavor, best used with Mexican, Latin American and Asian cuisine, rice, beans, fish, shellfish, poultry, vegetables, salsas and salads

- **Dill.** An herb with a mild sweet but tangy flavor, best used with seafood, chicken, yogurt, cucumbers, green beans, tomatoes, potatoes and beets
- **Ginger (dried).** A spice with a slightly sweet, citrus flavor, best used with squash, rice and chicken
- **Mace.** A spice with a sweet, warm flavor, best used with baked goods, fruit dishes, carrots, broccoli, brussels sprouts and cauliflower
- **Oregano.** An herb with a somewhat sweet and peppery flavor, best used with Italian and Greek cuisine, and meat and poultry dishes
- **Paprika.** A bright, brownish-orange spice that, depending on the variety, can add a mild, sweet flavor or a spicy flavor, best used with Spanish dishes, potatoes, soups, stews and baked fish
- **Rosemary.** An herb with a piney flavor, best used with mushrooms, roasted potatoes, stuffing, ripe melon, poultry and meats, especially grilled
- **Sage.** An herb with a rich, musty flavor, best used with poultry stuffing, chicken, duck, pork, eggplant, and bean stews and soups
- **Thyme.** An herb with a strong minty, somewhat bitter flavor, best used with fish, poultry, tomatoes, beans, eggplant, mushrooms and potatoes

WEEK 8

DAY 3 MENU

Breakfast
1 c. whole-grain cereal *Carbohydrates* ● ●
1 c. skim milk *P/D* ●
* 1 small banana *Fruit* ●
Calorie-free beverage

Lunch
1 serving minted Mediterranean fruit mix *Fruit* ●,
Vegetables ●, *Fat* ● (See recipe on page A15.)
6 wheat crackers *Carbohydrates* ●
1 c. skim milk *P/D* ●
Calorie-free beverage

Dinner
3 oz. turkey *P/D* ●
1 serving wild rice pilaf with cranberries and
apples *Fruit* ●, *Carbohydrates* ●, *Fat* ●
* 2 c. mixed greens with 1 c. sliced mushrooms
and green peppers *Vegetables* ● ●
2 tbsp. reduced-calorie ranch dressing *Fat* ●
Calorie-free beverage

Snack
* 1 serving favorite vegetable *Vegetables* ●

* The serving size stated is the minimum amount.
Eat as much as you wish.

recipe serves 8

Wild rice pilaf with cranberries and apples

1½ c. wild rice
3 c. water
½ c. dried cranberries
2 tbsp. olive oil
1 tbsp. red wine vinegar
1 tbsp. sugar
2 Granny Smith apples, cored and diced
¼ c. slivered almonds, toasted

■ In a medium-sized bowl, rinse and drain the
wild rice. Bring the water to a boil in a medium
saucepan. Add the rice. Reduce heat and simmer,
covered, until tender, about 45 minutes. Stir in
the dried cranberries. Remove from heat and
let stand.

■ In a small bowl, mix together the oil, red wine
vinegar and sugar. In a large bowl, combine the
rice and the diced apples. Add the oil mixture
and toss. Serve warm or cold on individual plates.
Top with toasted slivered almonds.

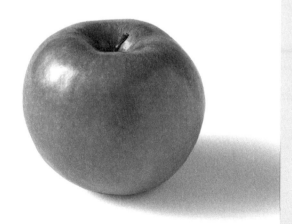

DAY 4 MENU

Breakfast
 1 egg fried in nonstick pan *P/D* ●
 1 slice whole-grain toast *Carbohydrates* ●
 1 tsp. margarine *Fat* ●
 ½ c. orange juice *Fruit* ●
 Calorie-free beverage

Lunch
 Tuna salad pita *Carbohydrates* ●, *P/D* ●, *Fat* ●
 Fill ½ whole-grain pita bread with mixture of 3 oz. water-packed tuna, chopped celery and onion, and 1 tbsp. reduced-calorie mayonnaise.
 * 1 medium bell pepper, sliced *Vegetables* ●
 * 1 small apple *Fruit* ●
 Calorie-free beverage

Dinner
 ¼ classic tomato-basil pizza *Carbohydrates* ● ●, *P/D* ●, *Vegetables* ●
 Top a prepared 12-inch pizza crust with 1 c. diced plum tomatoes, fresh basil, 1⅓ c. shredded low-fat mozzarella cheese. Bake at 400 F about 10 minutes.
 * 2 c. lettuce *Vegetables* ●
 2 tbsp. low-calorie dressing *Fat* ●
 * ¼ small cantaloupe *Fruit* ●
 Calorie-free beverage

Snack
 * 1 serving favorite vegetable *Vegetables* ●

 * The serving size stated is the minimum amount.
 Eat as much as you wish.

strategies

Maneuvering the menu: Avoiding hidden calories

When ordering food at a restaurant, do you know which items may be loaded with fat and calories? Unlike when you're grocery shopping, the foods in a restaurant don't have nutrition labels listing their fat and calorie content.

Hidden calories refer to the extra calories in many dishes that come from ingredients you may be unaware of. That's why they're such a problem for people grappling with weight control. Ingredients often are added to enhance the flavor, color or texture of food — for example, seasonings, sauces or dressings. And sometimes they're part of the process used to prepare the dish — for example, oil or butter for cooking. These calories add up in subtle ways.

When reviewing a restaurant menu, use these guidelines to help you steer clear of hidden fat and calories:

- **Appetizers.** If you're having an appetizer, choose one that contains vegetables, fruit or fish. Tomato juice, fresh fruit compote and shrimp cocktail served with lemon are healthy appetizers. Avoid fried or breaded appetizers, which are generally high in calories.

- **Soup.** The best choices are broth-based or tomato-based soups. Creamed soups, chowders, puréed soups and, occasionally, fruit soups can contain heavy cream or egg yolks.

- **Bread.** Muffins, garlic toast and croissants have more fat and calories than do whole-grain bread, breadsticks and crackers.

- **Salad.** Your best choice is a lettuce or spinach salad with a low-fat dressing on the side. Limit all of the add-ons, such as cheese and croutons. Chef salad and taco salad are usually high in fat and calories because of the meat, cheese and other extras — such as the taco salad's deep-fried shell.

- **Side dish.** Choose a baked potato, boiled new potatoes, steamed vegetables, rice or fresh fruits instead of higher calorie options, including french fries, potato chips and mayonnaise-based salads, such as potato salad.

- **Entrees.** You may want to skip pasta dishes with meat or cheese stuffing or dishes with sauces that contain bacon, butter, cream or eggs. The names of certain dishes indicate that they're high in fat, such as prime rib, veal parmigiana, stuffed shrimp, fried chicken, fried rice and fettuccine

DAY 5 MENU

Breakfast
 1 slice whole-grain toast *Carbohydrates* ●
 1 tsp. margarine *Fat* ●
* ½ large grapefruit *Fruit* ●
 1 c. skim milk *P/D* ●
 Calorie-free beverage

Lunch
 1 c. canned vegetable soup *Vegetables* ●
 6 wheat crackers *Carbohydrates* ●
 2 oz. low-fat cheddar cheese *P/D* ●
* 1 medium orange *Fruit* ●
 Calorie-free beverage

Dinner
 3 oz. grilled chicken breast *P/D* ●
 1 medium baked potato
  Carbohydrates ● ●
 3 tbsp. fat-free sour cream *Fat* ●
* 1½ c. green beans *Vegetables* ● ●
* 1 small wedge watermelon *Fruit* ●
 Calorie-free beverage

Snack
* 1 c. celery *Vegetables* ●
 1½ tbsp. peanut butter *Fat* ●

* The serving size stated is the minimum amount.
 Eat as much as you wish.

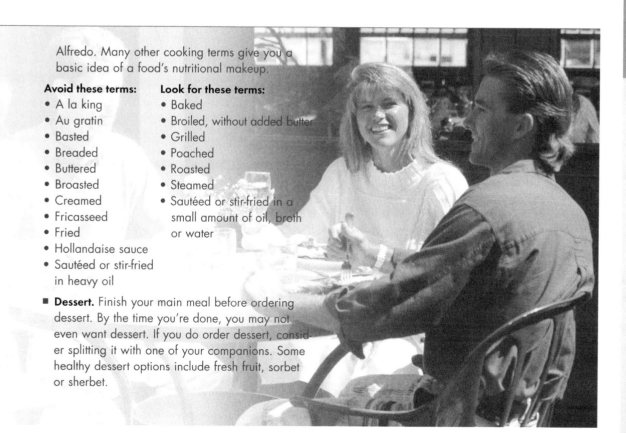

Alfredo. Many other cooking terms give you a
basic idea of a food's nutritional makeup.

Avoid these terms:
• A la king
• Au gratin
• Basted
• Breaded
• Buttered
• Broasted
• Creamed
• Fricasseed
• Fried
• Hollandaise sauce
• Sautéed or stir-fried
 in heavy oil

Look for these terms:
• Baked
• Broiled, without added butter
• Grilled
• Poached
• Roasted
• Steamed
• Sautéed or stir-fried in a
 small amount of oil, broth
 or water

■ **Dessert.** Finish your main meal before ordering
 dessert. By the time you're done, you may not
 even want dessert. If you do order dessert, consider splitting it with one of your companions. Some
 healthy dessert options include fresh fruit, sorbet
 or sherbet.

DAY 6 MENU

Breakfast

1 slice whole-grain toast *Carbohydrates* ●
1 ½ tsp. jam
* 1 large grapefruit *Fruit* ● ●
Calorie-free beverage

Lunch

Chicken ranch wrap *Carbohydrates* ●, *P/D* ●,
Fat ●

Combine 2 ½ oz. grilled chicken strips, shredded lettuce, sliced tomato and onion with 2 tbsp. reduced-
calorie ranch dressing. Wrap in a corn tortilla.
* 1 medium celery stalk *Vegetables* ●
* 1 small banana *Fruit* ●
Calorie-free beverage

Dinner

1 serving cornmeal-crusted sole with chili
vinaigrette *P/D* ● ●, *Fat* ●
1 medium baked potato *Carbohydrates* ● ●
3 tbsp. fat-free sour cream *Fat* ●
* 2 c. steamed broccoli *Vegetables* ● ●
Calorie-free beverage

Snack

1 serving favorite vegetable *Vegetables* ●

* The serving size stated is the minimum amount.
  Eat as much as you wish.

recipe serves 4

Cornmeal-crusted sole with chili vinaigrette

¼ c. all-purpose flour
¼ c. cornmeal, preferably stone-ground
¾ tsp. salt
4 sole fillets, 5 oz. each
3 tbsp. extra-virgin olive oil
2 tbsp. dry white wine
1 ½ tbsp. fresh lemon juice
1 ½ tbsp. vegetable stock or broth
¾ tsp. chili powder
¼ tsp. dry mustard
¼ tsp. ground cumin
1 tbsp. chopped fresh cilantro (fresh coriander)
1 tbsp. grated lemon zest

- In a shallow bowl, stir together the flour, cornmeal
  and ¼ tsp. of the salt. Dredge the fillets in the
  flour mixture, coating completely, and shake off
  the excess. In a large, nonstick frying pan, heat 1
  tbsp. of the olive oil over medium-high heat. Add
  the fish and cook, turning once, until the fish is
  opaque throughout when tested with the tip of a
  knife and the crust is golden brown, about 3 minutes on each side. Transfer to individual plates
  and keep warm.

- Add the wine and deglaze the pan, stirring to
  scrape up any browned bits. Cook to reduce by
  half. In a small bowl, combine the pan juices,
  lemon juice, vegetable stock, chili powder, mustard, cumin and the remaining ½ tsp. salt. Whisk
  in the remaining 2 tbsp. olive oil to make a thick
  vinaigrette.

- To serve, drizzle the vinaigrette over the fillets and
  sprinkle with the cilantro and lemon zest.

*This recipe is one of 150 recipes collected in "The New Mayo
Clinic Cookbook," published by Mayo Clinic Health Information
and Oxmoor House and available in bookstores in the United
States and Canada.*

DAY 7 MENU

Breakfast

1 breakfast burrito *Vegetables* ●,
Carbohydrates ● ●, *P/D* ●

Sauté ½ c. chopped tomato, 2 tbsp. chopped onion, ¼ c. canned corn and some liquid. Add ¼ c. egg substitute and scramble with the vegetables. Spread on 8-inch flour tortilla, roll up and top with 2 tbsp. salsa

* 1 medium orange *Fruit* ●

Calorie-free beverage

Lunch

Turkey pita *Carbohydrates* ●, *P/D* ●, *Fat* ●

Top ½ whole-grain pita with 3 oz. shredded turkey, ⅙ avocado, chopped lettuce, tomato and onion.

* ½ c. cubed pineapple *Fruit* ●

Calorie-free beverage

Dinner

"Beefed-up" salad *P/D* ●, *Vegetables* ● ●, *Fat* ● ●,
Carbohydrates ●

Assemble on large salad plate 2 c. spring greens, ½ c. sliced canned beets, 3 canned baby potatoes, 1 medium tomato cut into wedges, 1 ½ oz. thinly sliced marinated, grilled flank steak and 9 olives. Chill and top with 2 tbsp. reduced-calorie salad dressing.

Calorie-free beverage

Snack

* 1 serving favorite fruit *Fruit* ●

* The serving size stated is the minimum amount. Eat as much as you wish.

strategies

Assessing the salad bar

When dining out, you may think that eating at the salad bar is a healthy alternative to ordering from the menu. However, unless you make careful choices, you could end up with a plate filled with calories and fat.

Before you order, walk through the salad bar to see if it has ingredients you like to make a tasty yet healthy salad. Some salad bars look more like a delicatessen, with a lot of rich, high-fat options. Remember that just because a food is located in the salad bar doesn't automatically mean that it's healthy.

■ **Examine the greens.** Lettuce or fresh spinach is generally the foundation of a healthy salad. Do the greens look fresh and plentiful?

■ **Survey the fresh fruits and vegetables.** In addition to greens, you want to pile on fresh vegetables and fruits, such as tomatoes, mushrooms, carrots, broccoli, cauliflower, cucumbers, beets, radishes, bell peppers, mushrooms, pineapple, cantaloupe, watermelon, grapes and strawberries. Is there a good offering of these items?

■ **Acknowledge the extras.** Many people go wrong at salad bars by including too many high-fat ingredients. This includes items such as cheese, chopped eggs, bacon bits and buttery croutons, or other types of salads such as pasta salad or potato salad. Will you be able to go through the salad bar and take only very small amounts of these items or avoid them all together?

■ **Don't forget the dressings.** Look for fat-free or low-fat, low-calorie dressings, such as low-fat Italian or reduced-calorie French. Other options include vinegars. You can also add flavor to your salad with herbs and peppers. Check to see if any seasonings are available.

Week 9

Shopping and cooking

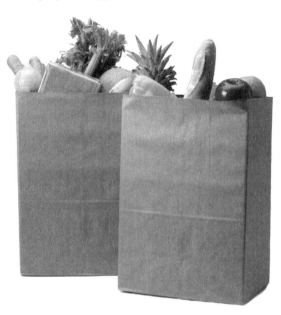

With everything that you have to do each day, making sure that you and your family eat a healthy meal every time you sit down at the table may seem like an impossible task. Perhaps your mother or grandmother had time to prepare delicious and healthy meals, but you don't. You have to work each day, or perhaps you're busy with community or service projects. Or it may be that you'd rather go golfing or spend time in the garden or with friends than in the kitchen.

When it comes to cooking, many people will claim that they just don't have the time. Lack of time is considered one of the most common obstacles to a healthy diet. That's because healthy eating is often associated with complicated recipes, time-consuming meal preparation and hours spent at the grocery store. That's simply not so. You can prepare a healthy meal just as quickly as you can an unhealthy one.

Healthy eating is all about having the right foods on hand and preparing them in a manner that won't add a lot of fat and calories to your diet. The key is planning. Healthy meals may come together in the kitchen, but they begin before you go to the grocery store. By taking the time to plan, you and your family can eat well without fuss and hassle. For more information, read Chapter 9.

If you really want to eat healthier, you can. And it doesn't have to cost you precious time. It's all a matter of priorities.

What are your shopping habits?

Smart shopping is a key factor in a healthier lifestyle. The following questions can help you judge whether your shopping habits are on track or could use some adjustment.

1. How often do you prepare a list before you shop?
   a. Every time
   b. Most of the time
   c. Occasionally
   d. Not very often or never

   A list is the best way to ensure you get everything you need in one grocery store trip. When you have everything, it's easier to prepare healthy meals and do it quickly.

2. What portion of your fruits and vegetables do you purchase fresh or frozen rather than canned?
   a. All
   b. More than half
   c. Less than half
   d. Just a few items or none

   Fresh or frozen produce typically is the tastiest and most nutritious.

3. How often do you read nutrition labels?
   a. All of the time
   b. Most of the time
   c. Some of the time
   d. Very infrequently or never

   Nutrition labels are the best way to assess how nutritious a product is or how it compares to a similar product.

4. How often do you purchase items with labels such as "reduced-fat," "fat-free," "low-calorie," "sugar-free" and "extra lean" rather than the regular items?
   a. All of the time
   b. Most of the time
   c. Some of the time
   d. Very infrequently or never

   Foods in which the fat or calories are reduced generally are healthier than their regular counterparts.

5. How often do you buy processed foods or prepackaged meals?
   a. Never
   b. Infrequently
   c. Some of the time
   d. Quite often or almost all of the time

   Processed or prepackaged foods are often, though not always, low in fiber and high in fat, calories, and ingredients such as sodium.

6. When do you typically shop?
   a. Early in the morning or in the evening
   b. During the day on a weekday
   c. On the weekend
   d. On the way home after work or right before a meal

   Stores tend to be busiest on weekends and in the late afternoons. You're also more likely to make an impulse purchase if you're hungry when you're shopping.

If your responses to most of the questions were *a* or *b,* you've already developed savvy shopping habits. If your responses to most of the questions were *b* or *c,* you're on the right track but could sharpen your skills even further. If your response to most of the questions was *d,* think of ways you can improve your shopping habits.

Week 9 shopping list

This shopping list includes many of the fresh ingredients and general grocery items you'll need on hand for the Week 9 menus. It does not include the kitchen staples listed on page 187 — make sure you have them in stock. If you replace any of the recipes with a selection of your own, you'll need to adjust the shopping list.

Fresh vegetables   QTY

- ❑ asparagus spears _____
- ❑ bell peppers, green and red _____
- ❑ broccoli _____
- ❑ carrots, regular and baby _____
- ❑ cauliflower
- ❑ celery _____
- ❑ cucumbers _____
- ❑ green beans _____
- ❑ lettuce, red and green leaf _____
- ❑ onions, red and yellow _____
- ❑ peppers, pepperoncini _____
- ❑ scallions _____

QTY

- ❑ squash, summer _____
- ❑ tomatoes, red and yellow _____
- ❑ zucchini _____
- ❑ favorite or seasonal vegetables _____

Fresh herbs

- ❑ basil _____
- ❑ cilantro _____
- ❑ garlic _____
- ❑ ginger or ginger root _____
- ❑ parsley, flat-leaf (Italian) _____
- ❑ thyme _____

Fresh fruits

- ❑ bananas _____
- ❑ blueberries _____
- ❑ grapefruit _____
- ❑ grapes _____

- ❑ oranges _____
- ❑ peaches _____
- ❑ strawberries _____
- ❑ favorite or seasonal fruit _____

Carbohydrates

- ❑ bagels, whole-grain _____
- ❑ bread, whole-grain _____
- ❑ buns, whole-grain _____
- ❑ couscous, whole-wheat _____

- ❑ graham crackers _____
- ❑ potatoes, baby, red-skinned _____
- ❑ rolls, whole-grain _____
- ❑ wheat bran, 100%, unprocessed _____

Protein & dairy

- ❑ chicken breast, boneless, skinless _____
- ❑ flank steak _____
- ❑ ground beef, extra-lean _____
- ❑ halibut or other fish fillet _____
- ❑ pork tenderloin _____
- ❑ shrimp _____
- ❑ turkey, smoked, sliced _____

- ❑ cheese, cheddar, low-fat _____
- ❑ cheese, feta, crumbled _____
- ❑ cheese, Parmesan, shredded _____
- ❑ eggs _____
- ❑ milk, skim _____
- ❑ yogurt, reduced-calorie, fat-free, _____
- ❑ yogurt, reduced-calorie, fat-free vanilla _____

Fats

- ❑ avocado _____
- ❑ cream cheese, fat-free _____
- ❑ olives, kalamata _____

- ❑ sour cream, fat-free _____
- ❑ vegetable dip, reduced-calorie _____

General groceries

- ❑ cocoa powder, unsweetened _____
- ❑ cranberry sauce _____
- ❑ curry powder _____
- ❑ pancake mix _____
- ❑ pineapple, crushed, canned _____

- ❑ pretzel sticks _____
- ❑ stir-fry sauce _____
- ❑ teriyaki sauce _____
- ❑ vanilla _____
- ❑ vegetable soup, canned _____

WEEK 9

DAY 1 MENU

Breakfast
1 c. reduced-calorie, fat-free yogurt *P/D* ●
* 1 large grapefruit *Fruit* ● ●
Calorie-free beverage

Lunch
Turkey sandwich *Carbohydrates* ● ●, *P/D* ●
Top 2 slices whole-grain bread with 3 oz. smoked turkey, Dijon mustard, lettuce and tomato slices.
* 2 c. mixed greens *Vegetables* ●
2 tbsp. reduced-calorie salad dressing *Fat* ●
Calorie-free beverage

Dinner
Pasta primavera *Carbohydrates* ● ●, *Vegetables* ● ●, *Fat* ●, *P/D* ●
1 c. cooked pasta topped with 1 c. steamed carrots, broccoli and cauliflower, sprinkled with 1 tsp. olive oil and 2 tbsp. shredded Parmesan cheese
* 1 medium orange *Fruit* ●
Calorie-free beverage

Snack
* 1 serving favorite vegetable *Vegetables* ●
2 tbsp. reduced-calorie vegetable dip *Fat* ●

* The serving size stated is the minimum amount. Eat as much as you wish.

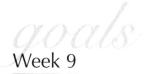

Week 9

You can adapt this week's goals or substitute different goals that are more to your liking. When you meet a goal, check the corresponding box.

❏ **Plan your meals for one week.** You can adapt the menu suggestions for this week or develop your own menus. Plan what you would like to eat for breakfast, lunch and dinner for an entire week. Adjust the number of servings from each food group to meet your daily calorie goals. Remember that vegetables, fruits and whole grains are the focus of a healthy diet. Write down your menus, even if you don't get around to preparing them.

❏ **Read nutrition labels.** When shopping, compare the nutrition labels of similar items to see if one is healthier than the others. You may find one has less fat or calories and more fiber or essential vitamins. For more information, see page 93.

❏ **Experiment with a recipe makeover.** Examine one of your favorite recipes and look for ways that you might make the recipe more nutritious. This might include reducing the sugar, using reduced-fat or fat-free products, or substituting legumes for meat. For more information, see page 91.

❏ **Update your Weight Record.** Weigh in and record the number of pounds gained or lost on the Weight Record. Whether you're meeting expectations or not, remember that sticking with the program for nine weeks is a major achievement in itself. Think about rewarding your efforts.

❏ **Use this week's healthy weight menu.** Try to follow the suggested menus in this unit. These menus are devised for a 1,200-calorie-a-day diet. If your calorie goal varies from the 1,200-calorie level, you need to adjust the menus accordingly. See page 185.

Daily recommended servings

Vegetables (no limit)	● ● ● ●
Fruits (no limit)	● ● ●
Carbohydrates	● ● ● ●
Protein & Dairy (P/D)	● ● ●
Fats	● ● ●

DAY 2 MENU

Breakfast

Fruit yogurt parfait *Fruit* ●, *P/D* ●
*Combine 1 c. reduced-calorie, fat-free vanilla yogurt
with 1 c. favorite fruit.*
½ whole-grain bagel *Carbohydrates* ●
3 tbsp. fat-free cream cheese *Fat* ●
Calorie-free beverage

Lunch

Chicken wrap *Fruit* ●, *Carbohydrates* ●, *P/D* ●
*Combine 2½ oz. shredded cooked chicken, 2 tbsp.
raisins, 3 tbsp. cranberry sauce and shredded lettuce.
Wrap in a 6-inch corn tortilla.*
1 sliced tomato *Vegetables* ●, *Fat* ●
*Drizzle tomato with 1 tsp. extra-virgin olive oil and
balsamic vinegar to taste.*
Calorie-free beverage

Dinner

2 oz. marinated pork tenderloin *P/D* ●
*Marinate whole pork tenderloin in ¼ c. teriyaki
sauce for 4 hours, turning frequently. Grill pork, turning
occasionally, until thermometer in center of pork reads
150 F. Tenderloin may also be browned and then
baked at 450 F about 15 minutes. Slice and serve.*
* 1 c. asparagus *Vegetables* ● ●
 3 red-skinned baby potatoes *Carbohydrates* ●
 1 small whole-grain roll *Carbohydrates* ●
 1 tsp. margarine *Fat* ●

Snack

* 1 serving favorite fruit *Fruit* ●

* The serving size stated is the minimum amount.
 Eat as much as you wish.

Dietitian's tips

*The following cooking techniques offer ways to cap-
ture the flavor and nutrients from your food without
adding excessive amounts of fat or salt. Choose these
techniques to prepare your favorite dishes.*

- **Baking.** Place the food in a pan or dish and put it
 in a hot oven. You may cook the food covered or
 uncovered. Baking generally doesn't require that
 you add fat to the food.
- **Braising.** Braising involves browning the ingredient
 first in an open or covered pan on top of the
 stove, and then slowly cooking it with a small
 quantity of liquid.
- **Enhancing.** Using spices and herbs is one of the
 best ways to add color, taste and aroma to foods.
 Choose fresh herbs that look bright and aren't
 wilted. Add them toward the end of cooking.
 Dried herbs should be added in the earlier stages
 of cooking. When substituting dried for fresh, use
 about one-third to one-half the amount.
- **Grilling and broiling.** These cooking methods
 expose fairly thin pieces of food to direct heat. To
 grill outdoors, place the food on a grill rack
 above a bed of charcoal embers or gas-heated

rocks. To broil indoors, place the food on a broiler rack below the oven's upper heat element. Both
methods allow fat to drip away from the food.
- **Poaching.** To poach foods, gently simmer the
 ingredients in water or a flavorful liquid such as
 broth or vinegar until they're cooked through and
 tender. You can also poach foods in foil packets
 in the oven or on the grill.
- **Roasting.** Place the food on a baking sheet or in a
 roasting pan and put it in the oven. For poultry,
 and meat, place a rack inside the roasting pan so
 that the fat can drip away during cooking.
- **Sautéing.** This method quickly cooks relatively
 small or thin pieces of food. With a good-quality
 nonstick pan, you can cook food without using
 fat. Depending on the recipe, use broth, nonstick
 cooking spray or water in place of oil.
- **Steaming.** Place the food in a perforated basket
 suspended above simmering liquid. Add seasonings to the water to flavor the food as it cooks.
- **Stir-frying.** Stir-frying quickly cooks small, uniform-
 sized pieces of food while they're rapidly stirred in
 a wok or large nonstick frying pan. You need only a
 small amount of oil or nonstick cooking spray.

DAY 3 MENU

Breakfast

½ c. whole-grain cereal *Carbohydrates* ●
1 c. skim milk *P/D* ●
* 1 medium orange *Fruit* ●
Calorie-free beverage

Lunch

2 oz. low-fat cheddar cheese *P/D* ●
5 round whole-grain snack crackers
 Carbohydrates ●
* ½ c. raw baby carrots *Vegetables* ●
2 tbsp. reduced-calorie ranch dressing *Fat* ●
* 1 c. grapes *Fruit* ●
Calorie-free beverage

Dinner

3 oz. halibut or other fish *P/D* ●
1 serving curried vegetable couscous
 Vegetables ● ● ●, *Carbohydrates* ●, *Fat* ●
* ³/₄ c. blueberries *Fruit* ●
Calorie-free beverage

Snack

30 pretzel sticks *Carbohydrates* ●
3 tbsp. fat-free sour cream dip *Fat* ●

* The serving size stated is the minimum amount.
 Eat as much as you wish.

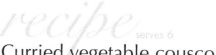

serves 6

Curried vegetable couscous

4-inch piece celery stalk, cut into 1-inch pieces
4-inch piece carrot, peeled and cut into 1-inch pieces
½ yellow onion, coarsely chopped
½ red bell pepper, seeded and coarsely chopped
⅓-inch piece fresh ginger, about 1 inch in diameter, peeled and thinly sliced
1 clove garlic
1 tbsp. extra-virgin olive oil
1 tsp. curry powder
1 c. whole-wheat (whole-meal) couscous
2 c. chicken stock, vegetable stock or broth
½ tsp. salt
2 tbsp. chopped fresh cilantro (fresh coriander)

■ In a food processor, combine the celery, carrot, onion, bell pepper, ginger, and garlic. Pulse until the vegetables are very finely minced. Don't puree. Set aside.

■ In a large nonstick saute or frying pan, heat the olive oil over medium heat. Add the minced vegetables and saute until they begin to soften, about 3 minutes. Add the curry powder and saute until fragrant, about 1 minute longer.

■ Add the couscous and stock and stir well. Bring the mixture to a boil over high heat. Reduce the heat to very low and cover the pan. After 5 minutes, remove from the heat.

■ Uncover and fluff the couscous with a fork. Add the salt and cilantro and toss to mix. Transfer to a serving bowl and serve immediately.

This recipe is one of 150 recipes collected in "The New Mayo Clinic Cookbook," published by Mayo Clinic Health Information and Oxmoor House and available in bookstores in the United States and Canada.

DAY 4 MENU

Breakfast
  ½ whole-grain bagel *Carbohydrates* ●
  1½ tbsp. jam
* 1 large grapefruit *Fruit* ● ●
  Calorie-free beverage

Lunch
  California burger *Vegetables* ●, *Carbohydrates* ● ●,
    P/D ● ●, *Fat* ● ●

Top 3 oz. cooked extra-lean ground beef patty with ½ grilled onion, lettuce and tomato slices. Serve on a small whole-grain bun spread with 2 tsp. mayonnaise.

* 1 medium orange *Fruit* ●
  Calorie-free beverage

Dinner
  1 serving Greek salad *Vegetables* ● ●,
    P/D ●, *Fat* ● (See recipe on page 236.)
  6 wheat crackers *Carbohydrates* ●
  Calorie-free beverage

Snack
* 1 serving favorite vegetable *Vegetables* ●

* The serving size stated is the minimum amount. Eat as much as you wish.

strategies

Planning a weekly menu

One of the best ways to ensure that you eat nutritious meals without a lot of time and effort is to plan your menus in advance. Set aside time each week — before going to the grocery store — to plan your menu for the next seven days. The more times you can do this, the more this practice will become routine. With experience, the task may take only a half-hour of your time.

Based on your daily calorie goal, the table on page 185 will show you how many daily servings should come from each of the food groups.

■ **Keep the menus practical and simple.** But, at the same time, don't exclude good flavor and fun. Remember that you need to enjoy your meals if you're expecting to stick with your plan.

■ **Aim for balance.** Try to include at least one serving from most food groups in most meals. To get plenty of vegetables each day, build lunches and dinners that incorporate two vegetable servings each, or have them for snacks during the day.

■ **Don't make meat the focus.** Build the main part of your meal around vegetables and fruits, in addition to rice, noodles or other grains.

■ **Be flexible.** Don't get hung up on hitting exact daily serving totals. Think in terms of the week as well as day-to-day. If on Monday you don't reach your target for fruit servings, you can add an extra serving or two on Tuesday. If you exceed your sweets limit on one day, you can cut out sweets on the following day.

■ **Include your favorites.** It's OK to include your favorite foods in your weekly menus on occasion. But you may need to adapt the recipes slightly to make them more healthy. Look for ways to reduce the fat and calories without significantly affecting the taste or texture.

DAY 5 MENU

Breakfast

Blueberry pancake *Fruit* ●, *Carbohydrates* ●, *Fat* ●
Top a 4-inch-diameter pancake with ³/₄ c. blueberries,
1 tsp. margarine and 1 ¹/₂ tbsp. syrup.
1 c. skim milk *P/D* ●
Calorie-free beverage

Lunch

Banana and peanut butter bagel *Fruit* ●,
    Carbohydrates ● ●, *Fat* ● ●
Spread 1 tbsp. of peanut butter on whole-grain bagel
and top with 1 small banana, sliced.
1 c. fat-free, reduced-calorie yogurt *P/D* ●
* 1 c. grapes *Fruit* ●
Calorie-free beverage

Dinner

¹/₄ recipe beef stir-fry *Vegetables* ●, *P/D* ●
Sauté chopped garlic and ginger root in 1 tsp. oil.
Add ¹/₂ pound thin strips of flank steak, scallions,
green beans sliced diagonally, and ¹/₄ c. stir-fry sauce.
Use cornstarch to thicken.
¹/₃ c. cooked brown rice *Carbohydrates* ●
* 12 steamed asparagus spears *Vegetables* ● ●
Calorie-free beverage

Snack

* 1 serving favorite vegetable *Vegetables* ●

* The serving size stated is the minimum amount.
  Eat as much as you wish.

strategies

Adapting recipes

The recipes in this book are a starting point toward
a healthier lifestyle. As you become more comfortable with changes in your diet, you'll likely want to
experiment with other foods and recipes.

But just because you're eating more healthfully
doesn't mean that you can't enjoy your favorite "less
healthy" foods on occasion. You can do this by looking for ways to make some of your traditional dishes
more nutritious. Chances are, you can reduce the
calories and fat without greatly affecting the taste.

Here's an example of how a simple recipe for a
tuna salad sandwich was modified. The original
recipe contains 625 calories and 50 grams of fat.
The modified version contains 250 calories and 2
grams of fat and is healthier overall. For more about
adapting recipe ingredients, see page 91.

Original	Modified
1 can oil-packed tuna, drained	1 can water-packed, unsalted tuna, drained
¹/₂ c. diced celery	¹/₂ c. diced celery
1 tsp. lemon juice	1 tsp. lemon juice, optional
1 c. mayonnaise	¹/₂ c. fat-free mayonnaise
4 lettuce leaves	4 lettuce leaves
8 slices white bread	8 slices whole-wheat bread

DAY 6 MENU

Breakfast

1 whole-grain bagel *Carbohydrates* ● ●
3 tsp. peanut butter *Fat* ● ●
* 1 medium orange *Fruit* ●
Calorie-free beverage

Lunch

1 c. canned vegetable soup *Vegetables* ●
6 wheat crackers *Carbohydrates* ●
2 oz. low-fat cheddar cheese *P/D* ●
* 1 medium sliced pepper, any color *Vegetables* ●
* 1 c. grapes *Fruit* ●
Calorie-free beverage

Dinner

1 serving grilled chicken breast with roasted
yellow tomato sauce *Vegetables* ●, *P/D* ● ●
3 red-skinned baby potatoes with fresh parsley
Carbohydrates ●
1 tsp. margarine *Fat* ●
* 3/4 c. green beans *Vegetables* ●
Calorie-free beverage

Snack

* 1 serving favorite fruit *Fruit* ●

* The serving size stated is the minimum amount.
Eat as much as you wish.

---

recipe *serves 4*

Grilled chicken breast with roasted yellow tomato sauce

4 yellow tomatoes, halved crosswise and seeded
1 1/2 tbsp. extra-virgin olive oil
2 cloves garlic, minced
1 tbsp. balsamic vinegar
3 tbsp. fresh basil, chopped
3/4 tsp. salt
1/4 tsp. freshly ground pepper
4 skinless, boneless chicken breast halves,
about 5 oz. each
2 tbsp. chopped fresh flat-leaf (Italian) parsley
1 tbsp. chopped fresh thyme

■ Prepare a hot fire in a charcoal grill or preheat a gas grill or broiler. Away from the heat source, lightly coat the grill rack or broiler pan with cooking spray. Position the rack or pan 4 to 6 inches from the heat source.

■ Arrange the tomatoes skin-side down on a grill rack or skin-side up on a broiler pan lined with aluminum foil. Grill or broil until the skins begin to blacken, about 5 minutes. Remove the tomatoes from the rack or pan. Transfer them to a bowl. Cover the bowl with plastic wrap and let the steam loosen the skins, about 10 minutes.

■ In a small frying pan, heat the olive oil over medium heat. Add the garlic and sauté until softened, about 1 minute. Remove from the heat and set aside.

■ Core and peel the tomatoes. In a blender or food processor, combine the tomatoes, the garlic with the oil, and the vinegar. Pulse until well blended. Stir in 1 tbsp. of the basil, 1/2 tsp. of the salt and 1/8 tsp. of the pepper.

■ Sprinkle the chicken breasts with the remaining 1/4 tsp. salt and 1/8 tsp. pepper. In a shallow dish, stir together the parsley, thyme, and the remaining 2 tbsp. basil. Dredge the chicken in the herb mixture, coating completely. Grill or broil the chicken, turning once, until browned on both sides and no longer pink on the inside, about 4 minutes on each side.

■ Transfer the chicken breasts to warmed individual plates. Spoon the tomato sauce on top, dividing evenly, and serve immediately.

This recipe is one of 150 recipes collected in "The New Mayo Clinic Cookbook," published by Mayo Clinic Health Information and Oxmoor House and available in bookstores in the United States and Canada.

DAY 7 MENU

Breakfast

* ½ large grapefruit *Fruit* ●
  1 slice whole-wheat toast *Carbohydrates* ●
  1 tsp. margarine *Fat* ●
  Calorie-free beverage

Lunch

Southwestern salad *Fruit* ●, *Vegetables* ●●,
  P/D ●, *Fat* ●●

*Top 2 c. shredded lettuce with 2½ oz. shredded
cooked chicken, 1 c. chopped green peppers and
onions, ½ c. crushed pineapple, ⅙ avocado, and 2
tbsp. reduced-calorie Western-style salad dressing.*
Calorie-free beverage

Dinner

3 oz. large shrimp, steamed *P/D* ●
⅔ c. cooked brown rice *Carbohydrates* ●●
* 1½ c. zucchini and summer squash,
  steamed *Vegetables* ●●
* 1 large peach *Fruit* ●
  Calorie-free beverage

Snack

1 serving chocolate pudding pie *P/D* ●,
  Carbohydrates ● (See recipe on page A16.)

* The serving size stated is the minimum amount.
  Eat as much as you wish.

strategies

Healthy cooking techniques

*One of the most important changes you can make to
your kitchen technique is learning to prepare foods
with little or no oil.*

- Trim visible fat from meat before cooking. Broil,
  roast or bake the meat on a rack to allow remaining fat to drip away. After cooking, drain off
  fat drippings.
- Remove fat from soups, stews, sauces and gravies
  by chilling them and skimming it off.
- When you need oil, choose olive, peanut and
  canola oils, which are low in saturated fat.
- Use nonstick cookware or vegetable cooking
  sprays, which minimize the need for oil or butter.
- Sauté vegetables, such as onions, mushrooms or
  celery, in a small amount of water, broth or wine.
- Cook fish in paper parchment packets (*en papillote*). You can buy parchment paper at supermar-
  kets. You can also use aluminum foil. Both types
  of packets seal in flavors and juices.
- Poach fish or skinless poultry in broth, vegetable
  juice, flavored vinegar or dry wine.
- Season meat and poultry with herbs and spices to
  add flavor.

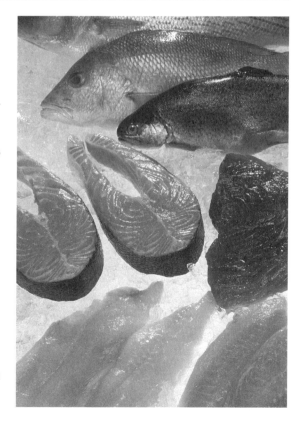

Week 10

Staying motivated

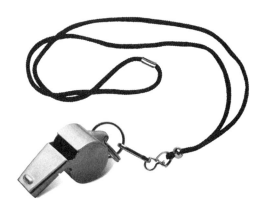

Starting a weight-control program takes energy and initiative. Sticking with the program takes commitment. You may have had boundless enthusiasm at the start of your program because you were dedicated to making changes in your life and you couldn't wait for a new, thinner "you" to happen.

Now, several weeks into the program, it feels like your enthusiasm is waning. You're pleased with what you've been able to accomplish — the weight you've lost — but the luster of your new challenge is wearing off.

Perhaps the new routine that you're trying to follow still isn't as comfortable as your old one had been. You miss some favorite foods that you've had to limit. You miss being able to just sit and read the newspaper after work instead of having to go for your daily walk. You worry that your desire to reach a healthy weight is losing out to your desire to return to the "good ol' days."

Successful weight control is a lifetime commitment. How do you stay motivated once that initial burst of energy at the start of your program has diminished? How do you stay enthusiastic if things don't happen quite as you'd planned? How do you keep from gradually falling back into old behaviors and ways of thinking that contributed to your weight problem in the first place?

Read Chapter 11 for strategies that may help renew your vigor and keep you on course. Now may also be the time to reassess your original goals and review your daily routine. Perhaps it's time to make some adjustments. Change sometimes can provide the spark you need to maintain your weight-control program.

Are you still motivated to lose weight?

The following questions can help you assess your levels of enthusiasm and motivation now that you're well into the program. Do you still have the motivational commitment to achieve a healthy weight or are you finding the task is becoming more difficult?

1. How would you describe your motivation to lose weight at this point?
   a. Extremely motivated
   b. Quite motivated
   c. Somewhat motivated
   d. Slightly motivated or not at all

2. To what extent are you able to focus on losing weight and making lifestyle changes?
   a. Can focus easily
   b. Can focus pretty well
   c. It's becoming more difficult
   d. Can focus only somewhat or not at all

3. How have your weight-loss expectations compared with the amount of weight you've actually lost?
   a. Somewhat or very realistic
   b. Moderately realistic
   c. Somewhat unrealistic
   d. Very unrealistic

4. Since beginning the program, have you run into situations in which you were unable to control your eating?
   a. No
   b. Yes

5. If you answered *yes* to question 4, how often has it happened?
   a. Only once
   b. A few times
   c. About once a week
   d. About twice a week or more

6. Have you been able to exercise regularly?
   a. Daily
   b. Most days of the week
   c. Occasionally
   d. Not at all

7. Since you began eating more healthy foods have you felt deprived?
   a. Never
   b. Rarely
   c. Occasionally
   d. Frequently

If your responses to most of these questions are *a* and *b,* you're doing fine. Keep going with the routine that you have in place and keep up the good work.

If your responses to most of these questions are *b* and *c,* you may need to re-energize your commitment to losing weight. Review the strategies in this week's program on ways to keep motivated.

If your responses to most of these questions is *d,* you definitely need a motivation boost. Review the reasons that prompted you to start on the program in the first place. Are they still valid? If you feel they are, use them to reinvigorate your effort.

Week 10 shopping list

This shopping list includes many of the fresh ingredients and general grocery items you'll need on hand for the Week 10 menus. It does not include the kitchen staples listed on page 187 — make sure you have them in stock. If you replace any of the recipes with a selection of your own, you'll need to adjust the shopping list.

Fresh vegetables   QTY

☐ asparagus spears   _____
☐ beets, red and yellow, baby   _____
☐ bell peppers, green and red   _____
☐ broccoli, fresh and frozen   _____
☐ carrots, baby   _____
☐ cauliflower   _____
☐ celery   _____
☐ corn on the cob, fresh or frozen   _____
☐ cucumbers   _____
☐ green peas, fresh or frozen   _____
☐ lettuce or mixed greens   _____

Fresh fruits

☐ apple   _____
☐ bananas   _____
☐ berries   _____
☐ grapefruit   _____

Carbohydrates

☐ bagels, whole-grain   _____
☐ bread, whole-grain   _____
☐ breadstick, large   _____
☐ bulgur wheat   _____
☐ buns, whole-grain   _____

Protein & dairy

☐ chicken breast, boneless, skinless   _____
☐ flank steak, lean   _____
☐ ham, lean   _____
☐ pork, lean   _____
☐ tuna or other fish fillet   _____
☐ turkey   _____
☐ cheese, American, reduced-fat   _____

Fats

☐ butter   _____
☐ sour cream, fat-free   _____

General groceries

☐ imitation seafood, frozen   _____
☐ lemon juice   _____
☐ marinara sauce   _____

QTY

☐ mushrooms   _____
☐ onions, yellow and red   _____
☐ spinach leaves   _____
☐ tomatoes, regular and cherry   _____
☐ zucchini   _____
☐ favorite or seasonal vegetables   _____

Fresh herbs

☐ dill   _____
☐ garlic   _____
☐ parsley, flat-leaf (Italian)   _____

☐ honeydew melon   _____
☐ pear   _____
☐ pineapple   _____
☐ favorite or seasonal fruit   _____

☐ English muffins, whole-grain   _____
☐ muffins, small, any flavor   _____
☐ potatoes, baking   _____
☐ sweet potatoes   _____

☐ cheese, cheddar, low-fat   _____
☐ cheese, mozzarella, part-skim   _____
☐ cheese, Swiss   _____
☐ cottage cheese, low-fat   _____
☐ milk, skim   _____
☐ yogurt, fat-free, reduced-calorie   _____
☐ yogurt, frozen, fat-free   _____

☐ vegetable dip, low-calorie   _____
☐ whipped topping, nondairy   _____

☐ orange juice   _____
☐ orzo pasta   _____

WEEK 10

WEEK 10

DAY 1 MENU

Breakfast
1 c. whole-grain cereal *Carbohydrates* ● ●
1 c. skim milk *P/D* ●
* 1 small banana *Fruit* ●
Calorie-free beverage

Lunch
Chef salad *Vegetables* ● ●, *P/D* ●
Top 2 c. mixed greens with 1 oz. low-fat cheddar
cheese strips, 1 ½ oz. turkey strips, and 1 c. sliced
tomatoes, cucumbers, green peppers, broccoli florets
and red onion.
2 tbsp. reduced-calorie salad dressing *Fat* ●
6 wheat crackers *Carbohydrates* ●
* 1 apple *Fruit* ●
Calorie-free beverage

Dinner
2 oz. lean pork *P/D* ●
½ medium baked sweet potato *Carbohydrates* ●
1 tsp. margarine *Fat* ●
* ¼ c. green peas *Vegetables* ●
* 1 c. berries *Fruit* ●
Calorie-free beverage

Snack
* 4 celery sticks *Vegetables* ●
1 ½ tsp. peanut butter *Fat* ●

* The serving size stated is the minimum amount.
Eat as much as you wish.

goals

Week 10

*You can adapt this week's goals or substitute differ-
ent goals that are more to your liking. When you
meet a goal, check the corresponding box.*

❑ **Assess your motivation level.** The assessment in
this week's program can help you determine how
motivated you are to stick with your weight program. Remember that adapting new, healthy
habits and losing weight aren't simple tasks. Even
if you're committed for the long haul, your resolve
will be tested from time to time.

❑ **Take a menu detour.** To cut back on boredom
and add an element of change to your eating
plan, experiment with a new food this week.
Prepare a dish from a recipe that you haven't
tried before. If you've been eating most of your
meals at home, treat yourself and go out to eat.
Challenge yourself to find something new and
healthy at one of your favorite restaurants.

❑ **Take an activity detour.** At least once during the
week, try out an activity that you've never done
before. Instead of going for your daily walk, you
might go for a swim or go bowling or spend an
evening dancing.

❑ **Update your weight record.** Weigh in and record
the number of pounds gained or lost on your
weight record. Remember that gradual weight
loss of 1 or 2 pounds a week is the healthiest
weight loss.

❑ **Use Week 10's Healthy Weight menu.** Try to follow
the suggested menu in this unit. These menus are
devised for a 1,200-calorie-a-day diet. If your
calorie goal varies from the 1,200-calorie level,
you'll need to adjust the menus accordingly. See
page 185.

Daily recommended servings

Vegetables (no limit)	● ● ● ●
Fruits (no limit)	● ● ●
Carbohydrates	● ● ● ●
Protein & Dairy (P/D)	● ● ●
Fats	● ● ●

WEEK 10

DAY 2 MENU

Breakfast
* * 1 large grapefruit *Fruit* ●●
  1 small muffin *Carbohydrates* ●
  Calorie-free beverage

Lunch
  Bagel sandwich *Carbohydrates* ●●, *P/D* ●
  *Spread 1 whole-grain bagel with mustard. Top with
  2 oz. lean ham, lettuce, tomato and onion slices.*
* * 2 c. raw mixed vegetables *Vegetables* ●●
* * ¼ small honeydew melon *Fruit* ●
  Calorie-free beverage

Dinner
  3 oz. broiled flank steak *P/D* ●●
  ½ medium baked potato *Carbohydrates* ●
  1½ tbsp. sour cream, fat-free *Fat* ●
  1 serving baby beets and carrots with dill
      Vegetables ●, *Fat* ●
  Calorie-free beverage

Snack
* * 1 c. broccoli florets *Vegetables* ●
  2 tbsp. reduced-calorie vegetable dip *Fat* ●

* The serving size stated is the minimum amount.
Eat as much as you wish.

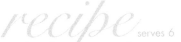

serves 6

Baby beets and carrots with dill

1 lb. red and yellow baby beets, about 1½ inches
in diameter
½ lb. baby carrots, peeled
2 tsp. butter
1 tbsp. extra-virgin olive oil
1½ tsp. fresh lemon juice
2 tsp. chopped fresh dill, plus sprigs for garnish

- If the beet greens are still attached, cut them off,
  leaving about an inch of the stem intact. In a
  large pot fitted with a steamer basket, bring an
  inch of water to a boil. Add the unpeeled beets,
  cover, and steam until tender, 20 to 25 minutes.
  Remove from the pot and let stand until cool
  enough to handle, then peel and cut into quarters.
  Set aside and keep warm.
- Check the pot, add water to a depth of an inch if
  necessary, and return to a boil. Add the baby carrots, cover, and steam until tender, 5 to 7 minutes.
  (If the carrots are varied sizes, cut the larger ones
  into halves or thirds for even cooking.) Remove
  from the pot.
- In a large bowl, toss the carrots with the butter,
  olive oil, lemon juice and chopped dill. Add the

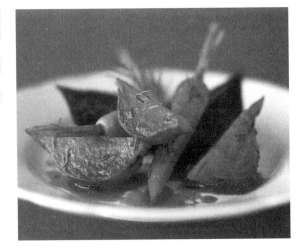

beets, toss gently to combine, and transfer to
a serving dish. Garnish with the dill sprigs
and serve.

*This recipe is one of 150 recipes collected in "The New Mayo
Clinic Cookbook," published by Mayo Clinic Health Information
and Oxmoor House and available in bookstores in the United
States and Canada.*

DAY 3 MENU

Breakfast
1 small muffin *Carbohydrates* ●
1 tbsp. honey
* 1 small banana *Fruit* ●
Calorie-free beverage

Lunch
1 serving pineapple chicken salad with
balsamic vinaigrette *Fruit* ●, *Vegetables* ● ●,
P/D ●, *Fat* ● ● (See recipe on page 206.)
4 crispy 6- to 8-inch breadsticks
Carbohydrates ● ●
* 1 c. raw baby carrots *Vegetables* ●
Calorie-free beverage

Dinner
3 oz. grilled tuna or other fish *P/D* ●
1 small ear corn on the cob *Carbohydrates* ●
1 tsp. margarine *Fat* ●
* Cucumber and tomato salad *Vegetables* ●
Combine ¹/₂ c. thinly sliced cucumber and 4 cherry
tomatoes, halved. Add balsamic, rice wine or herb-
flavored vinegar to taste.
* 1 apple *Fruit* ●
Calorie-free beverage

Snack
¹/₂ c. fat-free frozen yogurt *P/D* ●

* The serving size stated is the minimum amount.
Eat as much as you wish.

Dietitian's tips

*Here are suggestions to help you select the highest
quality fruits when shopping, and how to store them
once you get home.*

Selecting
- **Choose in-season fruits.** Generally, the closer you
  are to the growing source, the fresher the produce
  and the better it tastes.
- **Select fruits that feel heavy for their size.** Heaviness
  is a sign of juiciness.
- **Smell fruits for characteristic aromas.** Fruits should
  generally have their characteristic ripe scent but
  not smell overly ripe.
- **Test the texture.** An apple that feels mushy to the
  touch probably is too ripe. However, an avocado
  with a somewhat spongy texture is ideal.
- **Read the labels on packaged fruits.** Look for frozen
  fruits processed without added sugar. Choose fruit
  canned in water or fruit juice.

Storing
- **Keep fruits at room temperature to ripen them.**
  Fruits such as bananas, pears, nectarines and
  kiwi may be picked and sold at grocery stores

before they're ripe. To ripen, leave the fruit at
room temperature.
- **Store ripe fruits in the refrigerator.** The cool temperature slows the ripening process, giving you
  longer storage times. The length of time you can
  store fruit depends on the type of fruit and how
  ripe the fruit is at the time of purchase.
- **Throw away produce you've kept too long.**
  Discard fruit that's moldy or slimy, smells bad, or
  is past the "best if used by" date.
- **Freeze fruits for long-term storage.** You can freeze
  many types of fruit for up to one year. Grapes,
  cherries, berries and melon freeze particularly
  well. For best results, cut larger fruit into smaller
  chunks and remove the skin of peaches, apples
  and nectarines before freezing. Place in a single
  layer on a cookie sheet and put in the freezer.
  Once frozen, take the fruit off the cookie sheet
  and put into freezer bags for long-term storage.

DAY 4 MENU

Breakfast
1 slice whole-grain toast *Carbohydrates* ●
1 tsp. margarine *Fat* ●
* 1 large grapefruit *Fruit* ● ●
Calorie-free beverage

Lunch
Simple pizza *Vegetables* ● ●, *Carbohydrates* ● ●,
  P/D ● ●
*Top 2 English muffin halves each with ¼ c. marinara
sauce, ½ c. sliced onion and green pepper and
⅓ c. shredded part-skim mozzarella cheese. Broil
until cheese melts.*
Calorie-free beverage

Dinner
2½ oz. boneless, skinless chicken breast
  P/D ●
¼ c. cooked orzo pasta tossed with 1 tsp. extra-
  virgin olive oil *Carbohydrates* ●, *Fat* ●
* ½ c. peas *Vegetables* ● ●
* 1 small apple *Fruit* ●
Calorie-free beverage

Snack
1 c. berries *Fruit* ●
½ c. nondairy whipped topping *Fat* ●

* The serving size stated is the minimum amount.
  Eat as much as you wish.

strategies
Keeping it interesting

*People often stray from their weight plans because,
after a while, they get bored with their efforts. Having
to focus so much attention on diet and exercise day
after day becomes tiring and monotonous. Here are
suggestions to keep up your enthusiasm:*

- **Vary your menus.** Experiment with at least one
  new food or recipe each week. Explore world
  cuisines, or create a dish based on your own
  exotic-vegetable-of-the-week list. Dare yourself to
  eat something different!
- **Vary your activities.** Regularly change your activity
  routine. Walk a couple of days, swim on another
  and go for a bike ride on the weekend. Try out a
  new activity. On bad weather days, try mall walking or a new exercise videotape indoors.
- **Set weekly goals.** A good way to maintain your
  interest in your program and reinforce your sense
  of accomplishment is to set smaller goals that you
  can reasonably achieve each week. These weekly
  goals can be simple. Examples might include losing one pound, eating at least four vegetable servings each day, walking an extra three minutes
  each day or finding an exercise partner.

- **Get your family involved.** It's easier to make
  behavior changes and stick with them when your
  family can support you. Once a week, get the
  whole family together to prepare the evening
  meal, go for a hike or play a game of volleyball.
- **Focus on the positive.** Rather than dwelling on
  what you can't eat, focus on what you can.
  Granted, you may no longer be able to have a
  huge bowl of ice cream every evening, but you
  can have ice cream on occasion. And you can
  still enjoy an evening snack, provided it's something healthy.
- **Seek social support.** Having the support of one or
  more people can help keep you motivated. These
  are people whom you can turn to on bad days,
  and who will recognize your accomplishments.
  Spend time with people that you care about and
  who have a positive influence on you.

WEEK 10

DAY 5 MENU

Breakfast

Fruit yogurt parfait *P/D* ●, *Fruit* ●
*Mix 1 c. fat-free, reduced-calorie yogurt with 1
serving fruit.*
1 small muffin *Carbohydrates* ●
1 tsp. margarine *Fat* ●
Calorie-free beverage

Lunch

Chicken sandwich *Carbohydrates* ● ●, *P/D* ●
*Spread a whole-grain bun with honey mustard. Add
2½ oz. grilled boneless, skinless chicken breast, lettuce
and tomato slices.*
* 2 c. mixed greens *Vegetables* ●
2 tbsp. reduced-calorie salad dressing *Fat* ●
* 1 small apple *Fruit* ●
Calorie-free beverage

Dinner

⅙ recipe brown rice pilaf with vegetables
  P/D ●, *Carbohydrates* ●, *Vegetables* ● ●
*Over medium heat, stir 1 c. brown rice until golden.
Add 3 c. chicken broth, 1 chopped onion, 8 oz. sliced
mushrooms. Boil, reduce heat, simmer 30 minutes. Add
1½ c. asparagus pieces. Cook 5 minutes. Top with
grated Swiss cheese, ½ c. chopped parsley and serve.*
* ¼ small honeydew melon *Fruit* ●
Calorie-free beverage

Snack
* 1 serving favorite vegetable *Vegetables* ●
2 tbsp. reduced-calorie vegetable dip *Fat* ●

* The serving size stated is the minimum amount.
  Eat as much as you wish.

strategies
Get it on paper

If you're struggling to stay committed to your weight
program, here's one strategy that may help you
regain some of the enthusiasm you seem to have lost.
1. Make a list of all of the benefits of weight loss,
   such as having more energy, improving your
   health, wearing clothes that fit better, putting on a
   swimsuit without feeling self-conscious, and feeling better about yourself. Write down everything
   that you can think of, no matter how trivial, far-
   fetched or silly it may seem.
2. Now write down all of the obstacles you're facing,
   such as no time for exercise, not being able to eat
   foods you enjoy, having to plan what you eat, or
   other frustrations you may have experienced over
   these past few weeks. Again, write down everything that comes to mind. No issue is too minor.
3. Carefully compare the benefits list with the obstacles list. After assessing your entries, do you
   believe the positives of your weight program outweigh the negatives? Can you think of solutions
   you can work on to resolve these obstacles? This
   exercise, which was designed for people trying to
   stop smoking or problem drinking, is also successful at increasing your motivation for weight loss.

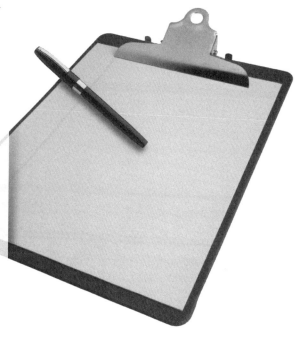

DAY 6 MENU

Breakfast

½ c. whole-grain cereal *Carbohydrates* ●
½ c. orange juice *Fruit* ●
1 c. skim milk *P/D* ●
Calorie-free beverage

Lunch

⅔ c. low-fat cottage cheese mixed with 2 pear halves *P/D* ●, *Fruit* ●
* 1 c. cauliflower florets *Vegetables* ●
1 slice whole-grain toast *Carbohydrate* ●
1½ tsp. peanut butter *Fat* ●
Calorie-free beverage

Dinner

1 serving broccoli seafood linguine
Carbohydrates ● ●, *P/D* ●, *Vegetables* ●
* 2 c. mixed greens *Vegetables* ●
2 tbsp. reduced-calorie salad dressing *Fat* ●
* 1 small pear *Fruit* ●
Calorie-free beverage

Snack

* 1 serving favorite vegetable *Vegetables* ●
2 tbsp. low-calorie vegetable dip *Fat* ●

* The serving size stated is the minimum amount. Eat as much as you wish.

recipe serves 4

Broccoli seafood linguine

1½ c. frozen broccoli cuts
2 c. cooked linguine
1 tsp. olive oil
1 garlic clove, minced
2 c. fresh tomatoes, chopped
¼ c. dry white wine
4 oz. shredded, reduced-fat American or mild cheddar cheese
1 8-oz. package imitation seafood, thawed

- Cook the broccoli until tender-crisp and cook the linguine.
- While broccoli and linguine are cooking, add olive oil to large skillet and sauté the minced garlic until golden. Stir in the tomatoes and wine. Simmer, uncovered, about 5 minutes or until the liquid is reduced by one-half. Stir frequently.
- Add the cheese to the tomato mixture, stirring until melted. Stir in the cooked broccoli and linguine and add the imitation seafood.
- Cook until thoroughly heated and serve.

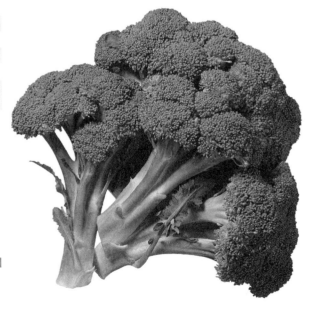

DAY 7 MENU

Breakfast
1 slice whole-grain toast *Carbohydrates* ●
1 tsp. margarine *Fat* ●
* ½ c. mixed fruit *Fruit* ●
1 c. skim milk *P/D* ●
Calorie-free beverage

Lunch
Grilled chicken salad *Vegetables* ● ●, *P/D* ●,
Fat ●

Combine 2 c. mixed greens with 2½ oz. grilled bone-less, skinless chicken breast strips and 1 c. sliced toma-toes, cucumbers, zucchini, bell peppers and onions. Top with 1 tsp. extra-virgin olive oil mixed with 2 tbsp. balsamic vinegar.
* 1 medium apple *Fruit* ●
Calorie-free beverage

Dinner
1 serving hearty grain-filled peppers
Vegetables ● ● ●, *Carbohydrates* ● ● ● (See recipe on page A12.)
* 1 c. honeydew melon, cubed *Fruit* ●
½ c. fat-free frozen yogurt *P/D* ●
Calorie-free beverage

Snack
7 whole almonds *Fat* ●

* The serving size stated is the minimum amount. Eat as much as you wish.

strategies

Staying on course

Here are two scenarios in which individuals were able to resolve problems that had been gradually eroding their motivation.

The office
Each day at work, Anne was bombarded with foods she was trying to avoid: the candy dish on a co-work-er's desk, the doughnuts at the morning meetings and the homemade goodies in the employee lounge.

Despite the success she was having at home, Anne realized that she was losing the battle at work. Instead of giving up, Anne thought of ways to make her workplace less of a dietary minefield.

- Anne asked her co-worker if she could include healthier items in the candy dish, such as pretzels and sugar-free candies.
- She decided to bring a bagel to the morning meetings so that she wouldn't grab a doughnut.
- During her break, Anne skips the employee lounge and goes for a short walk.
- She lets herself have a snack from the employee lounge but she waits until late afternoon to reduce the chance that she'll wander back for seconds.

Late night
At night, Bob gets a bad case of the munchies. Tired and worn out from the day's activities, he finds it hard to fight off the cravings. Worried that evening snack-ing was derailing his weight program, Bob decided he had to deal with the problem.

First, Bob tried to determine why he was so hungry at night. Was he eating dinner too early? Was he actually hungry or just plain bored? Was a snack part of his bedtime ritual? Bob decided it was proba-bly a combination of eating too early and needing food to help him sleep.

Bob then strategized ways to reduce his late-night snacking.

- Bob now eats dinner 30 minutes later in the evening.
- He sips on hot tea in the evening because it helps diminish his craving for food.
- Around 10 p.m. Bob eats a small snack of fruit or a piece of toast to help him sleep.
- Bob brushes his teeth as soon as he's finished his snack because he found a clean mouth discour-ages him from eating more.

Week 11

Coping with setbacks

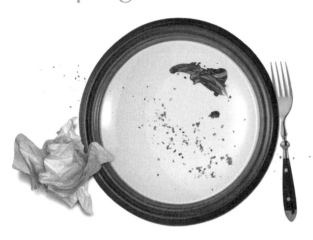

Sometimes, you make a minor slip that can trigger what seems like a downward spiral. You overeat at dinner or you skip a day of exercise. Guilt from the initial mistake can make you susceptible to more slips, which ultimately leads to a loss of control and an end to your commitment to reach a healthy weight.

This sequence is what's known as lapse, relapse and collapse. *Lapse* is the term that's commonly used for a minor slip. Lapses are commonplace and everyone trying to lose weight experiences them.

Relapse refers to a series of lapses that puts you off-track — a definite detour from your eating and exercise plan. It might be a vacation when weight control takes a back seat, or a busy week at work when you can't eat or exercise as you'd hoped to. Many people trying to lose weight will experience a relapse.

Collapse describes a total loss of control. Stress that has now extended over several weeks is threatening to overwhelm your ability to cope. You've given up on weight control, and you revert back to your old eating and exercise habits. Collapse is what you must avoid.

The important thing to keep in mind is that a lapse doesn't need to lead to a relapse, and a relapse doesn't need to result in full-blown collapse. The process is reversible and you can still get back on track!

Being ready to respond constructively can prevent a single slip from developing into something more sustained. Review some of the circumstances that may cause setbacks to occur, described on pages 110-113. Anticipation and planning for how to deal with setbacks is important to the success of your weight program.

What are your eating triggers?

One way to prevent a recurrence of overeating is to identify specific situations that may cause you trouble. Think about times when you've found yourself overeating. Were you eating because you were hungry, or were you eating in response to an event or emotion? For many people, food is a coping tool. It temporarily takes the edge off of stress and counteracts boredom.

There are many factors that can trigger overeating. Take a few minutes to consider what might be your eating triggers.

Time of day. Are there certain times of the day when you're more susceptible to overeating? Maybe you do well in the mornings and afternoons but have a tough time with food cravings in the evenings, when you're at home and relaxed. Or, perhaps, midafternoon is your difficult time. In that lull between lunch and dinner, you get a strong, uncontrollable urge to snack.

Emotions. Food is a common response to a negative mood. Do you find that certain feelings cause you to snack mindlessly? Do you tend to eat when you're bored, lonely or depressed? Is food a way to cope with anxiety or stress?

Activities. Do you find that you eat more when doing certain activities? Is reading the newspaper or sitting at the computer without food in hand a problem for you? Do you find yourself constantly snacking while watching television or preparing a meal? Is food how you deal with activities that you don't enjoy, such as paying bills or doing homework?

Social situations. Have you noticed that you eat more when you're around certain people? Maybe it's a good friend who likes to go out to eat or to invite you over for coffee and a "little snack." Maybe it's when your spouse gets the nibbles, and you find yourself eating, too. Maybe it's a family member who always seems to rile you up.

Foods. Does the sight or smell of certain foods tempt you to eat? Do you find that you just can't eat some foods in moderation, such as ice cream, chocolate or chips and salsa? Does the smell of pancakes and sausage or fresh cookies from the oven cause you to completely forget about your eating plan?

Physical factors. Do feelings cause you to overeat? You skipped breakfast and lunch, and now you can't control your hunger. When you're fatigued, do you turn to junk food as a source of energy? If you have chronic pain, do you use food to help distract you from the pain?

Assessing your eating triggers can help you predict situations that increase your risk of experiencing an overeating episode. By knowing ahead of time what your weaknesses are, you can plot strategies to avoid such encounters or lessen their effects.

Week 11 shopping list

This shopping list includes many of the fresh ingredients and general grocery items you'll need on hand for the Week 11 menus. It does not include the kitchen staples listed on page 187 — make sure you have them in stock. If you replace any of the recipes with a selection of your own, you'll need to adjust the shopping list.

Fresh vegetables   QTY   QTY
- ❏ asparagus spears   _____   ❏ tomatoes, regular and cherry   _____
- ❏ bell peppers, green, red and yellow   _____   ❏ favorite or seasonal vegetables   _____
- ❏ carrots, baby   _____
- ❏ celery   _____   *Fresh herbs*
- ❏ cucumbers   _____   ❏ basil   _____
- ❏ green peas, fresh or frozen   _____   ❏ chervil   _____
- ❏ lettuce or mixed greens   _____   ❏ dill   _____
- ❏ mushrooms   _____   ❏ garlic   _____
- ❏ onions, pearl and sweet   _____   ❏ ginger root   _____
- ❏ shallots   _____   ❏ parsley   _____
- ❏ snow peas   _____   ❏ rosemary   _____
- ❏ squash, summer   _____   ❏ tarragon   _____

Fresh fruits
- ❏ bananas   _____   ❏ limes   _____
- ❏ berries   _____   ❏ oranges   _____
- ❏ grapefruit   _____   ❏ pears   _____
- ❏ grapes   _____   ❏ strawberries   _____
- ❏ lemons   _____   ❏ favorite or seasonal fruits   _____

Carbohydrates
- ❏ bread, sourdough   _____   ❏ rolls, onion   _____
- ❏ bread, whole-grain   _____   ❏ potatoes, baking   _____
- ❏ pita bread, whole-grain   _____

Protein & dairy
- ❏ beef, lean   _____   ❏ salmon or other fish fillet   _____
- ❏ chicken, boneless, skinless   _____   ❏ turkey, breast   _____
- ❏ egg   _____   ❏ turkey, smoked, sliced   _____
- ❏ egg substitute   _____   ❏ cheese, cheddar, low-fat   _____
- ❏ flank steak   _____   ❏ cheese, Gouda, low-fat   _____
- ❏ pork tenderloin, trimmed   _____   ❏ milk, skim and soy   _____
- ❏ roast beef, lean   _____   ❏ yogurt, reduced-calorie, fat-free _____

Fats
- ❏ olives, black   _____   ❏ sour cream, fat-free   _____
- ❏ pecans   _____

General groceries
- ❏ applesauce   _____   ❏ pickles   _____
- ❏ artichoke hearts   _____   ❏ pineapple chunks, canned   _____
- ❏ beets, canned   _____   ❏ potatoes, baby, canned   _____
- ❏ fish stock, or bottled clam broth   _____   ❏ tuna, water-packed, canned   _____
- ❏ garbanzos, canned   _____   ❏ vegetable juice, canned   _____
- ❏ parchment paper   _____

WEEK 11

DAY 1 MENU

Breakfast

1 c. whole-grain cereal *Carbohydrates* ● ●
1 c. skim milk *P/D* ●
* 1 small pear *Fruit* ●
Calorie-free beverage

Lunch

Roast beef sandwich *Carbohydrates* ● ●, *P/D* ●
2 oz. lean roast beef, Dijon mustard, sweet onion, lettuce and tomato on onion roll.
* 1 c. sliced cucumber *Vegetables* ●
3 tbsp. fat-free sour cream *Fat* ●
* 1 medium orange *Fruit* ●
Calorie-free beverage

Dinner

¼ recipe ginger chicken stir-fry *P/D* ●,
   Vegetables ●
1 lb. boneless, skinless chicken cut into thin strips,
chopped garlic and ginger root sautéed in 1 tsp.
sesame oil, and a total of 2 c. snow peas, fresh
mushrooms and red peppers.
2 c. lettuce topped with 1 tbsp. sunflower seeds
   Vegetables ●, *Fat* ●
2 tbsp. reduced-calorie ranch dressing *Fat* ●
* 1 serving favorite fruit *Fruit* ●
Calorie-free beverage

Snack

* 1 serving favorite vegetable *Vegetables* ●

* The serving size stated is the minimum amount.
Eat as much as you wish.

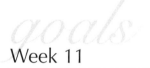

Week 11

You can adapt this week's goals or substitute different goals that are more to your liking. When you meet a goal, check the corresponding box.

❑ **Defuse a trigger.** Consider a problem situation that often seems to stand in the way of your efforts to eat better or to exercise. Create an action plan for handling this situation. For example, if paying bills or doing paperwork causes you to snack endlessly, look for alternate solutions. They may include munching on fresh fruits or vegetables instead, or doing your work other than at the kitchen table, where food is readily available.

❑ **De-stress your day.** Think about a situation that generally causes you stress and try to make one change that would reduce that stress. If getting to work on time is a source of stress, consider getting up a little earlier and eating a calming breakfast. Or do some early morning tasks the night before, such as packing your lunch.

❑ **Update your Weight Record.** Weigh in and record the number of pounds gained or lost on your Weight Record. Remember that gradual weight loss of 1 or 2 pounds a week is the healthiest weight loss.

❑ **Use Week 11's Healthy Weight menu.** Try to follow the suggested menu in this unit. These menus are devised for a 1,200-calorie-a-day diet. If your calorie goal varies from the 1,200-calorie level, you'll need to adjust the menus accordingly. See page 185.

Daily recommended servings

Vegetables (no limit)	● ● ● ●
Fruits (no limit)	● ● ●
Carbohydrates	● ● ● ●
Protein & Dairy (P/D)	● ● ●
Fats	● ● ●

DAY 2 MENU

Breakfast

Omelet *Vegetables* ●, *P/D* ●
Mix 1/2 c. egg substitute with 1/2 c. diced onions, tomatoes, peppers and mushrooms, and cook until set.
1 slice whole-grain toast *Carbohydrates* ●
1 tsp. margarine *Fat* ●
* 1 small banana *Fruit* ●
Calorie-free beverage

Lunch

Hummus pita *P/D* ●, *Fat* ●
Combine 1/3 c. mashed garbanzos with 1 tsp. extra-virgin olive oil. Add garlic, cumin, lemon and parsley to taste.
1 whole-grain pita *Carbohydrates* ● ●
* Cucumber and tomato salad *Vegetables* ●
Combine 1/2 c. thinly sliced cucumber and 4 cherry tomatoes, halved. Add balsamic, rice wine or herb-flavored vinegar to taste.
Calorie-free beverage

Dinner

1 serving salmon *en papillote P/D* ●, *Vegetables* ●
1/2 c. cooked lemon-peppered pasta *Carbohydrates* ●
* 3/4 c. summer squash *Vegetables* ●
* 1 small pear *Fruit* ●
Calorie-free beverage

Snack

* 1 serving favorite fruit *Fruit* ●

* The serving size stated is the minimum amount. Eat as much as you wish.

recipe serves 4

Salmon *en papillote*

Marinade:
1 clove garlic, chopped
1 tsp. shallots, chopped
1/8 tsp. black pepper
1 tbsp. fresh lime juice

1 lb. salmon (four 4-ounce fillets)
20 fresh asparagus spears
1 medium tomato, peeled and seeded
1 tbsp. tarragon, chopped
1 tsp. chervil, chopped
5 oz. fish stock (can substitute bottled clam broth)
2 oz. white wine
Parchment paper
Vegetable cooking spray

- Combine ingredients for marinade. Marinate salmon at room temperature for 20 to 30 minutes.
- Cut parchment paper into heart shape (about 12 inches). Spray one side lightly with vegetable cooking spray. Place the salmon on the paper and top with asparagus, tomato and herbs.
- Combine fish stock and white wine. Top salmon with the liquid. (Don't worry if a little liquid runs off the paper.) Fold parchment in half. Seal tightly. Fold edge of parchment in 1- to 2-inch segments from top to bottom of heart.
- Bake at 325 F for 8 to 10 minutes. Remove and serve in paper and garnish with tarragon.

WEEK 11

DAY 3 MENU

Breakfast

1 c. fat-free, reduced-calorie yogurt *P/D* ●
1 slice whole-grain toast *Carbohydrates* ●
1 ½ tbsp. jam
* 1 small banana *Fruit* ●
Calorie-free beverage

Lunch

Egg salad sandwich *Carbohydrates* ● ●, *P/D* ●,
   Fat ●
Mash one hard-boiled egg with a fork. Add chopped
onion and 1 tbsp. reduced-calorie mayonnaise. Serve
on 2 slices whole-grain bread.
* 1 small pear *Fruit* ●
½ c. vegetable juice *Vegetables* ●
Calorie-free beverage

Dinner

"Beefed-up" salad *P/D* ●, *Vegetables* ● ●,
   Fat ● ●, *Carbohydrates* ●
Assemble on large salad plate: 2 c. spring greens,
½ c. sliced canned beets, 3 canned baby potatoes,
1 medium tomato cut into wedges, 1 ½ oz. thinly sliced
marinated, grilled flank steak and 9 black olives. Chill
and top with 2 tbsp. reduced-calorie salad dressing.
* 1 c. grapes *Fruit* ●
Calorie-free beverage

Snack

* 1 serving favorite vegetable *Vegetables* ●

* The serving size stated is the minimum amount.
  Eat as much as you wish.

WEEK 11

Dietitian's tips

Calories from beverages can add up. To cut calories,
switch to low-fat or fat-free milk, drink lower calorie
juices and switch to diet soda. You can dilute juices
with plain or sparkling water to reduce calories,
too. Add a twist of lemon or lime to perk up
your water.

Beverage	Serving size	Calories*
Water	8 ounces	0
Coffee or tea (plain)	1 cup	0
Milk, whole	1 cup	150
Milk, 2%	1 cup	120
Milk, fat-free or skim	1 cup	90
Fruit juice, citrus or apple, unsweetened	6 ounces	80
Soda, regular	12 ounces	150
Soda, diet	12 ounces	0
Beer, regular	12 ounces	150
Beer, light	12 ounces	100
Wine, regular	5 ounces	100
Wine, light	5 ounces	80

* Average calories. Values for specific beverages may vary. Check the label.

DAY 4 MENU

Breakfast

1 pancake *Carbohydrates* ●, *Fruit* ●, *Fat* ●
Top 1 4-inch-diameter pancake with 1 c. berries,
1 tsp. margarine and 1 1/2 tbsp. maple syrup
* 1 medium orange *Fruit* ●
Calorie-free beverage

Lunch

Open-faced turkey sandwich *Carbohydrates* ●,
P/D ● ●, *Fat* ●
Spread 1 tbsp. reduced-calorie mayonnaise on 1 slice
sourdough bread. Top with 3 oz. smoked turkey,
2 oz. low-fat Gouda cheese, 1 slice tomato and
chopped basil.
* 2 c. raw vegetables *Vegetables* ● ●
Calorie-free beverage

Dinner

Beef fajita *Vegetables* ● ●, *P/D* ●, *Fat* ●
Sauté 1 1/2 oz. lean beef strips in 1 tsp. extra-virgin
olive oil. Add 1/2 c. sliced onion and 1/2 c. sliced
green, red and yellow bell peppers. Season with chili
powder and lime juice as desired.
2 corn tortillas *Carbohydrates* ● ●
* 1 1/2 c. strawberries *Fruit* ●
Calorie-free beverage

Snack

* 1 serving favorite fruit *Fruit* ●

* The serving size stated is the minimum amount.
Eat as much as you wish.

strategies

Stress and eating

Stress is what you experience when the responsibilities and demands placed on you at work or at home are beyond your ability to cope.

A fast-paced environment often leads to stress, which in turn can trigger overeating. Stress and overeating often are intertwined. People wanting to lose weight cite stress as one of the major obstacles in their battle to achieve a healthier weight. A stressful event may have led to their weight increase in the first place. And everyday stress keeps them from losing weight — when stressed, they nibble.

Are your eating habits influenced by stress? To find out, ask yourself these questions:

■ *When you're under pressure to complete something, are you pulled toward food ?*
■ *Do you, in general, have a high stress level?*
■ *When you feel stressed, do you lose track of your meal and exercise plans?*
■ *During stressful times, do you turn to food for comfort?*

If you answered yes to any of these questions, your eating habits may be affected to some degree — large or small — by stress.

So how do you keep stress from causing havoc with your eating plan? The answers are easy; implementing them takes more time and perseverance. To begin with, you want to look at ways that you can reduce stress in your life. And for those times when stress can't be avoided, it's important that you respond to it in a manner other than eating.

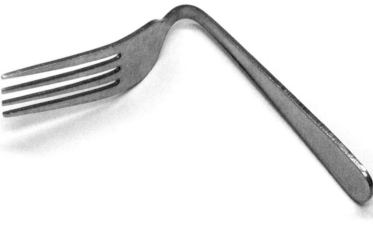

DAY 5 MENU

Breakfast
1 c. fat-free, reduced-calorie yogurt *P/D* ●
* 1 small banana *Fruit* ●
Calorie-free beverage

Lunch
Cheese wraps *Carbohydrates* ● ● ●, *P/D* ●
3 6-inch low-fat flour tortillas layered with 2 oz. shredded, low-fat cheddar cheese. Microwave to melt cheese.
* ½ c. raw baby carrots *Vegetables* ●
* 1 c. pineapple chunks *Fruit* ● ●
Calorie-free beverage

Dinner
Tuna-stuffed tomato *P/D* ●, *Vegetables* ●, *Fat* ● ●
Mix 3 oz. water-packed tuna (drained) with 2 tsp. reduced-calorie mayonnaise. Season with black pepper and a bit of chopped pickle, if desired. Core and partially quarter a tomato. Stuff it with tuna mixture.
* 4 medium celery sticks *Vegetables* ●
6 wheat crackers *Carbohydrates* ●
Calorie-free beverage

Snack
* 1 serving favorite vegetable *Vegetables* ●
2 tbsp. reduced-calorie salad dressing *Fat* ●

* The serving size stated is the minimum amount. Eat as much as you wish.

strategies

Put the brakes on stress

Stress can take a toll on your health, cause weight gain and create sleep troubles — all of which can lead to even more stress and derail your weight control program. To stay on track through stressful times, try this four-step strategy:

■ **Step 1: Take stock of your stressors.** When you're feeling overwhelmed or upset, jot down the particular circumstances in a notebook. Realize that stress can be caused by external factors — environment, family relations or unpredictable events — as well as by internal factors — negative attitudes, unrealistic expectations or perfectionism.

■ **Step 2: Examine your stressors.** Try to identify the problem at its root. Then ask yourself, "Can I change this situation?" or "Can I improve my ability to cope with this situation?" For example, if you always find yourself stressed when deciding what to wear to certain social events, ask yourself why that is. Is it because you don't like your clothes or because you're worried about how someone or some group will judge you? Once you know what's at the root of your stress, you can take steps to deal with it.

■ **Step 3: Evaluate your responsibilities.** Are you overcommitted, either at home, at work, or both? If so, can you delegate some of your tasks? Can others assist you? Can you say no to new responsibilities? Assess and monitor your daily and weekly responsibilities and do your best not to overextend yourself.

■ **Step 4: Learn to relax.** Develop a strategy that can help you relax when you find yourself becoming stressed. Proven stress-reduction strategies include exercise, deep breathing, and muscle relaxation techniques, as well as a good laugh. Any or all of these options generally provide a positive outlet for stress so that you can stay on track with your Healthy Weight Program.

DAY 6 MENU

Breakfast

1 c. fat-free, reduced-calorie yogurt mixed with
    4 chopped pecan halves *P/D* ●, *Fat* ●
* ½ large grapefruit *Fruit* ●
Calorie-free beverage

Lunch

Tuna salad sandwich *Carbohydrates* ● ●, *P/D* ●,
    Fat ●

Top 2 slices whole-grain bread with mixture of 3 oz. water-packed tuna, chopped celery and onion to taste, and 1 tbsp. reduced-calorie mayonnaise.
1 c. vegetable juice *Vegetables* ● ●
* 1 c. grapes *Fruit* ●
Calorie-free beverage

Dinner

3 oz. pork medallions with rosemary *P/D* ●
1 baked potato *Carbohydrates* ● ●
3 tbsp. fat-free sour cream *Fat* ●
* ¼ c. peas *Vegetables* ●
* ½ c. applesauce sprinkled with cinnamon
    Fruit ●
Calorie-free beverage

Snack

* 1 serving favorite vegetable *Vegetables* ●

* The serving size stated is the minimum amount.
   Eat as much as you wish.

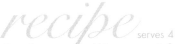 *serves 4*

Pork medallions with rosemary

1 lb. well-trimmed pork tenderloin
Freshly ground black pepper
1 tsp. rosemary, crushed
½ c. dry white wine

- Cut pork tenderloin crosswise into 12 pieces, each approximately 1-inch thick. Sprinkle the pieces of pork with pepper to taste.
- Place the pieces of pork between sheets of wax paper and pound them with a mallet until about ¼-inch thick.
- Brown pork medallions in large nonstick frying pan over medium-high heat, 2 to 3 minutes on each side. Remove and place on a heated platter. Sprinkle with rosemary and keep the medallions warm.
- Pour the wine into the skillet and boil. Scrape the brown bits from the bottom of the pan. Pour the sauce over the pork and serve hot.

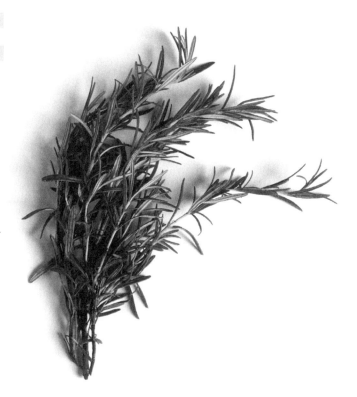

DAY 7 MENU

Breakfast
2 slices whole-grain toast *Carbohydrates* ● ●
1 tbsp. honey
* 1 small banana *Fruit* ●
Calorie-free beverage

Lunch
Chicken Caesar salad *Vegetables* ●, *P/D* ●,
    Fat ● ●
Combine 2 c. romaine lettuce with 2½ oz. grilled
boneless, skinless chicken breast strips, 2 tbsp.
reduced-calorie Caesar dressing, 9 black olives, and 1
tbsp. seasoned croutons.
* 1 medium tomato, sliced *Vegetables* ●
6 wheat crackers *Carbohydrates* ●
Calorie-free beverage

Dinner
1 serving turkey potpie with baby vegetables
    Vegetables ● ●, *P/D* ● ●, *Carbohydrates* ●, *Fat* ●
    (See recipe on page 220.)
* 1½ c. strawberries *Fruit* ●
Calorie-free beverage

Snack
* 1 serving favorite fruit *Fruit* ●

* The serving size stated is the minimum amount.
  Eat as much as you wish.

strategies

Healthy stress breaks

*Are you on stress overload? Some stressors you can
control, and others you can't. Concentrate on events
and circumstances that you can change. Here are
several ways that you might reduce daily stress:*

■ Go to bed 30 minutes earlier at night. Sleep gives
you energy to face the next day.
■ Eat properly and exercise regularly. Physical activity helps relieve emotional intensity.
■ Be positive. Spend time with people who have a
positive outlook and sense of humor.
■ Be patient. Realize that improvements in your
weight and overall health take time.
■ Organize your day to avoid conflicts or rushing
around at the last minute. Delay or delegate any
work that's optional.
■ Tackle unpleasant tasks early in the day. Get them
over with.
■ Go with the flow. Not every battle has to be
won — or even fought.
■ Simplify your schedule. Prioritize, plan and pace
yourself. Deal with only one thing at a time.
■ Ask a co-worker, friend or partner for help.

■ Create a change of pace. Make no plans for an
entire day. Read a good book or go to a thought-
ful or uplifting movie. Do volunteer work.
■ When you're fighting the urge to eat, look for a
distraction. Call a friend, put on music and dance
or exercise, clean the house, pull weeds in your
garden or organize the shelves in your garage.
With time, the urge to eat will pass.

Week 12

Lifetime commitment

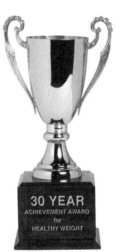
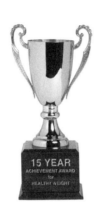
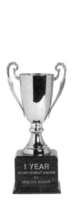

Think about the goals you set for yourself at the start of the Mayo Clinic Healthy Weight Program. Did the results of the program meet your expectations? Judging your progress in terms of the numbers — your weight when you started and your weight when you finished — may make you happy. But just as often it leads to disappointment and frustration — many people believe they can never lose enough weight.

Here's hoping that the Healthy Weight Program has provided you with much more. Weight control isn't only about the number of pounds you've lost. Consider that you're now eating better and that you're more active since you started the program. Think about the strategies you've tried and the new recipes you've prepared. All of this effort has made you healthier.

Remember that any weight loss, no matter how small, is a big step in the right direction because it makes you healthier. If you feel that you still need to lose more weight, continue what you're doing. With all that you've learned, you'll ultimately reach your goal.

One of the most difficult aspects of weight control may be how you come to terms emotionally with your weight. Sometimes, a lifetime commitment to weight control depends upon your ability to accept your body for what it is, with all of its imperfections (and perfections). Read Chapter 8 for more about the emotional aspects of weight control.

The strategies described in this last unit are directed toward helping you develop a healthier body image and boosting your self-confidence and self-esteem.

Strategies for a lifetime

Here are basic guidelines to help you transfer what you've learned in the Mayo Clinic Healthy Weight Program into a lifetime commitment to weight control:

Stick to basic principles

Continue to focus on maintaining a healthy lifestyle, and the weight will take care of itself. Stick with a balanced diet, moderate portions and daily physical activity. Get enough sleep and try to manage your stress level. Remember that these principles apply to everyone, not just to those individuals intent on losing weight. And they apply to any new situation.

Persistence pays off

Keep doing whatever worked for you in the program. You can adapt these strategies to new situations. You can vary them or add to them to keep your program interesting and challenging. Every step, every day, is important. Your ultimate goal is to incorporate the new, healthy behaviors that you learned into your routine — a natural part of your daily life. You don't want to set them aside after 12 weeks and revert to your old ways of doing things.

Make it enjoyable

The things you do to maintain your weight should be things you look forward to doing. You want them to be enjoyable and comforting, not unpleasant, tiresome or boring. If you start finding excuses or dragging your feet, these new behaviors will be quickly cast aside.

Keep a long-term perspective

Regardless of how many pounds you may have lost, the fact that you stayed with the program may be your most important achievement. Your health is improved and your self-esteem is stronger. It's important to consider weight control beyond a 12-week or 12-month or even 12-year period. It's for a lifetime. And no matter what your expectations are, by staying committed, you'll reach your goal — perhaps sooner than you think.

Give yourself credit

Acknowledge the vital role you played in making this program a success. It was your commitment to losing weight that got you started. It was your energy and focus that kept you moving through the weeks. You should now have the tools and experience to continue on. Giving yourself credit for what you've accomplished helps to improve your confidence level so that you can manage whatever challenges may come along in the future.

Week 12 shopping list

This shopping list includes many of the fresh ingredients and general grocery items you'll need on hand for the Week 12 menus. It does not include the kitchen staples listed on page 187 — make sure you have them in stock. If you replace any of the recipes with a selection of your own, you'll need to adjust the shopping list.

Fresh vegetables   QTY

- ❏ bell peppers, red and yellow _____
- ❏ broccoli _____
- ❏ carrots, regular and baby _____
- ❏ cucumbers _____
- ❏ eggplant _____
- ❏ lettuce or mixed greens _____
- ❏ mushrooms _____
- ❏ onions, green, red and yellow _____
- ❏ spinach leaves _____

    QTY

- ❏ summer squash, yellow _____
- ❏ tomatoes, regular and cherry _____
- ❏ zucchini _____
- ❏ favorite or seasonal vegetables _____

Fresh herbs

- ❏ basil _____
- ❏ garlic _____
- ❏ ginger _____
- ❏ mint _____

Fresh fruits

- ❏ apples _____
- ❏ bananas _____
- ❏ blueberries _____
- ❏ grapefruit _____
- ❏ honeydew melon _____

- ❏ kiwi fruits _____
- ❏ oranges _____
- ❏ pears _____
- ❏ favorite or seasonal fruits _____

Carbohydrates

- ❏ bread, whole-grain _____
- ❏ buns, whole-grain _____

- ❏ pita bread, whole-grain _____

Protein & dairy

- ❏ chicken breast, boneless, skinless _____
- ❏ ground beef, extra-lean _____
- ❏ egg _____
- ❏ egg substitute _____
- ❏ orange roughy or other fish fillet _____
- ❏ shrimp or other fish fillet _____
- ❏ ham, lean, sliced _____

- ❏ roast beef, lean, sliced _____
- ❏ turkey, sliced or shredded _____
- ❏ cheese, Parmesan _____
- ❏ cottage cheese, low-fat _____
- ❏ milk, skim _____
- ❏ soy milk, low-fat, vanilla _____
- ❏ yogurt, plain, fat-free, reduced-calorie _____

Fats

- ❏ avocado _____
- ❏ pecans _____

- ❏ vegetable dip, reduced-calorie _____
- ❏ whipped topping, nondairy _____

General groceries

- ❏ Cajun spices _____
- ❏ cheese pizza, thin-crust, frozen _____
- ❏ corn, canned or frozen _____
- ❏ pineapple rings, canned _____
- ❏ popcorn, microwave, low-fat _____

- ❏ salsa _____
- ❏ spaghetti sauce, meatless _____
- ❏ tomato soup, canned _____
- ❏ tuna, water-packed, canned _____

DAY 1 MENU

Breakfast
  1 c. whole-grain cereal *Carbohydrates* ●●
  1 c. skim milk *P/D* ●
* 1 small banana *Fruit* ●
  Calorie-free beverage

Lunch
  2/3 c. low-fat cottage cheese mixed with 2 pear
    halves *P/D* ●, *Fruit* ●
* 1 c. broccoli florets *Vegetables* ●
  2 tbsp. reduced-calorie vegetable dip *Fat* ●
  Calorie-free beverage

Dinner
  3 oz. orange roughy or other fish *P/D* ●
  2/3 c. cooked brown rice *Carbohydrates* ●●
  Spinach salad *Vegetables* ●●, *Fat* ●●
  *Combine 2 c. fresh spinach with 8 cherry tomatoes,
  halved. Top with 1 tbsp. sunflower seeds and 2 tbsp.
  reduced-calorie ranch dressing.*
* 1 c. berries *Fruit* ●
  Calorie-free beverage

Snack
* 1 serving favorite vegetable *Vegetables* ●

* The serving size stated is the minimum amount.
  Eat as much as you wish.

goals

Week 12

*The following goals are for you to try in this week's
Healthy Weight Program. You can adapt them or
substitute a different goal that's more to your liking.
Continue the practice of setting small, achievable
goals for yourself after the completion of this program to help maintain your lifetime commitment to
weight control:*

❑ **Reward yourself.** Celebrate your completion of the
12-week Mayo Clinic Healthy Weight Program and
acknowledge the hard work you've done. You might
reward yourself with a trip, new clothes or new
hobby. To signal that this is a new "you," plan something that incorporates aspects of your new, healthier
life. Consider involving people who may have
helped and supported you through the program.

❑ **Assess your outlook.** Do you feel like you can continue your lifestyle changes indefinitely, or do you
feel like it's an ongoing struggle? If you're still
struggling, you may want to review some of the
chapters in the book and the obstacles listed in
the Action Guide.

❑ **Pursue a goal.** Identify something in your life that
you chose to delay or avoid, thinking you'd hold

off until you'd lost enough weight. Now may be
the time to reconsider pursuing that goal.

❑ **Update your Weight Record.** Weigh in and record
the number of pounds gained or lost on your
Weight Record. After this final week of the
Healthy Weight Program, continue to weigh in
and update your record. You'll still want to follow
a regular weigh-in schedule, although this may
change from your original schedule, according to
your new weight goals.

❑ **Use Week 12's Healthy Weight menu.** Try to follow
the suggested menu in this unit. These menus are
devised for a 1,200-calorie-a-day diet. If your calorie goal varies from the 1,200-calorie level, adjust
the menus accordingly (see page 185).

Daily recommended servings

Vegetables (no limit)	●●●●
Fruits (no limit)	●●●
Carbohydrates	●●●●
Protein & Dairy (P/D)	●●●
Fats	●●●

DAY 2 MENU

Breakfast

1 c. fat-free, reduced-calorie yogurt mixed with 4 chopped pecan halves *P/D* ●, *Fat* ●

* 1 small banana *Fruit* ●

Calorie-free beverage

Lunch

Chicken ranch wrap *Carbohydrates* ●, *P/D* ●, *Fat* ●

Combine 2½ oz. grilled chicken strips, shredded lettuce, sliced tomato and onion. Top with 2 tbsp. reduced-calorie ranch dressing. Wrap in a corn tortilla.

* Cucumber and tomato salad *Vegetables* ●

Combine ½ c. thinly sliced cucumber and 4 cherry tomatoes, halved. Add balsamic, rice wine or herb-flavored vinegar to taste.

* 1 small apple *Fruit* ●

Calorie-free beverage

Dinner

Spaghetti with tomato sauce *Carbohydrates* ● ●, *P/D* ●, *Vegetables* ● ●

Top 1 c. cooked whole-grain spaghetti with ½ c. meatless spaghetti sauce from a jar and 4 tbsp. Parmesan cheese.

* 2 c. lettuce *Vegetables* ●

2 tbsp. reduced-calorie salad dressing *Fat* ●

* ¼ small honeydew melon *Fruit* ●

Calorie-free beverage

Snack

2 c. low-fat microwave popcorn *Carbohydrates* ●

* The serving size stated is the minimum amount. Eat as much as you wish.

Dietitian's tips

Snack suggestions

Snacking on vegetables and fruits is one way to make sure that you get your daily servings of these nutritious foods. A good piece of fresh fruit, in particular, is the ideal snack — it's low in calories, satisfying and healthy. You can eat virtually unlimited amounts of fresh vegetables and fruit, and have you ever noticed that they always taste better than what you anticipated? Here are suggestions for different ways that you can enjoy vegetables and fruits as snacks:

- Make a fruit smoothie by blending fruit with low-fat yogurt or skim milk.
- Cut fruit in slices or halves and dip the pieces in low-fat cottage cheese or yogurt.
- Make frozen fruit chips. Purée or crush fruit and then freeze it.
- Freeze fresh grapes and enjoy them when the weather is warm.
- Use chunks of fresh fruit to make fruit kebabs on skewers.
- Dip partially cooked vegetables (carrots, green beans, broccoli, cauliflower) in cottage cheese, hummus, low-fat ranch dressing or yogurt dip.

- Place a light coat of peanut butter or low-fat cream cheese on bell pepper slices, zucchini chunks or tomato wedges.
- Spread peanut butter on celery slices and top the peanut butter with raisins.
- Mix low-fat ricotta cheese with unsweetened pineapple and spread on celery strips.
- Make vegetable kebabs with bell pepper strips, mushrooms, cherry tomatoes and zucchini chunks.

Other kinds of food offer snack options. Nuts are a good choice as long as the portion size is reasonable — a little goes a long way in terms of making you feel full. If you prefer carbohydrates, stick to whole-grain products that have little saturated fat, trans fat, sodium and other additives. Check out a local bakery and enjoy a slice of dense, whole-grain bread. Different kinds of brown-rice and wild-rice cakes are low in calories. Some whole-grain crackers and cereal fit the bill as well.

When having a snack, eat a little less than what you think you'll need. You'll often end up feeling satisfied and will have saved a few calories. While you're at it, why not make the snack "healthy?" You'll feel a whole lot better about your choices.

DAY 3 MENU

Breakfast

1 medium hard-boiled egg *P/D* ●
1 slice whole-grain toast *Carbohydrates* ●
1 tsp. margarine *Fat* ●
* 1 medium orange *Fruit* ●
Calorie-free beverage

Lunch

Open-faced roast beef sandwich *P/D* ●,
   Carbohydrates ●
*Top 1 slice whole-grain bread with Dijon mustard and
2 oz. sliced lean roast beef.*
* 8 cherry tomatoes *Vegetables* ●
* 1 small apple *Fruit* ●
Calorie-free beverage

Dinner

$^1/_4$ recipe pasta with marinara sauce and grilled
   vegetables *Carbohydrates* ● ●, *Vegetables* ● ● ●,
   Fat ●
$^3/_4$ c. blueberries with $^1/_2$ c. nondairy whipped
   topping *Fruit* ●, *Fat* ●

Snack

1 c. fat-free, reduced-calorie yogurt *P/D* ●

* The serving size stated is the minimum amount.
Eat as much as you wish.

recipe serves 4

Pasta with marinara sauce and grilled vegetables

2 tbsp. olive oil
10 large fresh tomatoes, peeled and diced
1 tsp. salt
$^1/_2$ tsp. minced garlic
2 tbsp. chopped onion
1 tsp. dried basil
1 tsp. sugar
$^1/_2$ tsp. oregano
Black pepper, to taste
2 red peppers, sliced into chunks
1 yellow summer squash, sliced lengthwise
1 zucchini, sliced lengthwise
1 sweet onion, sliced into $^1/_4$–inch rounds
8 oz. package of whole-wheat spaghetti

- Heat oil in a heavy skillet. Add tomatoes, salt,
  garlic, onions, basil, sugar, oregano and black
  pepper. Cook slowly, uncovered, for 30 minutes
  or until sauce is thickened.
- Brush peppers, squash, zucchini and onion with
  oil. Place under broiler and cook, turning frequently until browned and tender. Remove to bowl.
- Cook spaghetti until al dente. Drain well and portion onto plates. Cover with equal amounts of

sauce. Top with equal amounts of vegetables.
Serve immediately.

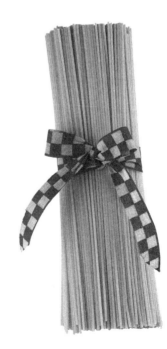

WEEK 12

DAY 4 MENU

Breakfast
1 c. reduced-calorie, fat-free yogurt *P/D* ●
* ½ large grapefruit *Fruit* ●
Calorie-free beverage

Lunch
1 c. cream of tomato soup *Vegetables* ●
6 saltine crackers *Carbohydrates* ●
* 1 small apple *Fruit* ●
Calorie-free beverage

Dinner
California burger *Vegetables* ●, *Carbohydrates* ● ●, *P/D* ● ●, *Fat* ● ●
Top 3 oz. cooked extra-lean ground beef patty with grilled onion, lettuce and tomato slices. Serve on a small whole-grain bun spread with 1 tbsp. reduced-calorie mayonnaise.
* 2 c. lettuce with ½ c. sliced tomatoes, red onions and mushrooms *Vegetables* ● ●
2 tbsp. reduced-calorie salad dressing *Fat* ●
* 1 small banana *Fruit* ●
Calorie-free beverage

Snack
2 c. low-fat microwave popcorn *Carbohydrates* ●

* The serving size stated is the minimum amount. Eat as much as you wish.

strategies
Bolstering your body image

A sad fact is that only about one in seven adult Americans — both men and women — is happy with his or her body. Dissatisfaction with body size or shape can cause feelings of disappointment or disgust, distort self-image and trigger overeating and weight gain. Consider these suggestions for being more accepting of yourself:

■ **Appreciate the body you have.** Write a list of your strengths and best features.
■ **Make a list of the people you most admire.** This may include anyone from your parents or your children to educators, scientists and world leaders. Do they have perfect bodies? Does it matter?
■ **Don't take yourself for granted.** Take care of yourself each day. Eat well, be physically active and get plenty of rest.
■ **Exercise.** Individuals who regularly exercise generally report improved body image. Exercise helps improve flexibility, build muscle and tone your body. All of these can improve body image.
■ **Continue to focus on your health.** If you'd like a healthier body shape or weight, set small, realistic goals and work to meet them.

■ **Get support.** Surround yourself with friends who don't focus on body size or appearance. If you're so preoccupied with your body image that it interferes with your life and prevents you from pursuing your goals, talk to a licensed mental health professional.

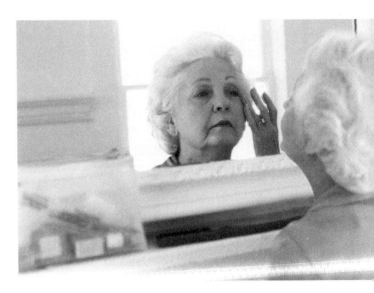

DAY 5 MENU

Breakfast

Fruit yogurt parfait *P/D* ●, *Fruit* ●
Combine 1 c. reduced-calorie, fat-free yogurt with
1 serving of fruit.
* 1 small apple *Fruit* ●
Calorie-free beverage

Lunch

1/4 recipe tuna and pasta salad
Carbohydrates ● ●, *Vegetables* ●, *P/D* ●, *Fat* ●
Combine 1 can tuna in spring water, 4 c. cooked shell
pasta, 2 c. diced carrots and zucchini, and 4 tbsp.
reduced-calorie mayonnaise.
Calorie-free beverage

Dinner

1/2 10-inch, thin-crust cheese pizza
Carbohydrates ● ●, *Vegetables* ●, *P/D* ●
Lettuce salad *Vegetables* ● ●, *Fat* ●
Top 2 c. lettuce with 1/2 c. sliced tomatoes, red onions
and mushrooms, and 1 tbsp. sunflower seeds.
2 tbsp. reduced-calorie salad dressing *Fat* ●
Calorie-free beverage

Snack
* 1 serving favorite fruit *Fruit* ●

* The serving size stated is the minimum amount.
Eat as much as you wish.

strategies

Self-esteem boosters

*How do you feel about yourself? Your answer to that
question expresses your level of self-esteem. Here are
ways to help you boost your self-esteem and keep a
positive attitude:*

- **Stay social.** People need a certain amount of interaction with others to feel a sense of belonging,
which can build self-esteem.
- **Set realistic expectations.** Setting your expectations
too high can lead to feelings of failure. Realistic
expectations, on the other hand, can provide you
with a sense of accomplishment.
- **Learn to celebrate.** Congratulate yourself when
you succeed. Give yourself nonfood rewards.
- **Change your perspective.** Think about the things
you do well instead of focusing on what you're
not able to do.
- **Take care of yourself.** Pay attention to both your
physical and emotional needs. Set aside time for
regular meals, rest and personal hygiene. If you
value yourself, others will value you as well.
- **Exercise.** Setting and accomplishing a physical
goal can give you an emotional boost, as well as
help you achieve a healthy weight.

- **Be involved in activities you enjoy.** Take advantage
of your own special talents and interests to build
self-confidence. At the same time, don't avoid
opportunities to try something new when these
opportunities arise.
- **Do something nice for someone else.** Offer assis-
tance when someone needs help. Send a card or
flowers to a friend on special occasions such as
birthdays or anniversaries. Do volunteer work in
your community or for a worthy organization.
- **Accomplish something.** Establish small, realistic
goals for yourself and accomplish them. Then build
on that success.

DAY 6 MENU

Breakfast

· 1 slice whole-grain toast *Carbohydrates* ●
1½ tbsp. jam
* 1 large grapefruit *Fruit* ●●
Calorie-free beverage

Lunch

Ham sandwich *P/D* ●, *Carbohydrates* ●●,
Vegetables ●

Between 2 slices whole-grain bread, top 2 oz. lean ham with lettuce, tomato slices and Dijon mustard.

* ½ c. raw baby carrots *Vegetables* ●
2 tbsp. reduced-calorie ranch dressing *Fat* ●
Calorie-free beverage

Dinner

1 serving chicken stir-fry with eggplant and basil
Vegetables ●●●, *P/D* ●, *Fat* ● (See recipe on page 210.)
⅓ c. cooked brown rice *Carbohydrates* ●
* 2 pineapple rings *Fruit* ●
Calorie-free beverage

Snack

1 serving yogurt-almond ice cream *P/D* ●, *Fat* ●

* The serving size stated is the minimum amount.
Eat as much as you wish.

recipe *serves 6*

Yogurt-almond ice cream

2 c. fat-free plain yogurt, without gum additives or stabilizers
1 c. low-fat vanilla soy milk, chilled
⅓ c. honey
1 tbsp. canola oil
¼ c. coarsely chopped almonds

■ Place a bowl in freezer to chill.
■ In another bowl, whisk together the yogurt, soy milk, honey and canola oil until well blended. Pour mixture in ice cream maker and freeze according to the manufacturer's instructions.
■ When ice cream is firm, transfer to chilled bowl and add the nuts. Stir gently to distribute evenly. Serve immediately or freeze until ready to serve.

This recipe is one of 150 recipes collected in "The New Mayo Clinic Cookbook," published by Mayo Clinic Health Information and Oxmoor House and available in bookstores in the United States and Canada.

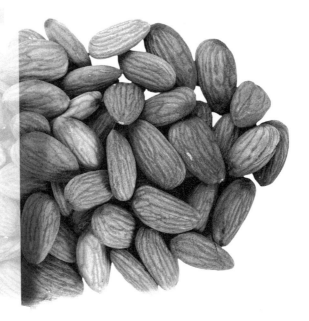

WEEK 12

DAY 7 MENU

Breakfast

1 breakfast burrito *Vegetables ●,*
  Carbohydrates ● ● ●, P/D ●

*Sauté 1/2 c. chopped tomato, 2 tbsp. chopped onion,
1/4 c. canned corn and some liquid. Add 1/4 c. egg substitute and scramble with the vegetables. Spread mixture on a tortilla, roll up and top with 2 tbsp. salsa.*

* 1 small banana *Fruit ●*
Calorie-free beverage

Lunch

Turkey pita sandwich *Carbohydrates ●, P/D ●,*
  Fat ●

*Top 1/2 whole-grain pita with 3 oz. shredded turkey,
1/6 avocado, chopped lettuce, tomato and onion.*

* 1 small apple *Fruit ●*
Calorie-free beverage

Dinner

3 oz. broiled shrimp *P/D ●*
  Season with Cajun spices.
2 c. lettuce with 4 cherry tomatoes, 1/4 c. red
  onion and 1 tbsp. sunflower seeds
  Vegetables ● ●, Fat ●
2 tbsp. low-calorie salad dressing *Fat ●*

* 1 large kiwi *Fruit ●*
Calorie-free beverage

Snack

* 1 serving favorite vegetable *Vegetables ●*

* The serving size stated is the minimum amount.
Eat as much as you wish.

review

Week 12

- **Evaluate your progress.** Write down some of the benefits that you feel you've received from participating in the Mayo Clinic Healthy Weight Program. Do you feel healthier? Do you feel better about yourself? Do you feel more in control? Do you feel a sense of accomplishment? How does your current weight compare with the weight goal that you established at the start? Hopefully, the results will reveal how much you've accomplished in a short amount of time, and inspire you to continue working toward a healthy weight.

- **Review the program.** The 12 topics highlighted in the Healthy Weight Program are intended to help you develop your own personalized weight program. Reflect on how these separate topics are so essential to weight control. Consider what strategies worked or didn't work for you. As you move forward, you'll want to make the healthy behaviors that you've learned part of your daily routine.

- **Your weight record.** You've used weigh-ins throughout the 12 weeks of the Healthy Weight Program to track your progress and keep you motivated. You should continue to maintain a weight record now that the program has ended.

But remember that the scale is not the only way to measure success. Consider going for the next week without weighing yourself. Test how confident you are that the new, healthier behaviors and routines you've established can still keep you on track. Then re-establish a regular schedule for weigh-ins, which may change slightly, according to your needs, from the schedule you maintained during the program.

- **Looking forward.** In the months and years ahead, occasionally take time to reconfirm your commitment to weight control. Review your reasons for wanting a healthy weight and the benefits you receive from following a healthier lifestyle. Don't ignore any negative feelings or emotions that you may have regarding your efforts — try to determine their cause and look for solutions. Over time, you may adapt your program or include different strategies in light of changing needs and circumstances.

Index